The Diffusion of
Medical Innovations

An Applied Network Analysis

ENVIRONMENT, DEVELOPMENT, AND PUBLIC POLICY

A series of volumes under the general editorship of
Lawrence Susskind, *Massachusetts Institute of Technology, Cambridge, Massachusetts*

PUBLIC POLICY AND SOCIAL SERVICES
Series Editor:
Gary Marx, *Massachusetts Institute of Technology, Cambridge, Massachusetts*

Other subseries:

ENVIRONMENTAL POLICY AND PLANNING
Series Editor:
Lawrence Susskind, *Massachusetts Institute of Technology, Cambridge, Massachusetts*

CITIES AND DEVELOPMENT
Series Editor:
Lloyd Rodwin, *Massachusetts Institute of Technology, Cambridge, Massachusetts*

The Diffusion of Medical Innovations

An Applied Network Analysis

Mary L. Fennell

The Pennsylvania State University
University Park, Pennsylvania

and

Richard B. Warnecke

University of Illinois at Chicago
Chicago, Illinois

Plenum Press • New York and London

Library of Congress Cataloging in Publication Data

Fennell, Mary L.
   The diffusion of medical innovations: an applied network analysis / Mary L. Fennell
and Richard B. Warnecke.
   p.   cm.—(Environment, development, and public policy.   Public policy and
social services.)
   Bibliography: p.
   Includes index.
   ISBN 0-306-42752-4
   1. Cancer—Treatment—United States—Technological innovations. 2. Diffusion of
innovations—United States. 3. Cancer—Hospitals—United States. 4. Network analysis
(Planning) I. Warnecke, Richard B. II. Title. III. Series. [DNLM: 1. Communication. 2.
Interinstitutional Relations. 3. Research. W 20.5 F335d]
RC270.8.F46   1988
616.99′406—dc19   88-2475
                                                                              CIP

© 1988 Plenum Press, New York
A Division of Plenum Publishing Corporation
233 Spring Street, New York, N.Y. 10013

Printed in the United States of America

For Dennis and Barbara

Preface

This book has several objectives. Most basically it presents an approach to assessing interorganizational innovation diffusion. To do this we have tried to link contemporary organizational theory with more person-centered diffusion theory. We have also combined contingency theory with the resource dependence perspective to explain why organizations might choose to initially consider an innovation, redefine it to suit their particular environmental context, and then implement it.

Another objective has been to examine how environmental constraints can limit the ways in which diffusion channels form, and can determine when diffusion can be truly organizational and when it will depend upon individuals. In doing so, we have tried to indicate how organizational structures emerge to manage resources in ways that are consistent with those environmental constraints. We have borrowed the notion of boundary management from resource dependence, and we have used it to examine how organizations use various boundary management strategies to preserve their autonomy in exchange relationships with other organizations. We have done this both at the network level and at the level of individual organizations.

When we conducted this study (in the late 1970s and early 1980s), the "network" strategy had just been adopted by the National Cancer Institute as a method for disseminating state-of-the-art cancer treatment strategies. The data we present and the observations we have made provide a view of a strategy just beginning to unfold. This early vantage point has given us what we believe is a unique view of a major organizational effort sponsored by the NCI to disseminate scientific information from research centers to community practitioners and community hospitals. By viewing the system at this early timepoint we have been able to show how performance gaps were identified by various parties in this process, and how they influenced agenda setting at the local, regional, and national levels as part of the "War on Cancer." We were also able to examine closely how early network strategies were implemented in various types of environments.

Because these were very large organizational systems, and the networking approach was at an experimental stage, we adopted a combined qualitative/quantitative methodology to chronicle the development of these cancer networks. Those social scientists who see the word *network* will probably immediately see *blockmodel-*

ing and other quantitative techniques that have developed in social network analysis. These data do not lend themselves to this type of analysis, and with the exception of Chapter 5, readers will find very little of it here. However, we hope you will bear with us, because we believe the reader will find considerable empirical evidence in support of the diffusion model we present.

Another type of caution is also pertinent. Because the diffusion strategy described here was new and had not been tested elsewhere, it would be easy to conclude that the system was largely ineffective. This would be an error. Although there were factors in this program that inhibited the NCI in attaining some of its stated objectives, the results of this initial effort had far-reaching consequences for the national cancer program and for all of the institutions that participated.

The results of this first effort greatly influenced subsequent diffusion efforts. Many different forms of diffusion networks followed this first attempt, each with a different focus or set of objectives. But all of them were designed to somehow strengthen the ties linking community hospitals to the objectives of the NCI. In each instance the objective was to increase the access of cancer patients to newly developed treatment strategies, and to provide newly trained oncologists who chose to practice in community hospitals with better access to state-of-the-art treatment methods. In most instances the source of the state of the art was a university research center, or in some cases the NCI. However, as these programs developed, the community physician increasingly became a partner in both the development of that knowledge and its implementation.

Thus, this book is really a first look at an ongoing program of diffusion. We hope that it will stimulate others to apply the concepts discussed here in the examination of other attempts at diffusion of state-of-the-art treatment or patient care strategies for other diseases and in other contexts. This was another purpose in writing the book: We have tried to develop a methodology and conceptual framework to be used by other health services researchers in conducting such studies.

Overall, then, we view this book as an attempt to examine organizational change in the delivery of cancer treatment resulting from the introduction of new treatment strategies and patient management techniques. If we have been successful, it might provide guidance about when such strategies can be effectively applied and when they cannot. It might also be useful in identifying the limits of such strategies and what impact the diffusion efforts themselves are likely to have on the form of the technology that is ultimately diffused. We have taken the position that the social and organizational context of diffusion itself forces changes in the form of the innovation. This is particularly likely when the innovation is a *set of concepts about treatment*, rather than a particular treatment technology based solely on particular hardware. How this change occurs and what might be done to promote consistency in the diffusion of new treatment strategies are important issues, but difficult to discuss given the data we have. Nevertheless, we have made an attempt.

Acknowledgments

In a project of this size and length, many individuals make contributions. The actual project was carried out under a contract with the NCI (NO1-CN-95446-46). However, this book represents an interpretation of the data from that contract that is our responsibility and does not reflect the opinions or policies of the NCI. Moreover, the reader should be aware that these data were collected from 1978 through 1982, and they therefore do not reflect current activities at any of the programs or institutions discussed.

In addition to the NCI contract support, Dr. Fennell was provided support in the form of release-time from teaching, computer facilities, and staff support from the Department of Sociology at the University of Illinois at Chicago. Dr. Warnecke's time was also supported under two grants from the NCI, Cancer Control Science Program (CA34886) and Community Interventions for Cancer Prevention (PO1-CA42760).

Rosemary Yancik was the project officer on the initial contract from the NCI and provided considerable assistance in completing the initial research. She also critically read drafts of the materials developed under that contract and provided good feedback. However, the content of this book in no way reflects the opinions of Dr. Yancik.

We are also indebted to the principal investigators of the individual network projects who generously and graciously made available the materials and other information necessary to conduct this research. Again, the interpretation of these materials is ours, but the original resources came from these programs. Specifically, we would like to thank James Y. Suen (University of Arkansas for Medical Sciences), James H. Brandenburg (University of Wisconsin), Donald Shedd (Roswell Park Memorial Institute), John M. Lore (State University of New York at Buffalo), Sol Silverman (University of California at San Francisco), Luther Brady (Hahnemann Medical Center), Frank Hendrickson (Rush University), George Sisson (Northwestern University), and Emmanual M. Skolnick (University of Illinois).

A special note of thanks is due Jerellyn Logemann (Northwestern University), who was a coinvestigator on the original evaluation contract and who had also been a major participant in the rehabilitation program of the network. Her observations and insights were most helpful in enhancing our understanding of these networks.

As our project coordinator and Number One Research Assistant, Penny L. Havlicek performed yeoman's work throughout the research project and completed a most impressive doctoral thesis using the project data. Her efforts and input were not restricted to Chapter 6.

Of our many colleagues at the University of Illinois at Chicago, Chris Ross was extremely helpful in the network analysis of our survey data. He is a patient teacher as well as a good friend.

Dorothy Young assisted us throughout the project, typing early manuscripts and all tables for the final manuscript. The library of Bowdoin College in Brunswick, Maine, was most generous in providing library resources and a study carrel to Dr. Fennell for two summers. Major portions of this manuscript were drafted in those cool, restful environs. The final word processing of the manuscript could not have been accomplished without Dennis Hogan's IBM-XT and his Laser-Jet printer.

Finally, our respective families provided support and listened to endless discussions about this book. Special thanks to Dennis Hogan and Barbara Warnecke for their support and encouragement throughout the project.

Mary L. Fennell
Richard B. Warnecke

Contents

CHAPTER 4

CONSIDERING THE ENVIRONMENT: ENVIRONMENTAL CONTEXT AND NETWORK FORM

CHAPTER 5

NETWORK FORM, NETWORK STRUCTURE, AND BOUNDARY MANAGEMENT

CHAPTER 6

VARIATION ACROSS HOSPITALS IN NETWORK PROGRAM PARTICIPATION

PENNY L. HAVLICEK

CHAPTER 7

DEFINITION AND DIFFUSION OF THE INNOVATION

CHAPTER 8

NETWORK OUTCOMES: TRANSFORMATION, SURVIVAL, AND INSTITUTIONALIZATION

APPENDIXES

Medical Innovations and Interorganizational Diffusion

INTRODUCTION

Throughout their history as sponsors of biomedical research, the National Institutes of Health (NIH) have mainly emphasized basic research and have allotted few resources to the translation of research findings into clinical applications. This policy was based on the assumption that medical education sufficiently equips the physician to keep abreast of new medical developments. Subscription to medical journals, attendance at professional meetings and continuing medical education symposia, and talking with colleagues are presumed to provide access to up-to-date information on how to deliver state-of-the-art care to patients (Breslow, 1977; Kaluzny et al., 1976; Tilson et al., 1975).

When we think about advances in medical technology and how medical innovations become known and used, two very familiar images come to mind. The first image is of the lone scientist, hard at work in his lab, surrounded by an array of test tubes, bunsen burners, cages of mice, and petri dishes with strange things growing in them. This is, after all, where scientific breakthroughs in medicine take place. Once in a while these very harried fellows are accosted by the news media, usually following publication of such a breakthrough. The ensuing television news interview usually takes place in the scientist's lab or in his library (suitably surrounded by books), and this white-jacketed individual with glasses pushed up on his forehead describes the significance of his new findings, and usually cautions the reporter that many more tests are needed before the new drug/machine/artificial-whatever will be ready for general clinical application.

Here is introduced the second image of the trusted family physician hard at work in his office/library (suitably surrounded by books), late at night, absorbed in the most recent medical journal, reading the paper that was the subject of the scientist's press conference and deciding for himself whether to use it to treat Mrs. Smith's arthritis/liver/heart problem.

After the Coleman et al. (1966) study of medical innovation diffusion, our sociological understanding of the way in which the physician-practitioner learns about and decides to use new medical procedures and technology changed somewhat. In light of the insights from that study, we now recognize that physicians learn and evaluate as they interact with other physicians through informal networks that develop around consultation, referral, and collegial exchange. However, the basic image of the key points in the diffusion process remain unchanged; the lone scientist and the individual physician are still considered to be the major actors in the development and diffusion of medical innovations.

The level and rapidity of scientific development and progress attained by organized medical research over the past several decades belies the image of the physician-scientist as a lone investigator. Sociological research has established that the organizational context of scientific research is a crucial aspect of research creativity and productivity (Kornhauser, 1962; Pelz and Andrews, 1966). Management of the scientist's laboratory, the organizational and resource commitments required of universities and free-standing laboratories, the relationship between the scientist and his/her funding sources, evaluators, clients, colleagues, and co-workers all have important effects on creativity and successful research. Finally, very often the complexity of the subject matter and the research technology requires interdisciplinary collaboration. What is more often observed in reality is the physician-investigator as a member of a multidisciplinary team of scientists and highly trained research technicians who work in interlocking laboratories and whose workscope includes the process of data collection, publication of results, and preparation of new research proposals to ensure that the funding is available for the next round of studies. Thus, the scientist is also a team member and entrepreneur.

The image of the physician-practitioner also requires modification; a growing body of research documents the complex organizational base in which most physicians practice. Increasingly, physicians are drawn to group practice because it provides access to patients and a secure opportunity to practice in their specialty field. Even if physicians remain solo practitioners, the hospital is increasingly their primary delivery point for medical care. The hospital often controls access to most of the technology physicians need to treat their patients. Moreover, if solo practitioners are specialists, they are usually part of referral networks in order to obtain sufficient patients to practice their specialties. Such networks often arise out of common affiliations of attending staff at a given hospital. Also, the complexity of most specialty fields is such that physicians are able to keep abreast of the literature only in their own fields. Thus, keeping up with the whole body of medical literature is probably beyond the technical capabilities of most physicians.

Finally, between the practicing physician and the physician-scientist there is often a complex infrastructure that filters and interprets information and constrains the adoption of new treatment innovations directly by the physician. First, there are various professional gatekeepers who evaluate the information before it is disseminated. These include journal reviewers, grant study sections, and the professional leadership who in many ways formulate a consensus on the meaning and relevance of new scientific breakthroughs. Often these individuals establish the criteria and define what is ready for dissemination through their positions on various advisory panels.

The viability of new technologies must be established scientifically. This usually is done in large-scale experimental evaluations or clinical trials. In these multi-institutional, national studies, new treatment strategies are evaluated against existing treatment procedures. Often one trial leads to questions that must then be evaluated in subsequent trials. The trials can take several years to complete, and the results are often debated in the literature and by various review panels for more years before they become accepted for general application in the clinical setting. Although community physicians may participate in these trials, access to the new treatment is usually restricted to investigational purposes, and the drugs or procedures being evaluated are not made available to nonparticipants.

When the results of such studies are equivocal or controversial, or require major alternation of accepted medical practice, they are often reviewed by a panel of experts drawn from clinical medicine, the relevant basic sciences, and biostatistics. Called "consensus conferences," these panels are convened by the Office of Medical Applications and Research (OMAR), which is a branch of the National Institutes of Health. They are open to a wide audience, which also often includes practitioners, basic scientists, statisticians, and consumer groups. In these conferences the data are reviewed and the panel and audience attempt to arrive at a consensus as to whether the procedure or technology in question is ready for general dissemination. The results of the conferences are published in a report, and an executive summary is distributed to the major medical journals and to relevant specialty journals. Thus, the outcomes of the consensus conference often represent the first step in the innovation diffusion process.

Another aspect of the filtering process between scientist and practitioner is the regulatory system. When a new treatment involves a drug, approval for general use in treatment must be secured from the Food and Drug Administration. Usually this follows the successful conclusion of the clinical trial, but until the trial data are reviewed, access for noninvestigational use may be limited. When the new treatment approach requires expensive equipment or other capital expenditure, approval from a local health systems agency or state regulatory program may be necessary before the hospital can purchase the equipment, and before the individual practitioner can begin to incorporate the technology into the treatment process.

Finally, the level of technology required for implementation often requires major commitment on the part of the hospital or other health care agency where the physicians see and treat their patients. In such instances the hospital administration and frequently other medical care providers who are responsible for the delivery of ancillary treatment are involved in the decision, and they may make it without consulting the physicians who actually decide whether or not to refer patients for treatment. An example of this type of technology would be radiation therapy, where the equipment and the treatment are under the control of a radiation therapist, who makes the decision as to what kind of equipment is to be purchased by the hospital (Greer, 1986). However, the radiation therapist depends upon other physicians to refer patients to him/her for the treatment.

In sum, the underlying assumptions of the traditional diffusion model—(1) that knowledge flows from the scientist to the practitioner via the medical journal, professional meeting, and/or contact with other professionals, and (2) that the physician makes an individual decision to adopt or reject a new idea on the basis of that information—are inconsistent with the state of modern research and modern medical practice. The traditional images stem from an era when medical technology was less complex, when it could be carried in the physician's black bag, when the information needed to practice medicine was carried in the physician's head, and the scientist could easily communicate new ideas because they were based on a minimal level of technological complexity. This is now an archaic picture.

Given the persistence of the traditional images of the physician as researcher and as practitioner, it is not surprising that much of the existing research on the diffusion of medical innovation focuses on individuals (Rogers, 1983). Moreover, as we have noted, the policies regarding the dissemination of new procedures established by the NIH also reflect this orientation. When organizations are incorporated into the research, the emphasis is on how the innovation is adopted *within an organization* (Zaltman *et al.*, 1973). For the most part, the type of question addressed tends to be of the form "Why do specific physicians/specific hospitals choose to adopt specific innovations?"

Innovation studies in organizations have not usually addressed the process of innovation diffusion across organizations, nor have they considered the special case of diffusion among professional organizations like hospitals, where two classes of actors (doctors and administrators) are involved in the decision to adopt and/or implement an innovation (Greer, 1984). There is little or no information on how "networks" of health organizations, which link individual professionals but take into account organizational constraints, function as vehicles for the spread and use of new medical technologies. There is little understanding of the processes by which such networks develop in response to the need to implement new technologies or treatments, and how strategies are devised to meet the particular needs and characteristics of local communities. Such organizational networks develop within the context of social communities. Their shape and character reflect the nature of that context. For networks of health organizations this means that the health-related characteristics of the community's populace, the levels of resources available for health care, how these resources are distributed among existing medical care organizations, and the preexisting patterns of interaction among medical professionals and organizations are all important factors that influence how innovation diffusion occurs.

Within these contexts the formation of networks constitutes a statement or "signal" by network actors to other segments of the community of the intent to alter in some way the existing patterns of health care delivery. The success of the network effort depends on the ability of the organizers of the network to convince the larger community of two things: (1) that a need exists within the community for change in extant patterns, and (2) that the organizational network is an appropriate response. It follows, then, that both the way in which organizational needs are defined and the form in which the innovation diffusion process takes place will be critical to the success of the network as a diffusion channel.

There is almost no information about how successful such networks are as vehicles for diffusing new technologies. The issue of network performance and influence on the diffusion of new technology is particularly thorny because various levels of analysis are possible in defining diffusion outcomes, and because multiple levels of linkage are involved in medical organizational networks. Where should we look to find the results of network diffusion of medical innovation? Should we look at the level of patient care and patient outcomes defined by changes in mortality or morbidity rates? Should we focus on the hospital, and look at changes in hospital structure or changes in the care process? Or, should we look at the regional level and try to identify changes in referral patterns or resource availability? Or finally, should we look at the national level and ask: Is change directly evident in the national policies by which medical technology diffusion is promoted?

Second, what aspects of medical networks should be emphasized for evaluation? One option is to examine the performance of various linkages in the network. Another might be to examine the performance of the particular organizations involved in the diffusion network. Finally, the performance of the interorganizational structure or of the coordinating system that links individuals and organizations could be examined. These important issues will be addressed in the following chapters.

The purpose of this book is to explore the emergence and development of the organizational network and its role in the diffusion of modern medical technology. In this exploration we will use both recent organizational theory and diffusion theory to analyze data from a case study of seven networks. These networks were established to promote the diffusion of "state-of-the-art" treatment for head and neck cancer to community practitioners in seven different regions of the United States. This volume is a comparative and descriptive study of how these networks emerged, achieved their specific character, and functioned for a period of three to four years. We have examined the diffusion process by looking at the development, structure, process, and performance of these seven networks. Our analysis is based on a combination of contingency theory and the resource dependence perspective on organizations to determine how these seven programs adapted a single innovation to address particular problems in their own regions. The story of these seven networks shows clearly, in fact, that the classic innovation diffusion theory consistent with the two images of the physician as lone scientist and as solo practitioner is inadequate for understanding innovation diffusion in the modern medical setting. Today, decisions about medical innovation are contingent upon a complex set of factors related to the innovation, the environment, and the organizations in which health care is practiced.

HISTORICAL BACKGROUND OF NETWORKS IN THE HEALTH SECTOR

The history of the network concept in health care is rife with contradictions. The network idea is basically a very simple one: By the linking of health care providers, whether physicians, clinics, hospitals, or other institutions, through cooperative exchanges of patients, personnel, programs, or facilities, the quality of care in an area should improve, and costs should decrease (through the reduction of facility/service duplication). This is essentially the argument advanced to explain the recent explosion in the number of sharing arrangements among hospitals, and the upswing in the number of multihospital systems. As monitored by the American Hospital Association surveys, the number of hospitals participating in sharing arrangements of all types (from clinical services to administrative functions and purchasing agreements) increased 100% from 1965 to 1975 (Taylor, 1977) and has continued an upward curve into the 1980s. Similarly, many researchers have noted the steady increase in multihospital systems, in which two or more hospitals are owned, leased, or contract-managed by a single corporate office (DeVries, 1978;

Mullner *et al.*, 1981; Zuckerman, 1979). The American Hospital Association's 1985 Directory of Multihospital Systems lists 267 such systems, representing 35% of all U.S. community hospitals operating in 1984. Both sharing arrangements and multihospital systems are expected to become even more prevalent in the future.

Government Intervention in Regional Planning

These figures would seem to suggest that cooperation among health care providers is definitely on the rise, and that cooperative networks are an idea whose time has come. Although that might now be true, the road leading to these developments has been extremely rocky, and progress was impeded by the twin obstacles of professional autonomy and hospital independence (Starr, 1982). Cooperation among hospitals and the emergence of cooperative hospital networks have only recently become possible, thanks primarily to the federal government's "carrot and stick" approach to fostering hospital cooperation during the 1960s and 1970s. An appreciation of the history behind this forced trend is necessary in order to understand both the story of the networks studied in this volume and the future of such networks given an environment with fewer and fewer federal carrots.

The period from 1940 to 1965 marked an era of expansive growth for the hospital industry, and particularly for community general hospitals. Private, third-party insurance plans had been introduced in the 1930s and were now well established, increasing access to voluntary hospital care among working- and middle-class subscribers. The demand for hospital services grew with increased population and higher personal incomes. With the passage in 1948 of the Hill-Burton Act, the federal government acted to stimulate capital improvements in nonprofit community hospitals. Hill-Burton signaled the beginning of large-scale government intervention in the health sector. Both the government and health care providers emphasized the need to eliminate deficiencies in the nation's bed supply and to improve hospital facilities across the board, so that every community hospital could become a "center for the integration of medical specialties and expansive technologies" (Zald and Hair, 1972, p. 58). The remarkable growth of these facilities during this time, however, contributed to the development of autonomous, local hospital delivery systems in which every community hospital operated independently, seeking to augment its domain and prestige vis-à-vis other hospitals.

With the passage of Titles 18 and 19 (Medicare and Medicaid) in 1966, however, several important trends converged, adding to the escalation of hospital costs, which had begun as early as the 1950s (Feldstein and Taylor, 1977). With the opening of access to hospital care to the two groups left uninsured by most private plans, the elderly and the poor, the demand for care increased considerably (Feldstein, 1979). Second, incentives to keep costs down did not keep pace with increases in the quality and quantity of services provided in this early period. As medical knowledge and technology expanded, hospitals competed with each other to have all of the most "up-to-date" facilities that physicians could want or use. Following Medicare/Medicaid, the government was forced to become involved in hospital regulation in a big way. Although both quality (licensure) and cost control were the focus of regulation, cost control was probably the dominant concern.

In the 1960s the federal government began to emphasize coordination, comprehensive health planning, and reduction of service duplication, albeit in rather limited and indirect ways. Many of these initial efforts were based on the principle of fostering cooperation and interorganizational linkages between academic medicine and the local community, among heretofore independent health organizations. For example, through President Johnson's Community Action Programs, neighborhood health centers were established as satellite facilities of medical schools and teaching hospitals in the community. Their mission was to relieve the deplorable health care access problems experienced in the inner cities. Medicare/Medicaid regulations required extended-care facilities to enact "transfer agreements," or interfacility cooperation with one or more other hospitals to participate in these programs (Greenfield, 1975). Also, in 1966 Congress passed Public Law 89-785, the "sharing law," which allowed (and actually encouraged) Veterans Administration hospitals to share medical resources with private sector and other governmental facilities. None of these programs, however, could effectively get community hospitals to coordinate their facility expansion projects, or to share resources with other hospitals in their communities. In fact, much of this cooperative activity involved interaction between academic medical centers and community health planning agencies.

The Comprehensive Health Planning Act in 1966 also introduced incentives for community-based, regional planning through the establishment of Regional Medical Programs (RMPs). These programs were to plan for the provision of health services in the regions where they were established. It was assumed that through such programs both medical and nonmedical groups would increase their commitments to equitable access to health care and, thus, decrease waste. The quality and emphasis of the RMPs varied. Often they were unable to manage competing interest groups within their regions. As a result, special-interest groups within communities often pressured the RMPs to meet their particular needs at the cost of truly comprehensive regional planning. Consequently, the RMPs and the concept of regional planning proved to be less than totally successful.

The 1974 National Health Planning and Development Act replaced RMPs with the Health System Agencies (HSAs). These new agencies were also responsible for regional health planning, but they did not have the implementation funds for planning activities that had been available to the RMPs. The HSAs were primarily planning groups, but they did have authority over final approval of large expenditures that would appreciably affect health costs in their regions. One of the most important provisions of the 1974 act was to vest the authority for administration of certificate-of-need (CON) programs in state health planning and development agencies created by the act. These programs have been adopted by 48 states, and they represent the federal government's most aggressive effort to influence the local supply of hospital services and facilities. When hospitals plan capital expenditure programs exceeding $150,000, they must obtain a permit and satisfy a set of need criteria. In many states certificate-of-need programs have been supplemented by agreements within the federal government under Section 1122 of the Social Security Act, whereby the federal government can deny Medicare/Medicaid reimbursements to hospitals that have invested in unapproved facilities. Some Blue Cross plans have adopted similar reimbursement policies.

Thus, hospitals moved out of the Hill-Burton era, which promoted individual growth, into an era of constraints on growth, in which active consideration of the local hospital market by an external agency is required before decisions about individual hospital expansion can be implemented. Clearly, however, this shift in emphasis from the autonomous hospital to the interdependent local market was made possible only with the pressure of government regulation affecting health care.

As the government attempted to control costs through regulation that required individual hospitals to consider other hospitals in the area and the community's need for expanded facilities, it also tried to improve the quality of care by promoting hospital and provider "networks" for the diffusion of innovations in medical technology and treatment. As can be seen in the following passages of the 1974 Health Planning and Development Act, the focus of the act was to foster actual interaction and cooperation at the local level among hospitals, through

> —Development of multi-institutional systems for coordination or consolidation of institutional health services (including obstetric, pediatric, emergency medical, intensive and coronary care, and radiation therapy services);
> —Development of medical group practices (particularly those whose services are coordinated or integrated appropriately with institutional health services), health maintenance organizations, and other organized systems for the provision of health care;
> —Development of health service institutions that have the capacity to provide various levels of care (including intensive care, acute general care, and extended care) on a geographically integrated basis;
> —Development of multi-institutional arrangements for the sharing of support services necessary to all health service institutions.

The institutions of regional oversight by law represented a radical departure from earlier efforts at promoting cooperation focused on the voluntary sharing of new medical technology and information through professional interaction and the medical literature. Historically, as we have noted, the model used to promote medical innovation diffusion centered on the individual physician-practitioner and the individual physician-scientist.

Government Regulation and the Diffusion of Medical Innovations

In fact, the diffusion of medical information and technology from the academic medical center to the community treatment center through the individual practitioner was originally formulated by Abraham Flexner (1910). Flexner believed that professional socialization was the way to ensure that practitioners remained current. He proposed a system of professional education designed to motivate physicians to keep abreast of new medical discoveries and techniques. With the educational background this system would provide, the physician would be able to implement basic principles in everyday practice, and to determine whether to adopt new concepts introduced through continuing educational programs and medical journals.

The influence of Flexner's recommendations was pervasive and is apparent in policies developed later by the National Institutes of Health concerning the support of research, medical education, and community outreach. Following the Flexner model, general research support to be incorporated into new medical education programs was given to medical schools. Such support was contingent upon publication of resulting research findings. Federal funds even supported the publication of specialty journals (such as the *Journal of the National Cancer Institute*) in order to ensure that new information resulting from research was made available to community-based practitioners (Breslow, 1977; Kaluzny *et al.*, 1976; Tilson *et al.*, 1975).

After publication of the 1964 report of the President's Commission on Heart Disease, Cancer, and Stroke, however, Congress demanded more efforts to disseminate research to the community. The traditional orientation based on the Flexner model began to change and to reflect the increasingly important role of the hospital in diffusing innovations for treatment and management of chronic diseases. This new approach recognized that adoption decisions were contingent decisions that could go forward only if both physicians and hospitals were convinced of the innovation's worth. Moreover, it was further recognized that the decision to adopt new, expensive technologies requiring capital investment on the hospital's part rested upon the shoulders of hospital administrators, not the doctor. Thus, the traditional approaches to medical innovation diffusion that emphasized only the physician's role were no longer adequate.

The federal government's most recent attack on escalating hospital costs concentrates on the method of hospital reimbursement for patients covered by Medicare. Prospective, per case payment based on diagnosis-related groupings (DRGs) was established as the national Medicare payment system under the 1983 Social Security Amendments (Public Law 98-21) and was implemented in October of 1983. Although ostensibly focused on the issue of per case hospital costs, DRGs will probably have rather far-reaching effects on both the development/adoption of new hospital technology and the structure of local hospital delivery systems. The nature of those effects, however, is at this point difficult to predict.

Prospective payment means that hospitals are given fixed reimbursement schedules at the beginning of each fiscal year. If the hospital's actual costs exceed the prospectively set reimbursement schedule, the hospital loses money. This method of payment stands in sharp contrast to the traditional method of retrospective payment, in which essentially all costs are recovered, retrospectively, at a year's-end accounting that sets reimbursements on the basis of actual costs. Obviously, prospective payment creates incentives for hospitals to reduce costs—incentives not present in retrospective payment. Further, reimbursing on a per case basis effectively focuses cost reduction on the process of inpatient care itself. Payment is set at a specific amount for each patient, depending upon the diagnostic category he/she falls into, regardless of the actual number or types of services the patient has received. Cost savings for the hospital can be found, then, in both reducing the length of stay for each patient and carefully evaluating the benefits of additional services against the likelihood of incurring nonreimbursable costs. The assumption behind DRG reimbursement schemes is that both physicians and hospitals will modify their traditional no-holds-barred approach to service-intensive patient care if a substantial proportion of the hospital case load is covered by DRG payment. It is important to remember, however, that so far only hospital costs fall under the Medicare DRG program; physician fees and outpatient services are still reimbursed in the pre-1983 fashion.

In a technical memorandum on the implications of DRGs for medical technology (1983), the Office of Technology Assessment (OTA) concluded that DRGs would probably affect both the use of current technology and future patterns of technological change in medicine. Unfortunately, since such effects were inadequately evaluated prior to the implementation of DRGs, and the DRG program is itself relatively new, our discussion will of course be to some extent hypothetical. Nonetheless, DRGs represent an additional complexity in the process of adoption and diffusion of medical innovations. As pointed out by the OTA memorandum, DRGs will influence hopsitals' decisions to adopt new technologies, and they could affect the rate and direction of technological change in medicine. Clearly, technologies that can be labeled as cost-reducing will be encouraged, while cost-raising technologies will be discouraged. However, classification of innovations as cost-effective and/or conducive to better treatment outcomes *prior to their development* and adoption is itself problematic. Furthermore, technologies are neither cost-saving nor cost-raising in an absolute sense; such assessments cannot be made independent of an understanding of the context in which adoption would be made. Thus, in their attempts to adopt new technologies in a cost-effective fashion, hospitals cannot be expected to proceed in only one direction: What might be cost-effective for one hospital might be cost-raising for another.

Although it is too soon to know exactly how DRGs will affect technological change in medicine, we do have some evidence of how hospitals react to the sorts of incentives imposed by prospective payment programs. Studies by Joskow (1982) and Cromwell and Kanak (1982), for example, suggest that rate setting generally decreases the availability of complex, costly services, but this is dependent upon both the overall design and the stringency of the payment system itself. With the Medicare DRG program, this means we should probably pay considerable attention to the methods and procedures available to make adjustments to average payment levels, relative DRG rates, and the definition of DRG categories themselves. Built into the DRG payment system are a number of possible procedures for updating DRG rates and categories to take into consideration reestimation of relative DRG costs, the application of a general "technology factor" to increase rates annually, central policy decisions to change DRG rates, provider-initiated appeals for rate adjustments, and the creation of new DRGs reflecting the use of specific technological innovations. Each of these adjustment mechanisms will have different effects on the program's cost incentives and the program's ability to encourage the adoption of "appropriate," i.e., cost-reducing, technologies. Each of them, however, requires detailed information about new technologies and their readiness for adoption and coverage. Thus, technology assessment becomes a crucial aspect of the DRG program and its ability to adjust to medical progress.

Finally, there is some reason to believe that the use of DRG payment programs will also affect the shape or structure of hospital delivery systems in the future. A common expectation is that the kinds of coordinative mechanisms we have seen expanding in recent years among hospitals in local areas could become even more likely. It is possible that DRGs will lead to greater specialization of services among hospitals. As a result of the greater incentives to reduce costs per case, DRGs may encourage the concentration of capital-intensive technologies in a few regional institutions, where high volume and experience levels could increase profits and lead to better health outcomes. Concomitantly, unprofitable services may be abandoned, but the hospital industry's long history of comprehensive service availability may block this side of the story. Services that are important, either symbolically or actually, to physicians or patients may be kept, even if they are unprofitable or infrequently used. Again, it is still too early to tell. DRGs may change the structure of service delivery to what some have labeled high-volume, for-profit medicine, delivered by corporate hospital chains (Salomon, 1984; Starr, 1982). Then again, inertia has always been an important characteristic of the hospital industry (Fennell, 1980, 1982).

BACKGROUND OF THE HEAD AND NECK CANCER DEMONSTRATION NETWORKS

The history of federal efforts to control cancer can provide a particularly useful example of the change from a physician-centered to a hospital-inclusive approach to medical innovation diffusion, as well as of the increasing importance of the federal carrot in encouraging interhospital or regional cooperation. Before 1971, the NIH approach to cancer control was consistent with the Flexner model. Programs emphasized educating the physician rather than direct intervention in the community. After 1971, however, the National Cancer Act contained a "line item" in the budget to design and implement cancer control programs that would disseminate new research findings into community treatment centers.

Community-based outreach networks were among the first cancer control programs initiated. The director of the Division of Cancer Control and Rehabilitation, who had responsibility for these programs during their initiation period, noted several reasons why the time seemed appropriate to begin network programs. In addition to the mandate from Congress, evidence indicated that standard treatment was not uniformly available at many community hospitals where the most prevalent cancers were frequently treated. Outdated or inadequate procedures were often being performed at institutions in the same cities or regions where institutions renowned for their excellence in cancer treatment were located. Also, the results of ongoing clinical trials indicated that new treatment procedures were likely to require multidisciplinary inputs; thus, treatment guidelines had to be developed that emphasized the collaboration of several medical disciplines (such as surgery, radiation therapy, and chemotherapy). The development of networks composed of both university and community hospitals was seen as an opportunity for hospitals that did not have the necessary multidisciplinary staff to have access to those institutions that did.

The experience with these networks was generally positive, although some difficulties were encountered from the outset. One persistent problem arose from the uneven distribution of treatment facilities among participating hospitals, particularly in those networks located in rural areas. A second difficulty arose when local practitioners in one network service area challenged the government's right to support treatment programs in community hospitals. These challenges reflected the skepticism among private physicians and the AMA regarding the propriety of federal funding for treatment interventions in community settings, and their fear that such programs would interfere with professional autonomy (Breslow, 1977).

Following the cancer network experience, similar network programs were initiated by the NIH in the areas of heart disease, end-stage renal disease, maternal and neonatal care, and emergency medical services. In fact, implicitly or explicitly, the network concept became the heart of many programs with the objective of transferring information or technology.

Despite the ubiquity of the network concept in planning such programs, the issue of how networks of health care facilities affect the delivery of services has not been intensively studied. Although there are references in the organizational literature to "action-sets," defined as temporary interorganizational collaborations created by external agencies (like the federal government) for the purpose of promoting cooperation in specified areas (Aldrich and Whetten, 1981), very few studies have documented the effects of these created programs. (Notable exceptions are the studies by Aiken *et al.*, 1975, of federally funded coordination of mental health services, Rushing's 1971 study of medical intervention assistance programs, and Lehman's 1975 study of coordination among health care facilities.) Further, the value of network programs in actually improving the dissemination of new treatment technologies or disease management has not been adequately explored, on either a theoretical or an applied level. Accordingly, we turn now to the central issues of this book: an analysis of organizational networks as a method of diffusing medical innovations in cancer care. We begin with a brief discussion of the role of innovation diffusion within the NCI's philosophy of cancer control, followed by a description of the innovation studied here.

Cancer Control and Diffusion Networks

The cancer control philosophy at the NCI before the 1971 National Cancer Act was heavily influenced by the Flexner model. As such, cancer control *per se* was not a separately established component of the overall scientific program. This created problems when, after 1971, the NCI attempted to institute such a program.

A former program head at the NCI responsible for cancer control expressed the policies of the NCI prior to 1971 in the following description of the mission:

> Major emphasis in cancer control is placed on programs to aid physicians, by improving professional undergraduate, graduate and postgraduate education, and by providing diagnostic and other aid to help the physician be effective. (Kaiser, 1955)

This philosophy was reflected operationally within the institute by the separation of cancer control activities from the natural scientific bases being developed in other program areas. For example, epidemiology, which had provided the scientific basis for infectious disease control, developed at the NCI in a separate division and had no formal linkage or responsibilities for cancer control. Similarly, although the initial network concepts came from the clinical science program, when they were transferred to the cancer control program, responsibility and interest disappeared. Thus, when the cancer control program was formally established, it lacked scientific sponsorship within the NCI that could lend legitimacy to cancer control activities and provide a scientifically sound basis from which community interventions could be launched.

The formal initiation of cancer control programs within the NCI came with the passage of the 1971 National Cancer Act, which expressly directed the NCI to address cancer control as a specific program area and included a line item in the budget for this purpose. The act also specifically authorized the creation of comprehensive cancer centers that were to implement research and demonstration programs in clinical research, epidemiology, biomedical science outreach, and cancer control. However, there was no precedent at the NCI, or in the NIH more generally, for programs geared toward information dissemination rather than for information creation. Initially, the NCI insisted that all of its programs were concerned with cancer control (Breslow, 1977).

However, as we have noted, publication of the report from the President's Commission on Heart Disease, Cancer, and Stroke raised public awareness and concern about chronic disease control. As more of the population reached middle and old age, chronic disease supplanted infectious disease as the major cause of death. In addition to its recommendations for establishment of regional centers for multidisciplinary management of chronic disease in community settings, the commission noted that strategies for information dissemination and community-based health care delivery were lacking at the NIH.

It soon became clear that the mandate from Congress incorporated in the National Cancer Act required effective and well-designed programs in cancer control. This in turn meant that accountability to Congress had to be established. A special division and planning structure to design and implement cancer control programs that would disseminate new research findings into the community was established.

This expansion and shift in emphasis to focus on information and technology diffusion through community demonstration programs rather than through traditional channels of physician education required a new orientation for the NCI staff. Since there was no recent history of successful cancer control planning that could provide guidance for development of these new programs, between 1972 and 1974 a series of planning conferences was organized to determine the strategy for the new cancer control programs. Those attending were drawn primarily from academic medicine and from the staff of the NCI that shared the academic orientation. Given the experience and organizational affiliations of the attendees, it is not surprising that the program format eventually decided upon once again reflects the influence of the Flexner model. Medical innovation was to be defined and established at academic medical centers and then communicated to, and implemented by, community practitioners.

In recognition of the potential institutional influence of the hospital, a new dimension was added: In the proposed workscope it was indicated that diffusion of innovation was to take place through interorganizational networks that linked community hospitals (which had limited medical resources and few specialized staff) with academic centers (which had a broad spectrum of resources and personnel). But, following the Flexner model, the linkages limited participation to community practitioners, and the programs were to be designed, developed, and directed by the academic staff at the teaching center. Participation by organizational leaders (administrators) was not included in the plan, nor was there any practical recognition of the limitations on diffusion presented by gaps in the organizational capacity of any particular hospital. It was assumed that the community doctor would simply decide to adopt the innovation in the hospital setting where he/she practiced, without any impediments from the organization. Moreover, the new model did not allow for any participation by the community physicians in the formulation of the innovations to be introduced.

One of the outcomes of these first planning conferences was the program description for community-based demonstration networks. The overall objectives of these projects were to

1. Establish regional collaboration among the colleges, medical schools, cancer centers, and those community hospitals with facilities and staff that meet the minimum standards established by the Commission on Cancer of the American College of Surgeons for a clinical cancer program
2. Develop treatment guidelines through multidisciplinary collaboration
3. Establish an effective data system for evaluation of the implementation of the guidelines (U.S. DHEW, 1973)

Implementing network programs on the basis of these objectives assumed two conditions. First, it was assumed that state of the art for managing these cancers was sufficiently well established that it could be expressed in a communicable format. Second, it was assumed that the hospitals in the network had the necessary staff and equipment to implement these defined treatment procedures. In the absence of such staff and equipment, patients would presumably be referred to the academic center for those aspects of treatment that could not be delivered in the community hospital. The planning groups also stressed the need to integrate the leadership in cancer control, diagnosis, and treatment at major medical centers with the professional staff at community treatment centers, primary care providers, the lay public, and local government. Although this more inclusive conception of cancer control in some ways went beyond the Flexner model, the key nexus in all these early cancer control programs was still the old linkage between the academic physician-researcher and the community-based physician-practitioner.

Community-based outreach networks were first initiated for cancer control by the Division of Cancer Treatment with the NCI. The Division of Cancer Control and Rehabilitation (now the Division of Cancer Prevention and Control) had not yet been established but would later assume responsibility for the expanding network demonstration programs. The initial project was organized to disseminate the results of successful clinical research on new approaches for the chemotherapeutic management of acute lymphocytic lymphomas (ALL) among children, and for Hodgkin's disease and other lymphomas in adults. It was designed according to the pattern recommended by the cancer control planning group. Every institution involved in the networks established by this project had to implement a common set of ALL chemotherapy protocols, and six networks adopted additional protocols for treating adult lymphomas.

Following this initial experiment, the network concept was extended to the management of two additional disease sites, cancer of the breast and cancer of the head and neck. These sites were selected as early targets because it was believed that state-of-the-art treatment for them was sufficiently advanced and well defined to permit dissemination to community practitioners. The validity of this assumption, however, was questionable, as will be discussed in Chapter 3. In any case, the breast cancer and head and neck cancer network demonstration projects were to implement "proven" multidisciplinary treatment procedures in community settings and to conduct educational programs for medical professionals and the lay public.

The initial request for proposals from the NCI for head and neck cancer networks specified seven objectives:

1. To deliver standardized, modern care to all head and neck cancer patients in each network service region
2. To develop standard treatment and continuing care management guidelines
3. To establish and implement rehabilitation procedures for all patients
4. To establish a standard data system
5. To conduct regional educational programs directed at the medical and lay communities dealing with prevention, detection, diagnosis, and treatment, rehabilitation, and continuing care
6. To provide a vehicle for sharing specialized personnel and facilities among community hospitals to effect the highest quality and cost-effective multidisciplinary care for head and neck cancer patients
7. To evaluate each project in terms of its activity, process, and impact as prescribed by the evaluation guidelines of the NCI

Five academic centers were originally awarded contracts to develop network programs: Rush-Presbyterian-St. Luke's Medical Center and Northwestern University in Chicago, Illinois; the University of Wisconsin in Madison, Wisconsin; Roswell Park Memorial Institute and the State University of New York in Buffalo, New York. Applicants from Chicago indicated an intention to merge their programs and to add the University of Illinois and the University of Chicago. The two Buffalo applicants also planned cooperative programs. Funds were proffered to these institutions for the planning year, during which the two projects in Chicago merged and the two in Buffalo did the same. The three resulting networks received full implementation funds in 1975–1976. The NCI then initiated a second request for proposals in 1975 and awarded four additional contracts to Hahnemann Medical Center in Philadelphia, Pennsylvania; the Northern California Cancer Program in San Francisco, California; the University for Medical Sciences in Little Rock, Arkansas; and the University of Mississippi Medical Center in Jackson, Mississippi.

The concept of a multihospital network as the diffusion channel was explicitly incorporated into the contracts awarded to these seven academic centers to develop head and neck cancer programs. However, nowhere in the proposals submitted or in the contracts awarded was the operational nature of the concept specified, nor were there any specific instructions provided for how the regional hospital networks should develop. Thus, the network forms that developed in the seven regions varied considerably in structure, process, content, and, ultimately, outcome.

Innovation in the Management of Head and Neck Cancer

First of all, cancers of the head and neck include malignant tumors in a number of different sites: the oral cavity (including tongue, floor of the mouth, gingiva, buccal mucosa, palate, and lips), major salivary glands, nasal fossa, paranasal sinuses, nasopharynx, oropharynx, hypopharynx, larynx, cervical esophagus, and cervical trachea. Not included are cancers of the eye, ear, or brain, or skin cancers that occur on the face, neck, or scalp. Thyroid cancers were originally excluded in the NCI request for proposals, but because of the interests of one of the principal investigators who joined the project in the second year, it was later included.

In 1975, when these demonstration projects were initiated, the total number of newly diagnosed cases of head and neck cancer in the United States was estimated to be 33,000, or an incidence rate of 15 per 100,000 population. The incidence of all cancers for the same year was estimated to be 665,000, so these cancers represented 5% of the total cancer incidence (U.S. DHEW, 1976). The relative frequency of cancers by the various sites was as follows: oral cavity, 40%; larynx, 25%; oropharynx and hypopharynx, 15%; salivary gland, 7%; and the remaining sites, 13%.

Mortality during 1975 due to squamus cell cancers of the head and neck was estimated to be 12,000, which results in an incidence:mortality ratio of approximately 3 to 1. In general, about 50% of all head and neck cancer victims will survive for at least five years after diagnosis, but survival varies by tumor site and disease stage. Survival for five years was less than 10% for those with cancers of the cervical esophagus and for tumors diagnosed at an advanced stage (i.e., metastatic tumors). On the other hand, for early glottic tumors and for lip cancer, five-year survival was better than 90%.

A major reason for the poor prognosis for these tumors was the inability to detect them at an early stage of development, when treatment is least traumatic and when the prognosis for survival is likely to be best. The actual choice of treatment strategy is particularly important, too, even for those whose disease is likely to be terminal. Given the strategic location of these cancers, standard cancer treatment strategies such as radical surgery could result in a number of devastating side effects. For example, surgery can produce highly visible facial disfigurement, impairment of speech and swallowing, nutritional deficiencies that result from the inability to ingest food, and the social isolation that results from the inability to communicate.

Of course, there was considerable interest at that time in promoting management strategies that would improve survival. However, of even greater interest was the promotion of management techniques that would minimize these aftereffects of treatment and enhance the quality of life during whatever survival time remained for the patient.

The demonstration networks were intended, then, to diffuse a set of management guidelines that would enhance the likelihood of achieving these two objectives. The guidelines addressed strategies for early detection of head and neck cancers, management of precancerous lesions, therapeutic measures that are minimally disabling and disfiguring (such as a combination of minimal surgical incision with radiation therapy), early applications of effective rehabilitation procedures, and palliation for those who cannot be cured. The guidelines also contained a series of common errors in management of these patients.

ORGANIZATIONAL NETWORKS AND THE DIFFUSION OF INNOVATION

We have mentioned the limitations of exclusive reliance on classical theories of innovation diffusion that focus on the individual as both the target of the innovation and the controlling force in the adoption decision. In the medical sector new technologies may be adopted by the individual alone, by the individual using organizational resources, or by the organization. Depending upon the extent to which the resources of the medical organization, specifically the hospital, are involved, the decision to adopt an innovation can become increasingly complex and further removed from the control of the physician (Greer, 1986).

Researchers who have studied medical innovation diffusion in organizations have borrowed from organizational theory and incorporated into their logic some of the political aspects of decision making (Greer, 1977). The adoption process has been viewed as political behavior, reflecting the diverse values and goals of different constituencies within the organization, and their struggles for control over both resources and decision making. Alternatively, studies of organizational innovation have also sought to determine which aspects of organizational structure are most predictive of the decision to adopt or implement an innovation (Downs and Mohr, 1976). In either of these approaches, the focus of attention is on the decision to adopt an innovation *within a particular organization*. Little attention is paid in this literature to the influence on innovation diffusion of extraorganizational factors, or to the role of linkages among organizations in a particular environment that may promote or inhibit innovation diffusion.

Technology diffusion, however, must go beyond the individual organization and consider the organizational network or action-set as the diffusion model. Such an approach integrates traditional emphases of diffusion theory (the importance of individuals and/or organizational structures) with contemporary emphases from organizational theory that focus on the environment and interorganizational linkages within the environment. As we use the term here, *action sets* are groups of organizations, in this case hospitals or organizational actors, formed to meet the specific objective of disseminating an innovation, in this case state-of-the-art therapy for head and neck cancers, to community treatment centers.

The attempted utilization of action-sets, formed for the limited purpose of promoting this specific set of therapeutic interventions, introduced a higher level of organizational complexity into the diffusion process. Moreover, these complex organizational forms were initiated by an agency external to the communities in which they were established. Since the external agent that introduced the diffusion form was the federal government, it is important to take into account the type of signal that intervention gave to the participating communities (M. W. Meyer, 1979), and how those communities responded to that signal. Thus, the community's response (acceptance, indifference, hostility) becomes a key aspect of the social environment of the diffusion process. That response will influence the form of network to develop and the level of acceptance that will be encountered when the innovation is introduced. Thus, the success of such ventures will be contingent upon the environmental context in which they are introduced.

Contingency Theory and Innovation Diffusion

In considering how such interorganizational diffusion networks can be developed and how they perform, we have utilized contingency theory, because it provides a framework in which such environmental conditions are presumed to play a critical role in organizational design and formation. Contingency theory has also been used in organizational research to understand how the relationships among units in the organization's environment can influence performance and outcomes.

The basic premise of contingency theory is that organizational performance depends upon the meshing, or contingent nature, of environmental and technological constraints, and the organizational structures developed to match those constraints. Contingency theory is based on three assumptions: (1) There is no one best way to organize to achieve maximum performance; (2) different ways of organizing are not always equally effective; and (3) the most effective organizational plan depends upon the environment in which the organization exists. In short, good matching (strategic contingency) leads to good performance.

From the standpoint of innovation diffusion, Kaluzny and Hernandez (1983) argue that contingency theory draws special attention to the variation in internal organizational structures and processes that affect change. They also emphasize that variations in structure and process result from the nature of the organization's tasks, the attributes of the environment and of the innovation and their potential impact on acceptance, the type of organization initiating the change, and the nature of the change itself. In other words, the contingency model specifically addresses the interface between the characteristics of the innovation, the diffusion source, and the potential of the adopting group for incorporating the innovation (Aiken and Hage, 1968; Downs and Mohr, 1976). In this analysis, then, consideration will be given to the organization or class of organizations to which the innovation is targeted, the characteristics of the innovative technology as they potentially affect the target organizations, and the outcome or performance of the action-sets created to serve as diffusion channels.

Contingency theory has been criticized for many problems, but perhaps the most significant criticism has been the lack of a clear conceptualization of the central "matching" concept (Mohr, 1971; Pennings, 1975; Schoonhoven, 1981). However, the basic approach has been well accepted and provides the underpinnings for many contemporary analyses of organizational performance, growth, and survival (J. W. Meyer, 1978; VandeVen and Drazin, 1985). Moreover, it has been specifically tested with regard to organizational change by a variety of studies, all of which consistently show that environmental factors explain the preponderance of variance in different aspects of organizational change (Hage and Aiken, 1967; Lawrence and Lorsch, 1967; Schoonhoven, 1981). For our purposes, a contingency approach is ideal. It allows consideration of several crucial factors in the diffusion process: the characteristics of the technology at issue, the environment of the organizations in which the innovation is introduced, and the outcome or performance of the diffusion strategy. We will not be concerned here with developing anything like a definitive statement of the exact nature of the matching concept. Rather, we use the basic ideas of contingency theory as a general guide in our study of medical diffusion networks. In our analyses, matching will be assessed in terms of the organization's capacity to adopt the innovation (Is that capacity sufficient for direct adoption of the innovation?), the extent to which norms in the environment support change and organizational collaboration (Does the network project match or take advantage of preexisting linkages?), and by the form in which innovation diffusion finally occurred (Was the appropriate form implemented given environmental and organizational constraints?).

Starkweather and Cook (1983) and Scott (1987) have noted that natural selection or population ecology theory is a variant of contingency theory. The major postulate of natural selection models is that variation in organizational form stems from the constraints imposed by the environment that force the demise of organizations that do not "fit" those constraints (Hannan and Freeman, 1977; VandeVen and Drazin, 1985). However, innovation diffusion and organizational change following the adoption of innovation clearly imply an active response by the organization to environmental changes, and to the constraints imposed by these changes. Thus, it must be assumed that organizational structures can be modified through managerial decisions in ways that protect their core functions and ensure their survival. Although the environment does select or influence the survival of organizational forms, organizations can and do take purposive actions that shape their own futures and even change their environments (Aldrich and Pfeffer, 1976).

Kaluzny and Hernandez (1983) described three general forms of adjustive managerial change, each of which implies more control by the organization in responding to the environment. The three forms are these:

1. Technical change—modifications made to the way in which the normal or core activities of the organization are carried out
2. Adjustive change—modifications made in organizational goals but not in the normal or core activities
3. Adaptive change—modifications made in both the activities and the goals of the organization

With Starkweather and Cook (1983), we take the position that change at the level of organizational structure is not only possible but a likely response to the threat of complete organizational failure. Further, contingency theory is useful in explaining the environmental limitations on change; it emphasizes the need for potential change strategies consistent with critical environmental elements, such as resources, organizational forms, and norms governing interorganizational relationships within the environment. However, to understand the potential for organizational response to the environment, we need to go beyond contingency theory and introduce the resource dependence perspective.

Resource Dependence and Innovation Diffusion

Resource dependence begins from the premise that no single organization can generate all the resources it needs for survival; thus, it is necessary to take action to ensure access to necessary resouces (Aldrich and Pfeffer, 1976; Jacobs, 1974; Mindlin and Aldrich, 1975; Pfeffer and Salancik, 1978; Yuchtman and Seashore, 1967). Two strategies follow from the resource dependence perspective: As described by Starkweather and Cook, they are "buffering" and "linking" (Thompson, 1967). Through buffering, the organization protects its core activity from encroachment by the environment using boundary definition to limit interaction with other units in the environment. Through linking, the organization expands its boundaries to acquire a broader resource base and build linkages to other organizations.

Using the resource dependence perspective we consider innovation adoption as basically a response by an organization or group of organizations to environmental conditions that threaten its core functions. Acceptance of an innovation is an action taken by the organization to ensure access to resources. The diffusion process can employ either linking or buffering strategies. On the one hand, when the process of technology diffusion occurs through the formation of action-sets to promote diffusion, it can be conceived of as a linking response aimed at expanding the organization's resource base. This is done by distributing the innovation within the action-set, thereby establishing a broader base of action as a means of ensuring greater access. As we mentioned earlier, the formation of such linkages signals to the environment that the participants in the action-set are taking actions aimed at enhancing their access to resources in the environment. A major consideration, then, is the eventual impact of the innovation on the environment, and particularly on organizational relationships within the environment. On the other hand, a buffering strategy can be employed, in which the innovating organization internally elaborates its own resource base by adopting the innovation and protecting associated resources within its own boundaries. Then, by selectively marketing its new capabilities, the organization builds dependence relationships with other organizations in the environment who require access to the innovation. However, by buffering the innovation and the resources it represents, the organization maintains complete control over all its relationships with other organizations.

Performance Gaps and Innovation Diffusion

A key concept shared by resource dependence and contingency theory, and in fact technology diffusion more generally, is the idea of a "performance gap." Innovations are adopted by organizations only when it is acknowledged by decision makers within the organization that there is a deficiency in operation that in some manner threatens the performance by the organization of its key functions. Such a need can be generated by the presence of a specific problem, by the existence of a gap between desired and actual performance, or as a response to a need to acquire resources to protect central organizational functions.

The definitions and/or recognition of a performance gap is not limited to the concerns of individual organizations, or to a consideration of only "bottom-line" performance outcomes (cost/benefit ratios, profitability). For example, in medical care it is common to evaluate performance in terms of such patient outcomes as mortality or morbidity rates, or patient management concerns such as service intensity, length of stay, or staff qualifications. These sorts of performance criteria are fairly readily defined since it can easily be determined when a hospital's mortality experience or average length of stay for a specific disease varies from regional or national norms. Such performance measures are readily observable and can be generalized from the organizational to the interorganizational or regional level.

Hospital systems, local hospital consortia, and regional delivery systems are also subject to performance evaluation, however. Where the gap exists, i.e., which aspect of their performance is found wanting, is not always ascertainable solely from functional outcomes. When examining these more complex organizational forms other criteria may be needed. For example, ultimately all organizations must be successful in obtaining from their environments supplies of essential resources needed to survive. For community hospitals this means several things. Patients must be found to fill hospital beds. Skilled professional staff must be recruited and retained to treat the patients. The hospital must maintain a sufficient level of community standing (good standing, esteem, legitimacy) that patients are willing to be treated there. For research hospitals patients represent the key materials on which the core activities depend. Without patients, and patients of great variety, clinical research and professional education cannot function. In the absence of the ability to perform such essential activities, these institutions would lose their skilled professional staff and the support to maintain their facilities. Thus, patients, professional staff, and facilities represent different resources to these two types of organizations.

The importance of the resource dependence perspective is found in its explicit recognition that access to these sorts of resources is not completely controlled by any one hospital in any area. They exist in finite supply in a given community, and very often access to them requires interaction with other hospitals or even other kinds of community organizations. Often, too, access may require expansion of the boundaries of the "community."

A performance gap can exist in access to one or all of these core resources. The performance gap may be perceived by a single organization or by a consortium of organizations in the region. All organizations may recognize the same gap, or the perceived gaps may be different or complementary, depending upon the goals of each type of organization. In such a setting, the adoption and implementation of innovations by community hospitals are often the means of addressing performance inadequacies. Thus, a treatment innovation may expand the patient base available to the hospital, a new technology may attract specialists in areas where the hospital is weak, and new treatment capabilities and equipment can increase the visibility and esteem of the hospital in the region. All of these improvements in performance can ultimately affect patient care outcomes, although rarely are such direct effects actually verifiable or even needed to justify the adoption of many innovations.

For the teaching/research hospital, patients can be acquired directly or indirectly. Direct acquisition requires strategies similar to those used by community hospitals. However, since the research center is usually a tertiary facility, it is frequently dependent upon referrals from other primary and secondary providers in the region. If these organizations perceive the research center to be competing for the same scarce resources, then they may be less likely to refer patients, thereby depriving the research center of access to this resource. Hence, there is often a strong incentive for the teaching/research center to acquire resources by establishing linkages or exchange relationships with the community centers. Often an ensured rational allocation of patients is established in exchange for the development of joint training programs between the tertiary center and its community affiliates.

Organizational Environments and Innovation Diffusion

What contingency theory adds to this analysis of medical innovation diffusion, which has not been considered by most diffusion scholars, is the need for careful consideration of the impact of organizational environments on the diffusion of innovations among organizations. The decision by a hospital to adopt an innovation to address a perceived performance gap and the subsequent diffusion of the innovation to other organizations in the region occurs within the context of a specific environment. Indeed, the perceived performance gap may reflect the recognition by the organization of inadequacies resulting from changes in the environment, such as a declining population base, changing demographic character of the service area, decreasing revenues, or increased competition from other hospitals. On the other hand, it may result from misperception of these factors or misinterpretation of their meaning. Finally, the extent to which an innovation spreads throughout an area, and the channels through which the diffusion occurs, also depends upon the environmental constraints extant in the community or region.

As we have noted, an organization's environment is defined partly in terms of the supply and distribution of resources. These include patients, skilled professionals, community esteem, and legitimacy. However, the environment is also defined by its organizational components. Thus, the characteristics of those organizations competing for resources is important. Also important is the division of organizational activities: Which organizations produce, control, distribute, and use the resources? Once the patterns of resource development, allocation, and utilization are established, there is a need to understand the patterns of interaction among various organizations and/or key individuals. All of these factors will have some effect on types of diffusion channels that can develop within the region and how they operate.

Another aspect of particular concern in this study is the view of organizational development as occurring in a life cycle (Kimberly and Miles, 1980). The action sets that are the subject of this book were developed for a specific purpose: to promote technology diffusion. Using the life cycle approach, we intend to focus on the stages through which these organizations passed as they emerged, signaled a change to others in the environment, experienced initial success in establishing the interaction patterns that formed their identity, bureaucratized, and eventually evolved into more permanent organizational forms. These states are defined by Starkweather and Kisch (1971) as the search phase, success phase, bureaucratic phase, and succession phase. Others have characterized these phases more simply as initiation and implementation, but they have identified similar patterns of activity and structural variation and personnel requirements as an innovation is first considered and initiated, and later adopted and institutionalized.

In the current project, how the networks initiated their activity during the initial start-up, or "search and success," phase had a great deal of impact on their subsequent implementation and ultimate success as innovation diffusion networks. As noted by Starkweather and Cook (1983), it is necessary to consider different organizational constituencies at the start-up and inplementation phases of the organizational life cycle. During start-up, input constituencies are important and are cultivated to provide the resources needed for initial survival and growth. Once initial survival is assured and there is some stability to the organization, output constituencies are established that are more directly related to the organization's functions. These are basically client relationships and reflect the organization's service objectives. In our analysis of the effects of the environment on the various types of network forms to emerge, we will consider the input and output constituencies as these networks moved from planning to implementation stages. Thus, focusing on the life cycle as a component of contingency theory provides a developmental or dynamic focus to the analysis.

FOCUS OF THIS STUDY

In summary, the focus of this study is not individual organizations but patterns of relationships among organizations in a given area. In other words, the patterns of growth and the performance of the diffusion networks are our central concerns. Using the basic assumptions of contingency theory and resource dependence, we are interested in examining how the "fit" or meshing of environmental contingencies and network structure can affect network performance or outcomes.

We have three broad hypotheses that will be explored in the remainder of the book. The first hypothesis is based on the assumption that the acceptance of new technologies by hospitals (either as single units or as networks) is a response to a perceived performance gap, or threat to the adopting unit's access to essential resources (patients, skilled professionals, or research support). Thus, acceptance does not occur unless a performance gap can be identified and the innovation defined as a legitimate solution.

A second hypothesis is that the environment within which organizations exist circumscribes both the extent of diffusion and the form of diffusion channel through which the process occurs. In other words, resource capacity and uneven distribution can limit the interorganizational diffusion of medical innovations.

The third hypothesis is that "fit" or mesh between environmental contingencies and the form of diffusion network will affect network performance. We expect a broad range of performance and outcome criteria to be affected by the level of "fit," including how the performance gap is defined, variation in actual implementation of the proposed innovation, changes in organizational structure and relationships resulting from the diffusion of the innovation, and the survival of the network after the initial innovation has been introduced and either accepted or rejected in the region.

To evaluate these broad hypotheses we will consider the following specific research questions. For each question we have indicated the chapter or chapters where answers are developed.

1. How does the nature of the environment affect the perceptions and definition of a performance gap that could lead to consideration of an innovation? What factors stimulate initial interest in the innovation among the target audience? (Chapter 3)

2. How are performance gap perceptions related to agenda setting within the networks? (Chapter 3)

3. How does the environment influence the formation of channels through which the innovation is diffused? Under what circumstances will diffusion occur through interpersonal or interorganizational channels? (Chapter 4)

Also, what is the relationship involving network enviornment, network form (interpersonal vs. interorganizational channels), and network structure (patterns of linkage and linkage characteristics)? (Chapter 5)

4. Within various network forms, what explains variation in participation levels by individual organizations? (Chapter 6)

5. How do both the environment and channel form affect the way in which the innovation is introduced and initially tried? (Chapter 7)

6. How does the form of network interaction relate to the institutionalization or abandonment of the innovation? In other words, what outcomes can be predicted from the context and structure of the networks that develop? (Chapter 8)

These questions will be investigated using the data from our study of seven network demonstration projects initiated by the NCI to transmit the concepts of modern patient management for head and neck cancer from university research centers to community treatment settings. These networks were developed on the premise that the university medical setting had devised approaches to patient management that reflected the state of the art for the care of head and neck cancer patients. It was further assumed that with appropriate motivation and support, these strategies could be disseminated to community treatment settings through linking community hospitals to academic medical centers, and to each other.

Earlier in this chapter we traced the development of the network concept in health planning in general terms. In the chapters to follow we will examine differences in application of the network concept in detail. Chapter 2 describes our data and methodology, and presents brief thumbnail sketches of each network.

Chapter 3 begins our substantive analysis with a consideration of environmental uncertainty and the perception of performance gaps in organizations and innovations as solutions to those gaps. In Chapter 4 we will argue that the environment of the social system constrains and promotes the formation of diffusion channels, and strongly influences whether diffusion occurs through interpersonal or interorganizational channels. Since the focus of this book is diffusion among organizational actors who are members of a social system of organizations, this analysis will consider the effects of the characteristics of the organizational environment on the diffusion process, particularly the development of boundary-spanning roles and strategies.

In Chapter 5 the focus will shift from the form of the channels to the interaction of the actors through the channels. We will analyze how network form creates and addresses basic problems of boundary definition and maintenance. We will also consider how these problems influence the more formal characteristics of network structure, such as linkage density, formalization, and complexity.

In Chapter 6 we will shift levels of analysis from the networks to the individual community hospitals and consider question 4, how the characteristics of the individual network participants influenced their participation in the diffusion process. At this level we will consider how hospital participation is constrained by organizational characteristics, particularly those factors that limit the potential dependence of community hospitals upon the headquarters institutions, or ensure that community hospital interests are represented.

Chapter 7 will address question 5. We will examine how the environment affects the way innovations are defined. Using the concept of "reinvention" (Rogers, 1983), we will show how contingent relationships influence the specific forms of the innovation that occurred in the different settings. The discussion will focus on the actual definition and dissemination of the innovation in various networks. We will explore how the diffusion process works in social systems with varying environmental characteristics, and the way in which the innovation is introduced in these different environments.

Our final chapter, Chapter 8, examines various outcomes of these network diffusion programs at the hospital, regional, and national levels, and discusses the policy implications for health care delivery of diffusion networks. We also consider the utility of network models as the basis of innovation diffusion in other contexts.

2

Data and Methods

INTRODUCTION: PROCESS EVALUATION AND RETROSPECTIVE CASE STUDIES

Our basic approach for tracing the development of the seven head and neck cancer networks involved placing the networks within a historical context. The fact that the seven networks (each funded for five or six years prior to the award of our contract) were about to be terminated as we began our study limited the observation of the network programs to a retrospective view. Our research problem suggested two methodologies simultaneously: (1) a descriptive historical case study of each network, and (2) a comparative analysis of the networks. Through the first analysis, the foci for the latter analysis emerged. The latter analysis, in turn, confirmed the conclusions reached through the first. Since the comparative analysis presented in this report is based on case studies, the methods followed to compile those studies need to be described. These case studies are available upon request; however, thumbnail sketches of each network based on these comprehensive case studies are included in this chapter.

A standard, comprehensive outline was followed for each historical case study. This outline was derived from the theoretical framework of the study and thus depicted each network as a response to the conditions in its environment or context. The outline was designed so that the analysis would first focus on an assessment of the geographical region of the network, and then on the network and its various parts. The outline was also constructed to capture both the static and the dynamic features of the network.

The detailed outline is presented as Appendix A. It is divided into three parts corresponding to three major factors affecting network development. First, the general context within which each network developed and the relevant resources immediately available to it are considered. This context is described in terms of the sociodemographic characteristics and mortality rates of its patient population, the availability of medical personnel, and the characteristics and availability of hospitals. The resources immediately available to the network are examined by focusing on the institutional members of the network. Two elements characterize these institutions: their resources and the links among them that preexisted the network. The resources examined include medical staff, treatment facilities, beds, and patients.

The second aspect of network development concerns how these institutions combined into a network organization. The establishment of new linkages between participants is examined, and the new structure designed to conduct the network activities is described. Finally, the procedures adopted to develop and implement programs are considered.

Applying the outline to two time periods in each network's existence provides a comprehensive, longitudinal analysis. The prenetwork period and the funded planning year constitute the first time period. The second time period covers the implementation years of network operation. Thus, when the outline was applied to the first time period, the resulting descriptions of network organization and procedures are largely descriptions of plans and proposed strategies. The descriptions written for the second time period are accounts of actual events. This approach allowed us to trace how proposed programs actually evolved into implemented programs.

These two periods differ slightly for the networks according to when their contracts were issued. The National Cancer Institute issued the first group of contracts in 1974 to the Wisconsin Head and Neck Cancer Control Network, Rush-Presbyterian-St. Luke's Medical Center and Northwestern University in Chicago, and Roswell Park Memorial Institute and the State University of New York in Buffalo, New York. The two Chicago applicants originally planned to collaborate, and the two Buffalo applicants also planned cooperative programs. The second set of contracts was awarded in 1975 to Hahnemann Medical Center in Philadelphia, Pennsylvania, the Northern California Cancer Program in San Francisco, California, the University of Arkansas for Medical Sciences in Little Rock, Arkansas, and the University of Mississippi Medical Center in Jackson, Mississippi. For the first group of networks, the first analytic time period extended from mid-1973 to mid-1975; for the last group of networks, from mid-1974 to mid-1976. Correspondingly, the second analytic time period extended from mid-1975 to mid-1980 for the first group, and from mid-1976 to mid-1980 for the second group, not including the Mississippi network, which terminated after one year of implementation. The funding ended for both groups at approximately the same time. The first group was funded for an extra year to collect follow-up patient data, but the second group was not.

Applying the outline to each network for both time periods required the use of a variety of data. Primary source data, or information gathered by the network, were supplemented by data from secondary sources. The primary sources included the documents produced by each network, interviews with key network participants, and a specially designed survey of the hospitals in each network. Secondary data were obtained from publications of the American Medical Association (AMA), the American Hospital Association (AHA), Marquis Who's Who, the U.S. Bureau of the Census, and the National Center for Health Statistics.

PRIMARY SOURCES

From the initiation of this study, we attempted to compile an entire set of network documents to serve as the central source of information about the networks. Those documents that proved most valuable included the written response to the NCI request for proposals to establish the demonstration projects, all annual and quarterly reports prepared by the networks, minutes of any committee and board meetings, the curriculum vitae of key network staff, the merit peer review reports prepared by each network for an NCI evaluation in 1977, all educational materials and scholarly papers the network produced, and the final reports submitted to the NCI by each network.

In addition to these documents, we requested each network to furnish information from their data bases on their patient population for analyses. These analyses included the following data for the initial and the 1978–1979 years of data collection:

1. The number of head and neck admissions in each hospital by site of disease
2. The number of head and neck admissions in each hospital by stage of the disease
3. The number of head and neck admissions by site and stage of disease
4. The number of head and neck admissions in each hospital by age, race, and sex
5. The treatment patterns for larynx and oral cavity cancers by disease stage

Information from the network data bases was also gathered on the completeness of the data base, or the number and type of data forms completed, by hospital. These data were used to assess the quality of data collected by each network.

The documents were grouped according to when they were produced. Thus, the information contained in the initial proposals and planning year annual reports pertained to the first analytic time period, while the bulk of the documents contained information pertaining to the implementation period, the second analytic time period.

These documents were limited sources of information in several respects. First, the types of documents collected and the amount of information they contained differed for each network. Second, since these documents were designed to report the activities and accomplishments of the network, they contained information about what programs were implemented, when they were implemented, and where they were implemented, but not about how they were organized. Network documents essentially portrayed finished end-products without the background of program development and process. Without this background information and with little or no account of the historical bases and context of network linkages, we could not trace the complete development of network programs. Also, given their purpose as activity reports, these documents were somewhat biased in favor of the networks.

To acquire information regarding backstage activity, personal interviews with key network participants were conducted between February and April of 1980. A basic interview protocol was developed (Appendix B), which addressed those categories or items of the outline generally omitted from network documents. This protocol was then adapted to each network. Project staff thoroughly studied the network documents to glean answers or partial answers posed in the basic protocol. This review also raised questions specifically about each network. Relevant information and new questions were then incorporated into the protocol for each network. When helpful, copies of portions of documents were appended to the protocol. By thus tailoring the interview to each network, the protocol served to brief the interviewing team before the site visits. The collection of duplicate information was then avoided, and a more detailed examination of each network project was permitted.

The design of this document helped to partially rectify a problem inherent in the interview method: a respondent's lapse in memory. Excerpts of network documents at hand in the protocol during the interviews sometimes helped to jog an interviewee's memory of past events. Some information was lost nevertheless, particularly when turnover in staff resulted in the departure of those persons with the most knowledge of certain events.

The documents provided little information on the historical basis of the formation of the network linkages between the participating hospitals, or on linkages established for reasons other than the head and neck cancer network. Some of this information was found in the original technical proposals submitted by network principal investigators, but it was often incomplete. A hospital questionnaire was designed to obtain this information (Appendix C). Completed by the chief executive officers (CEO) of each network hospital, this questionnaire contained items concerning the formation and history of various linkages, such as shared staff, shared service arrangements, and patient transfers between the hospital and other hospitals in the network, as well as other hospitals in the area.

This questionnaire was also tailored to each network by inserting the names of hospitals that were members of the network in all of the questions on linkages. It was sent to every hospital member in the six full-term networks. To help ensure their completion, the principal investigators of each network signed the cover letter for the questionnaires being sent to the hospitals in their project. Since these PIs were prominent in their fields and in their local regions, their association with our survey helped increase the importance attributed to our questionnaire by the hospital CEOs.

The initial response to our questionnaire varied by network. All of the nine hospitals in the Eastern Great Lakes Head and Neck Cancer Control Network and all of the nine institutions in the Greater Delaware Valley Head and Neck Cancer Network returned completed questionnaires. Nineteen of the 21 hospitals in the Illinois Head and Neck Cancer Network and 11 of the 12 Wisconsin Head and Neck Cancer Control Network participants responded to this questionnaire. The response from the hospitals in the Northern California Head and Neck Cancer Network and in the University of Arkansas for Medical Sciences Head and Neck Cancer Control Network was not nearly as good: 8 of the 15 California hospitals and 16 of the 22 Arkansas hospitals responded.

Complete data were eventually obtained from all network hospitals after telephone follow-up contact was made with expert informants in the CEO offices of each hospital.

The survey data were used primarily to measure the structure of general purpose linkages among network hospitals at the end of the funding period. This analysis is reported in Chapter 5, and a more technical description of the social network analysis performed with this data can be found in Fennell et al. (1987). Very briefly, the data on share service arrangements, the extension of staff privileges to staff of other hospitals, and formal arrangements for patient transfers were transformed into matrix form, and the following measures of network structure were developed:

1. Network density: the ratio of observed to potential linkages
2. Internal viability: the ratio of internal or within-set linkages to total linkages observed (counting both within-network and other hospital linkages)
3. Network complexity: using blockmodeling techniques, the ratio of the number of linkages between noncontiguous levels of actors within the network (using inclusion lattices to indicate levels) to the total number of linkages (Boorman and White, 1976; Light and Mullins, 1979)

SECONDARY SOURCES

Secondary data sources completed our information on the types and levels of resources relevant to medical care delivery systems in each network service region. These resources include hospital facilities, the availability of medical professionals, and patients.

A network's region was defined as those counties in which a member hospital was located. The application of this rule varied somewhat by network in order to take into account the unique characteristics of each region. For example, most members of the Illinois Head and Neck Cancer Network were located in Cook County, Illinois, which contains the city of Chicago. Because of the geographical expanse of the Chicago metropolitan area, the six counties constituting the Chicago Standard Metropolitan Statistical Area were chosen to represent this network's context.

Patients

The indices utilized to describe the potential patient population of each network are listed and described in Table 2.1. The sociodemographic information was obtained from various U.S. Bureau of the Census documents published in 1973. In addition, mortality data were obtained from vital statistics publications of the National Center for Health Statistics published in 1975 and 1976. Crude mortality rates were calculated because age-specific rates were not available. Although examined,

Table 2.1. Patient Characteristics

Variable	Calculation/definition
Median age	Median age of the county population
Percentage of the population over 65	Percentage of the county population over 65 years of age
Percentage white	Percentage of the county population that was white
Percentage urban	Percentage of the county population residing in urban areas (Urban areas are defined by the Bureau of the Census as places with 2500 or more inhabitants)
Median education	Median education of the county population 25 years of age and older
Median income	Median income of families and unrelated individuals residing in the county, i.e., median income of households

these rates are not particularly accurate descriptions of risk since they are affected by the age composition of the counties. They are thus not presented in this volume.

Health Personnel Resources

The availability of medical professionals is another resource in network service regions that is potentially important in network development. Three measures of this resource were developed focusing on physicians, as well as one measure of hospital labor intensity. These measures are shown in Table 2.2.

The indicator of the number of physicians per thousand population was derived from data published in 1974, 1975, and 1979 by the American Medical Association (1974, 1975, 1979) from their survey of all physicians in the United States (including graduates of foreign medical schools who are in the United States and meet U.S. education standards for primary recognition as physicians). The number of physi-

Table 2.2. Health Personnel Resources

Variable	Calculation/definition
Number of physicians per thousand population	Number of nonfederal physicians (excludes physicians associated with the United States Armed Services, the Public Health Service, and the Bureau of Indian Affairs) in the county, divided by the total population of that county, multiplied by 1000
Number of otolaryngologists per thousand population	Summation of the otolaryngologists listed in the county divided by the total population of that county, multiplied by 1000 (When the same physician practiced in two or more locations in the same county, he/she was counted only once. When the same physician was listed in two or more adjacent counties, he/she was counted as a fraction in each county. For example, when a physician was listed in two adjacent counties, he/she was counted as .5 in each.)
Number of radiologists per thousand population	Summation of the radiologists listed in the county, divided by the total population of that county, multiplied by 1000 (When the same physician practiced in two or more locations in the same county, he/she was counted only once. When the same physician was listed in two or more adjacent counties, he/she was counted as a fraction in each county.)
Ratio of personnel to hospitals	Summation of the number of personnel reported by each hospital in the county, divided by the number of hospitals in that county (The AHA defines personnel as the number of persons on the payroll as of September 30 of each year. It includes full-time equivalents of part-time personnel, calculated on the basis of two part-time persons equaling one full-time person. It excludes medical and dental residents and interns and other trainees.)

cians was calculated with revised 1973, 1974, and 1977 population estimates from the Bureau of the Census. This measure refers to nonfederal physicians only. Because this index excludes physicians associated with the United States Armed Services, the Public Health Service, and the Bureau of Indian Affairs, it slightly underestimates the physicians available in the network regions.*

Two other indices of professional resources were the number of otolaryngologists and the number of radiologists per thousand population. These two categories of physicians are especially relevant to the management of head and neck cancer. The sources of these measures were directories of medical specialists published by Marquis Who's Who in 1973 and 1977. The numbers were established by counting the specialists listed in each town of every county in all the network regions.

As with the first index described above, it is likely that these two measures underestimate the actual number of these specialists per thousand population. Although this document attempts to list all practicing physicians, the physicians themselves provide the biographical data on which our calculations are based. The percentage of physicians who chose to provide this information to the directory is unknown.

The last measure of health personnel resources is the average number of staff per hospital. The source of this information is described in the section on hospital facilities. It differs from other health personnel measures in that it includes nonphysicians based in hospitals.

Hospital Facilities

Since about 85 to 90% of all hospitals in the country respond to the yearly American Hospital Association survey of facilities and services, the publication series based on this survey, the *American Hospital Association Guide to the Health Care Field*, is considered a fairly complete source of information on hospital facilities. This publication contains basic, descriptive statistics on each responding hospital. We used these data to describe each network environment (all hospital facilities in the network regions), as well as each network's hospital facilities prior to the formation of the networks. The hospital resource indices listed in Table 2.3 use the county as the unit of analysis. County level data were calculated for the number of hospitals, number of beds, number of admissions, range of facilities, average occupancy, number of staff, and duplication of facilities.

The calculation of these indices depends on some inconstant factors. The number of reporting hospitals refers to those hospitals in each county that provided the AHA with all requested information. The calculation of the statistics shown, except for the number of beds per thousand population, was based on this number. The AHA had access to information on the number of beds in all hospitals, so this statistic is not limited by the occurrence of nonreporting hospitals.

Two of the indices used (number of beds and number of admissions) are rates. For their calculation, population estimates for the corresponding years were re-

---

*For a detailed description of the estimation procedures used, see U.S. Bureau of the Census (1978).

Table 2.3. Hospital Resources

Variable	Calculation/definition
Number of hospitals	Count of the hospitals in the county
Number of reporting hospitals	Count of the hospitals in the county that provided the AHA a full range of information
Number of admissions per thousand population	Summation of the number of admissions reported by each hospital in the county, divided by the total population of that county, multiplied by 1000 (The AHA defines admissions as the number of patients accepted for inpatient service during the reporting period, excluding newborns.)
Number of beds per thousand population	Summation of the number of beds reported by each hospital in the county, divided by the total population of that county, multiplied by 1000 (The AHA defines the number of beds as the average number of beds, cribs, and pediatric bassinets maintained for inpatients during the reporting period. The AHA derives this figure by adding up the total number of beds available each day during the hospital's reporting period and dividing by the total number of days in the reporting period.)
Average percentage occupancy	Average of the percentage occupancy of each hospital in the county (The AHA defines occupancy as the ratio of average daily census to the average number of beds maintained during the reporting period. The average daily census is defined as the average number of inpatients receiving care each day during the reporting period excluding newborns.)
Range of facilities	Number of unique facilities available in the county (If the service is available at more than one hospital, it is counted only once.)
Duplication of facilities	$1 - \dfrac{\text{range of facilities in the county}}{\text{total number of facilities in the county (including duplicates)}}$

quired. July 1 estimates of these years were obtained from the *Current Population Reports* published by the Bureau of the Census in 1976 and 1977.

Since not all hospitals in the United States respond to the AHA survey, the estimates we have calculated are probably somewhat different from the true measures. Depending on the types of hospitals for which data were unavailable and the statistic in question, our estimates may be either slightly greater or slightly less than the true values.

Underreporting is not the only factor influencing the accuracy of our calculated measures. The interpretation of the utilization statistics (admission and occupancy rates) is contingent upon the referrals to the hospitals in the region. The use of the county population statistics to calculate these rates assumes that all use of those facilities is limited to the population in the county. If the actual referral population is broader or smaller than the county population, then the numerator and denominator of the rate will not refer to the same population. This may result in inflated or deflated rates. For example, in places to which there are large numbers of referrals, the calculated rates may be inflated since the true denominator may have been larger than the county population.

The AHA data were also used to characterize each network hospital. These data supplemented the limited information provided in network documents about institutional participants.

When complete AHA information was available, each hospital was described by its number of beds, number of admissions, average percentage occupancy, number of personnel, and number of facilities for both its prenetwork year and the 1978 implementation year.

Particular attention was paid to the type of facilities these hospitals offered. The following 11 facilities considered relevant to the management of head and neck cancer were noted: X-ray, cobalt, and radium therapy facilities, diagnostic and therapeutic radioisotope facilities, histopathology laboratory, rehabilitation inpatient and outpatient units, social work services, dental services, and speech therapy services. Whether the institution had a cancer program approved by the American College of Surgeons was also noted.

THE PROCESS OF SYNTHESIS

These different sources of information were used to compose seven historical case studies. In turn, these descriptions served as the basic data for the comparative analysis. The seven networks were compared on a number of dimensions, corresponding to the major points in Chapter 1: sociodemographic context, the form of network organization and the structure of network linkages, and the approaches chosen to define the treatment innovation and implement network programs. This comparison identified general patterns that revealed a logic to, and permitted some tentative generalizations concerning, network context, structure, process, and outcomes.

A variety of data and methodologies provided a comprehensive description of the development and implementation of the seven head and neck cancer network demonstration projects. Although each method and source of data has its limitations, the diversity of methodologies and sources of information has served to check the validity of our data. We hope that, as a result, an accurate description of these networks has emerged. The comparative analysis has placed the experiences of the individual networks in a context that enhances and clarifies their meaning.

The remainder of this chapter comprises thumbnail sketches of each network project distilled from the seven comprehensive case histories. Each network sketch will describe the resources, the organizational milieu, and the preexisting linkages in each network area. We present these "mini case histories" in order to provide the reader with some background information on the individual networks. These vignettes are all based on actual data, as described above, but for reasons of space and production costs we present no tables; complete data on all indicators for all seven networks are available upon request from the authors. Although we believe these sketches are a useful vehicle for establishing the great variety represented by these seven demonstration projects, they are not crucial for an understanding of the more comparative analyses to be presented in the following chapters. In other words, if you are uninterested in details on the seven networks, you can skip ahead to the more analytic chapters. However, information presented in these cases will be referred to again, and sometimes repetition aids comprehension.

THUMBNAIL SKETCHES

University of Arkansas for Medical Sciences Head and Neck Cancer Control Network (UAMSHNCCN)

General Purpose and Objectives

The University of Arkansas for Medical Sciences Head and Neck Cancer Control Network (UAMSHNCCN) was established with the general purpose of developing a network of cooperating physicians through which comprehensive cancer control activities could be initiated. Although initially head and neck cancers would be the focus, and the principal investigator was an otolaryngologist, it was expected that the program would be a prototype for a broader range of cancer control programs. The geographic scope of the program was limited to central Arkansas, where UAMS was located.

Specific objectives were defined to meet the general goals. These included the following:

1. Educating medical professionals and the lay public about head and neck cancer
2. Training dental hygienists to detect head and neck cancers
3. Developing administrative linkages between the headquarters and participating members through use of the network data forms
4. Analyzing the data
5. Evaluating the network's effectiveness

Initially, membership was to include all hospitals in central Arkansas where head and neck cancers were treated. However, it became obvious that hospitals had no interest or reason to join, and the network members became the practicing physicians to whom the program was directed.

The resources for management of head and neck cancer in central Arkansas were centralized in the city of Little Rock and Pulaski County. The centralization of the resources in the region for treatment of these cancers was one of the most distinguishing features of the Arkansas network and influenced much of its development and operation.

Sociodemographic Characteristics

The Arkansas network region consisted of nine counties in central Arkansas. Census data on the sociodemographic characteristics of these counties prior to network funding reveals considerable variation in both median age and percentage of the population over age 65, the age category most at risk for this type of cancer. The range in median age across counties was 11.8 years. The lowest median age in a county was 25.4, the highest was 37.2, and the median for all counties was 30.5 years. The median percentgae of the population over age 65 in the nine counties was 11.6%, the smallest percentage in any county was 9.2%, and the greatest was 18.2%.

The predominant racial group in the region was Caucasian, but the percentage

Caucasian varied considerably among the nine counties. The range extended from a low of 59.3% to a high of 99.8%. The percentage of the population residing in urban areas also varied widely by county. The rural character of the area is evident in the median percentage of urban residents, which overall was 63.8%. The range varied between 84.5% in Pulaski County to 38.8% in the most rural county.

The sociodemographic character of the network service area showed very little variation and, given the measures we used, appeared low by national standards. The median level of education was 11.5 years, and the median annual income was $5365.

General Health Needs

The crude death rate in the network service area varied from 8.0 per thousand population to 15.4 per thousand and had a mean of 10.4, with a 2.06 standard deviation. The crude death rate seemed to be strongly correlated with the percent of the population over age 65. The crude cancer death rate varied from 1.4 per thousand to 3.2 per thousand, with a mean of 2.1 and a 0.56 standard deviation. It correlated strongly with the crude death rate. Deaths due to malignant neoplasms accounted for 19% of all deaths, which is somewhat below the national experience.

Professional Resources

In 1974 the number of physicians per 100,000 population in the network service area varied from 250 in Pulaski County, where UAMS is located, to 13 in the most rural of the counties. Otolaryngologists per 100,000 population varied from 5 to none. Therapeutic radiologists varied from 11 to none per 100,000. Finally, the ratio of specialists to generalists varied from 5.5 to 1.8. All of these rates reflect the centralization of medical professionals in one or two counties of the network region, particularly Pulaski County.

Hospital Resources

American Hospital Association data for each of the nine counties in 1974 showed that except for Pulaski County, the number of hospitals in each network county ranged from 1 to 4. Pulaski County had 12 hospitals, reflecting its centrality in the delivery of medical services to the region. By and large, admissions per 1000 population did not vary much by county. However, Pulaski County had substantially more beds per 1000 population than most of the other counties (13.4 compared to about 6) and maintained about the same occupancy rates (about 75%). These figures are consistent with the position of Little Rock as the center for health services in the region and reflect the high percentage of beds in Little Rock hospitals occupied by referrals from all over the region. Also significant are the extensive range of hospital facilities in Pulaski County (41 facilities, compared to about 22 elsewhere in the area) and the high rate of facility duplication (0.76). This pattern reflects the presence of several well-equipped hospitals in Pulaski County.

Resources of Network Institutions

Staff Resources. A nucleus of Little Rock head and neck practitioners affiliated with UAMS, the Veterans Administration Health Center in Little Rock, the Baptist

Medical Center, St. Vincent Infirmary, and the Central Arkansas Radiation Therapy Institute (CARTI) constituted the core staff for the network project. These hospitals were among the largest in Little Rock. The proposal specified that the staff would include a general surgeon, a radiotherapist, a nurse practitioner, a dentist, a facial prosthetist, a prosthodontist, and a head and neck surgeon. When the program was initiated, individuals with these backgrounds formed the core staff, and a social worker, a dental hygienist, and a statistician joined the staff.

As the network expanded, more physicians from the service area participated. All of these had been personally contacted by the principal investigator and came primarily from central Arkansas. Their specialties included otolaryngology, dentistry, surgery, oral surgery, radiation therapy, and plastic surgery.

Beds and Clinical Facilities. Although the hospital affiliated with the network headquarters institution (University Hospital) was not the largest in Little Rock (only 313 beds), it did offer an extensive range of hospital-based treatment facilities (25 of the 46 listed by the AHA in 1974). University Hospital offered 7 of the 11 facilities relevant to management of head and neck cancer: X-ray therapy, cobalt therapy, radium therapy, diagnostic radioisotope, therapeutic radioisotope, a histopathology lab, and a social work department. In addition, it had a cancer program approved by the American College of Surgeons Commission on Cancer, and 10 of its 313 beds were reserved for head and neck cancer patients.

The Veterans Administration Hospital in Little Rock was the largest of the original network-affiliated hospitals, with 1760 beds and 15,537 admissions in 1974. St. Vincent Infirmary had 522 beds and 24,498 admissions, and Baptist Medical Center had 437 beds and 20,661 admissions. Thus, as a consortium these hospitals represented a very large percentage of the total beds in the region. Moreover, among them they had most of the facilities necessary for treating head and neck patients. None of the hospitals in central Arkansas had inpatient rehabilitation facilities, and only the Veterans Administration Hospital had outpatient rehabilitation capabilities. However, among the consortium hospitals there were facilities for social work, dental services, and speech therapist services. As part of the network project the UAMS added dental services and speech therapy to its program. Thus, although there were other large and relatively well-equipped facilities in the region that were not part of the headquarters-consortium, none of these had the range of facilities available through the UAMS consortium, especially when the centralized radiation therapy facilities available through Central Arkansas Radiation Therapy Institute are considered.

Patients. During the first year of data collection a total of 297 head and neck cancer patients were seen at all reporting hospitals. Eighty-eight were treated at UAMS, 39 of which were seen at UAMS only, while 49 were seen at UAMS and the CARTI. Including those seen at UAMS, 190 patients, or 64% of all patients seen by the reporting hospitals in central Arkansas, were seen by the four original consortium hospitals and at CARTI. Clearly CARTI was an important resource that attracted head and neck cancer patients from the region for treatment in Little Rock.

Preexisting Linkages

Before the network project began, both individual and institutional relationships of a general nature linked the participants in the network. For example, physicians in the state were accustomed to referring cancer patients to the four hospitals in Little Rock that formed the headquarters, especially to UAMS. Over 50% of the patients at the UAMS and at the Veterans Administration Hospital were from outside the immediate area. Many physicians treating cancer patients either presented their patients at the UAMS tumor board or had personally contacted the principal investigator or other cancer specialists at UAMS.

A crucial general link predating the network was the implementation of CARTI. Although this radiation therapy center did not begin operation until 1976, plans for its creation were developed on the basis of prenetwork links. CARTI was a joint venture of radiation therapists from St. Vincent Infirmary, Baptist Medical Center, the VA Medical Center in Little Rock, and UAMS to combine personnel and resources into one central radiation therapy treatment center. All other hospitals in the area agreed to use the CARTI facilities rather than build their own. On the basis of these commitments, planning funds were obtained through the Regional Medical Program and construction money raised through a local bond issue.

A second major collaborative effort was the Area Health Education Center (AHEC). Like the CARTI, this program evolved at about the same time as the network, but plans for the program predated the network. The major thrust of AHEC was to place medical students in participating hospitals for training, internships, and residencies. As the AHEC developed it provided an important link between the UAMS and the community hospitals in the region.

Most of the links directly related to the treatment of head and neck cancer preceded the Head and Neck Cancer Control Network and were interpersonal rather than interorganizational. For instance, the principal investigator knew all the physicians in central Arkansas who treated head and neck cancer, either through his activity in the state otolaryngology society or because they were former students at UAMS or at M. D. Anderson Hospital and Tumor Institute in Houston, where he received his training. To further promote these ties, all specialists in head and neck cancer in central Arkansas were invited to become clinical staff at UAMS.

The network project grew out of a multidisciplinary head and neck oncology program at UAMS. This program involved several of the institutions in the network and was funded with support from UAMS and the Regional Medical Program. Naturally, the CARTI facility provided a major link for those treating head and neck cancer as well as for those treating other kinds of cancers.

Cooperative ventures beyond those described here were not considered useful or cost-effective owing to the small number of head and neck cancer patients seen in most regional hospitals. Given the size of this patient pool and the interpersonal links between the principal investigator and the other otolaryngologists in the region, centralization of treatment could be accomplished without further structure.

Eastern Great Lakes Head and Neck Cancer Control Network (EGLHNCCN)

General Purpose and Objective

The Eastern Great Lakes Head and Neck Cancer Control Network resulted from a merger following awards from the NCI to the two constituent organizations, Roswell Park Memorial Institute (RPMI) and the State University of New York at Buffalo (SUNYAB). From the outset, the two units in the EGLHNCCN agreed that the delivery of multidisciplinary care to patients in the region was their primary objective. They also concurred upon the mode by which this care should be delivered. Their approach had three elements: (1) Develop management protocols and model demonstration programs reflecting the multidisciplinary patient management philosophy, (2) document the impact of these programs, and (3) establish outreach and educational programs to communicate the multidisciplinary approach to participating institutions and professionals in the region. Individual physicians or institutions not part of the headquarters unit would not become funded participants, but rather would be the objects of the educational phase of activity and observers of the multidisciplinary treatment models.

Environment

When the EGLHNCCN was formed, the service area that was finally agreed upon reflected the characteristics of both SUNYAB and RPMI. The SUNYAB network concentrated in Buffalo and immediately adjacent towns. RPMI also described this as their service area but then added specific network units located in Rochester, New York, Erie, Pennsylvania, and Hamilton and Toronto, Ontario. Despite the intent to link to these other units, the geographic context and focal point for all network regions was the nine-county region of western New York and Pennsylvania. The resources for this program were centralized in Buffalo, the largest metropolitan center in the region. As with the Arkansas network, the centralization of treatment resources in the headquarters institutions was the prominent feature of the EGLHNCCN and, as already noted, was reflected in its primary objective and operational plan. Another prominent feature similar to the Arkansas program was the multihospital headquarters unit, which included all six hospitals capable of treating head and neck cancers in the region.

Sociodemographic Characteristics

There was considerable variation in median age across the nine counties of the network region. The median age range across counties was 6.1 years, and the average median age for all counties was 28.3 years. The median percentage of the population over age 65, the age group at greatest risk of head and neck cancer, was 10.9%.

A very small percentage of residents in the service area were nonwhite. Erie County, where Buffalo is located, had the highest percentage of nonwhite residents, 9.5%. One other county was more than 5% nonwhite; it contained a large Indian reservation. The region is quite rural. It had a median percentage of urban residents of 38.3%, but the individual counties ranged from 20.5% urban to 87.9%.

The socioeconomic character of the region is reflected in the median education and income by county. The range in median years of education was less than 1 year (0.8), and the median was slightly over 12 years. In only one county was the median below 12 years. A wide range in median income levels by county reflects two clusters. In one group of three very rural counties, median annual income ranged from $5232 to $7212. In a second group of six counties, the median annual income varied was higher: from $7788 to $8978.

General Health Needs

Three indices were examined to describe the general health status of the EGLHNCCN region. The crude death rate per thousand population in 1970 averaged 9.9 across the nine countes and had a standard deviation of 0.56, suggesting very little variation. The crude cancer death rate averaged 1.8 per thousand with a 0.14 standard deviation. The ratio of cancer deaths to total deaths was the same as found in Arkansas: 0.18, with a 0.02 standard deviation.

Professional Resources

The distributions of professional resources in 1973 generally reflected the importance of Buffalo as the center for medical care in this region. Erie County had 220 physicians per hundred thousand population, which is more than twice the number in any of the eight other counties. The mean number of otolaryngologists per hundred thousand was 2, with a 1.5 standard deviation. Although Erie County did not have the highest ratio on this indicator, it was among the highest. Similarly, the mean number of radiologists per hundred thousand within the nine counties was 3, with a 2.2 standard deviation. Erie County had six radiologists per hundred thousand, which was the second highest ratio. Overall, however, the ratio of office-based specialists to office-based general practitioners makes the concentration of specialists in Erie County apparent. Erie County's ratio was almost double that of the average for all nine counties.

Hospital Resources

The general pattern of resource centralization focused on Erie County is again reflected in the distribution of hospital facilities. Erie County contained three times as many hospitals as any other county in the region. The ratio of personnel to hospital in Erie County was almost twice the mean number for all counties. The 1973 American Hospital Association Guide to the Health Care Field listed 46 possible unique facilities; hospitals in Erie County had 45 of these facilities. The range and extent of duplication of facilities in Erie County was highest of all the nine counties. Overall, the picture that emerges in 1973 is that Erie County had more hospitals that were better staffed and equipped than the other counties in the region served by the network. Outside of Buffalo the typical hospital appeared to be small and equipped primarily for emergency care.

Resources of Network Institutions

Staff Resources. At both SUNYAB and RPMI the department responsible for the management of head and neck cancer patients initiated a proposal to launch the demonstration project. In each instance the initiator was the chief of the service or chair of the department. A broad multidisciplinary team was available at each center. However, notable gaps were filled when the two programs merged. At RPMI the proposed program contained no dentistry component. SUNYAB did not include rehabilitation services other than a speech therapist. With the merger, both of these gaps were filled.

Beds and Clinical Facilities. In general there was a fairly even distribution of facilities relevant to the treatment of head and neck cancer at the six headquarters institutions. Two of the hospitals, Millard Fillmore and Sisters of Charity, had no facilities for either X-ray therapy or cobalt therapy, and most of the network hospitals lacked rehabilitation facilities. The Sisters of Charity Hospital is of particular interest because it became the site of the headquarters of the SUNYAB program early in the project. However, since the principal investigator was chief of otolaryngology at several hospitals in the headquarters unit, he was able to arrange for radiation therapy at another hospital with facilities. By and large, the six hospitals that constituted the SUNYAB and RPMI headquarters were well equipped to manage head and neck cancer patients and to establish model programs as they proposed.

Patients. There were 435 head and neck cancer patients identified in the EGLHNCCN in the first year of data collection. Of these, 186 were seen at RPMI and 249 at SUNYAB. Within the SUNYAB component 88 patients came from Sisters of Charity Hospital, which was the main affiliation of the principal investigator. The other hospitals in the headquarters group contributed the remaining 161 patients.

Preexisting Linkages

The merger of the two successful proposal applicants constituted the key preexisting link of this network. Planning for the merger was facilitated by the number of preexisting linkages between SUNYAB and RPMI. The principal investigator from SUNYAB had a clinical appointment at RPMI, as did a surgeon and the maxillofacial prosthodontist. The latter was a member of the College of Dentistry at SUNYAB and was regarded as a regional asset. Each original application contained a letter from the other principal investigator indicating that the two institutions intended to cooperate regardless of the outcome of the competition for contracts.

Because both institutions were units of the State of New York, it might be expected that cooperation would be facilitated. However, the state bureaucracy did not work that way. RPMI was a unit of the Department of Health, and SUNYAB was part of the State University System controlled by its Board of Regents. It ultimately proved easier to award the contract to RPMI and then subcontract with SUNYAB.

RPMI was established as a state-supported cancer hospital in 1898. It had a long-standing research program that touched all aspects of cancer. Hence, it was among the first treatment and research centers to be recognized as a Comprehensive Cancer Center under the 1971 National Cancer Act, and it received its funding in 1974. Despite its national preeminence, or perhaps because of it, RPMI was unable to establish clinical interactions with other local institutions or with local clinicians in private practice. Normally, connections to medical institutions in the region occurred through teaching appointments, consulting relationships, or individual referrals. Accordingly, several factors worked against RPMI's establishing links in the area. First, staff at RPMI were full-time state employees, so they could not also be in private practice. Moreover, staff privileges at RPMI were not usually extended to local physicians. When patients were referred to RPMI, they became patients of the house staff and were required to undergo a complete medical and diagnostic work-up upon admission. Their records remained the property of the institute and were made available for staff research.

These policies met with considerable resistance among both the lay and professional communities in the immediate area. The public feared that referral to RPMI meant they would become guinea pigs for cancer research and would lose contact with their referring physician. These feelings were shared and, at times, fostered by local physicians who resented losing their patients.

In contrast, the clinical programs at SUNYAB were of necessity almost completely community based. Since the university did not have a teaching hospital, the clinical components of their educational programs depended upon contractual relationships between the university and local hospitals. These were for the most part multidisciplinary linkages, but they were established with various subsets of local hospitals, depending upon the clinical area. They involved faculty appointments and education, and the relevant house staff at contracting hospitals were frequently clinical faculty at the university. This arrangement proved mutually beneficial. Hospitals were able to obtain experienced senior staff and a guaranteed cadre of junior staff at minimal cost. Faculty at SUNYAB were able to continue their clinical practice and supplement their university salaries.

The Department of Otolaryngology at SUNYAB had a joint residency program with five hospitals, which formed the basis for their network program. The principal investigator at SUNYAB was chief of otolaryngology at four of these hospitals. The chief at the other hospital was a member of the SUNYAB faculty. However, although the SUNYAB program appeared to be a network with links between institutions, the links were themselves based on individuals since the same physicians staffed all of the key positions at all of the participating programs. Within SUNYAB, then, individuals crossed institutional boundaries and thus blurred the distinctions between units. What was a link between two separate institutions at one level actually represented the activities of a single individual at another level.

Other important links existed between SUNYAB, RPMI, and the other health programs in the area. One was the Lakes Area Regional Medical Program, which developed a telephone lecture program that was incorporated into the network project. Another was a link with the New York State Tumor Registry, which was to provide data support. Finally, RPMI had a long-standing relationship with the American Cancer Society, with which it sponsored continuing medical education programs that were widely attended by local practitioners. This program was one basis of the technology diffusion strategy of this network project.

It is significant that neither SUNYAB nor RPMI extended funded network membership beyond the core institutions that were already linked to and controlled by the principal investigators at the two centers. This strategy reflects the basic approach used by this network.

Mississippi Head and Neck Cancer Control Network (MHNCCN)

General Purpose and Objectives

The program proposed by the University of Mississippi Medical Center (UMMC) was organized to provide multidisciplinary approaches to management of all aspects of head and neck cancer. A second aspect of the program emphasized medical and lay education. The focus of the program was explicitly to be diffusion of state-of-the-art management. Early detection was particularly emphasized, and dental hygienists were to be trained to give patients complete head and neck examinations, and their performance was to be evaluated.

However, another stated objective of this program was to establish the UMMC as the principal tertiary treatment center for head and neck cancer in Mississippi. To this end, the structure of the program seemed to be twofold. First, UMMC proposed to establish a diffusion network, using existing referral networks and continuing education to provide links between the medical center and the community for rapid dissemination of information. At this stage, then, establishing a strong referral pattern to the newly established head and neck clinic at UMMC seemed to be the objective. However, their operational plan also incorporated the expectation that the multidisciplinary clinical activities developed at the clinic would eventually be disseminated to other participating hospitals. The remaining network activities were aimed at early detection of head and neck cancers by trained hygienists, identification and education of high-risk populations, and maintenance of a long-term data base that would allow follow-up treatment strategies. All of these latter activities reinforced the focus of the UMMC as the tertiary treatment center for the region for this disease.

Environment

As with the Arkansas and Eastern Great Lakes head and neck cancer control programs, the University of Mississippi Medical Center in Jackson was the central medical facility in Mississippi. Like Arkansas, it was the only medical school in the state. The network service area encompassed six counties in the central part of the state, and Jackson is also the major metropolitan area in Mississippi.

Sociodemographic Characteristics

Median age in the six county network region in 1970 was 24.8 and varied from 22.5 to 28.7 years. The percentage of the population over age 65 ranged from 7.8 to 12.5%, and the counties with the highest percentage of residents over age 65 also had the highest median age.

The network service region incorporated parts of Mississippi often described as the "black belt." Many of the largest cotton plantations were located in this region, and its soil contains a high concentration of black humus. The region also has a high percentage of black residents. Overall, the percent white in this area is the lowest of any of the seven network regions. By county the percentage ranges from 45.2% to 75.3%. The rural character is also indicated by the range of urban residents: from 37.3% urban to 83.9%.

Median education was less than 12 years (11.7) and varied from a low of 9.8 years to a high of 12.3 years. Excluding Hinds County, there is only slight variation across the six counties in median income, which was a rather low $4399. Hinds County had a median income of $6175.

General Health Needs

The crude death rate in this area per thousand population varied from 7.7 to 12.5 and averaged at 10. The standard deviation was 1.68 and reflects the rather high variation across counties. The crude cancer death rate varied less (1.2 to 1.8 per thousand). Overall, the mean ratio of cancer deaths to all deaths was 1.6.

Professional Resources

The number of physicians per hundred thousand in the six counties varied from 70 to 320. The mean number was 142, with a standard deviation of 82. Most physicians were located at UMMC. The number of otolaryngologists varied from 1 to 6 per hundred thousand. One county had more otolaryngologists per hundred thousand than Hinds, and another had an equal number. Hinds County had the most radiotherapists per hundred thousand population. The ratio of specialists to generalists was also highest in Hinds County. All of these rates reflect the centrality of Hinds County as the key source of medical care in the region.

Hospital Resources

As with physician resources, Hinds County had the most hospitals, the highest ratio of personnel to hospital, the most facilities, and the highest rate of facility duplication, indicating the extent of medical services available in the Jackson area. Although the next most populous county (Lauderdale) had some resources, they were not as extensive or as evenly distributed among the treatment facilities in that county.

Resources of the Network Institutions

Staff Resources. The core of the network staff was located at the UMMC and included a very broad range of skill and experience. The key staff of the project were clinicians associated with the Head and Neck Clinic at the UMCC and the Veterans Administration Center in Jackson.

Included in this group were two plastic surgeons, an oral pathologist, a health educator, a family practitioner, a radiation therapist, an otolaryngologist, a medical oncologist, and a chemosurgeon. Support staff were less available, and that created problems for the network.

However, unlike the Arkansas and Eastern Great Lakes Networks, there were qualified and relevant personnel in many of the participating hospitals. Of the six community hospitals that participated as network members, only one lacked a radiation therapist, and every institution had a participating otolaryngologist. Given the overall scarcity of resources in the region, the network institutions possessed significant resources. The key staff at the Veterans Administration Center in Jackson were also key staff at the UMMC.

Nonetheless, the absence of necessary support staff required for multidisciplinary management was evident. There were no oncology nurses at any of the institutions. There was no maxillofacial prosthodontist or other oral surgeon available to the staff of the network. The absence of such staff suggests that true multidisciplinary consultation was not a very high priority in this region.

Beds and Clinical Facilities. Among the facilities relevant to the management of head and neck cancer, rehabilitation facilities were completely lacking at all of the network hospitals, including the University Hospital. Aside from University Hospital and the Veterans Administration Hospital, there was only one approved cancer program and no dental or speech therapy available in the network. Thus, although several hospitals were well equipped for radiation therapy and nuclear medicine, there was a noticeable lack of support services for the patient with this cancer. There was, moreover, a general unevenness among the network hospitals, and three seemed to have few if any resources relevant to head and neck cancer. This distribution of resources is of interest in light of the network objectives to both promote referral and disseminate treatment protocols and capability out into the community setting.

Patients. Not much information was provided about the patients in this network. Patient registration was carried out for only one year and then only at the headquarters institutions, where 135 cases were registered in the first year of network operation. The Mississippi network voluntarily terminated activities following the second year of funding.

Preexisting Linkages

Two general categories of links existed before the establishment of the network: one linking physicians and another connecting the UMMC with service groups and medically related professionals not based in hospitals. The links with physicians occurred at two levels. A high percentage of physicians and dentists practicing in Mississippi were alumni of the UMMC. Thus, a natural pattern of consultation existed between the community physician and the UMMC in many areas of health care.

In addition, the complexities of managing head and neck cancer had already led to the implementation of referral relationships between some of the participating hospitals and the UMMC. When they were preparing the proposal for the project, administrative staff at the participating hospitals had already expressed an interest in the program and were easily signed on as participants.

Moreover, before the network model was even in place, the Department of Pediatrics at the UMMC had established newborn centers at several of the network hospitals. Programs in family planning and gynecologic screening were established by the Department of Obstetrics and Gynecology at some of the hospitals. Finally, an artificial kidney unit had been established and supported by the UMMC and a network of hospitals. Most of these programs included educational programs as well as service, and they were similar in form to the proposed head and neck network.

The staff at the UMMC had also worked closely with a variety of community service groups and voluntary associations that provided links to the community. Members of the head and neck clinic staff were active in both the local and state units of the American Cancer Society (ACS). These links facilitated the initiation of educational programs, smoking clinics, and other cancer prevention and detection programs. An ACS-sponsored speakers bureau provided an outlet for staff at the network to speak with lay groups about cancer management.

A second important link was between the UMMC and the Mississippi Educational Television Network. Shows on cancer, including head and neck cancer, were included in the health programming of the network.

A third important link was between the UMMC and the state social services. Since many of the head and neck cancer patients were eligible for state welfare support, the role of these agencies was to provide psychosocial counseling and rehabilitation.

Wisconsin Head and Neck Cancer Control Network (WHNCCN)

General Purpose and Objectives

Three broad objectives guided the organization of the Wisconsin Head and Neck Cancer Control Network: (1) to improve patient management by developing and disseminating guidelines or protocols for patient management, (2) to develop a data-abstracting, processing, and analytic center to monitor and evaluate the program, and (3) to conduct professional and public education aimed at promoting better diagnosis and earlier detection of the disease.

However, the WHNCCN was one of the initial statewide cancer control programs initiated by the Wisconsin Clinical Cancer Center (WCCC) at the University of Wisconsin, following its designation as one of the first comprehensive cancer centers authorized by the National Cancer Act of 1971. The head and neck project provided an opportunity and resources to begin to establish relationships with the Medical College of Wisconsin and other community hospitals in the state. Since cancer control outreach was required as a characteristic of these comprehensive centers, an outreach program had to be established if the designation was to be retained. Thus, as a second objective the network project provided an opportunity to launch a cooperative cancer control program with several community hospitals and enhance the visibility of the fledgling cancer center.

Environment

The WHNCCN was designed from the outset as a statewide program. Initially, hospitals from four areas of Wisconsin were included. Madison in Dane County, where the University of Wisconsin is located, is in the south central part of the state. Green Bay in Brown County is in northeast Wisconsin near Lake Michigan. Inland from Brown County is Outagamie and the cities of Appleton and Oshkosh. Finally, LaCrosse is located in southwestern Wisconsin near Iowa. In the initial application they were unable to include hospitals located in the north central and northwestern regions and in Milwaukee, the state's largest city. Eventually, three hospitals in Milwaukee joined the program, and in later years a clinic in Wausau in the north central part of the state was also included.

Unlike the networks in Arkansas, western New York, and Mississippi, the medical facilities in Wisconsin were not located exclusively in one area of the state. Rather, they were distributed in hospitals and clinics throughout Wisconsin. Thus, for the WCCC and the university to establish an effective network, it was necessary to obtain representation from most of these areas and institutions.

Sociodemographic Characteristics

The six counties covered by the WHNCCN (Brown, Dane, LaCrosse, Marathon, Milwaukee, and Outagamie) varied in age distribution. The median age for all participating counties was 25.3 years; however the range across counties on age was 5.5 years. Similarly, the average percentage of the population over age 65 in the six counties was 9.3%, but it ranged from 7.5% in Dane County to 11.5% in LaCrosse.

The racial character of the network service area was predominantly Caucasian. The median was 98.8% white, and only in Milwaukee was the nonwhite population more than 10% of the total. For the most part the population lived in urban areas. However, there was a broad range in this percentage: from 49.6% urban in Marathon County to 100% in Milwaukee County.

The socioeconomic character of the service area seemed relatively high. The median educational level across all counties was 12.2 years. In only one county was the median less than 12 years. The median income was $8417 and ranged from $6568 to $9040.

General Health Needs

As might be expected, the crude death rates paralleled the age pattern. The mean death rate in the areas where the network was located was 8 per thousand, with a 1.28 standard deviation. The mean crude cancer death rate was 1.5, with a 0.26 standard deviation. Cancer deaths amounted to 19% of all deaths in 1973 in these Wisconsin counties.

Professional Resources

Although there were qualified medical personnel in many parts of Wisconsin in 1973, Dane County was clearly a dominant center of health care providers in the state. The mean number of physicians per hundred thousand population for all six counties was 180, while Dane County had twice that average. Similarly, the number of otolaryngologists per hundred thousand was higher in Dane than in any other county, and although Marathon County had the same ratio of radiologists as Dane County, no county had a higher ratio. Finally, LaCrosse County had a higher ratio of specialists to generalists, but Dane County had the second highest ratio.

Hospital Resources

The numbers of hospitals correlated fairly well with the size of the county. Milwaukee with the largest population had the most hospitals (26), Dane County was next with 10, and LaCrosse with the smallest population had the fewest hospitals (2). The ratio of personnel to hospital also appeared to be associated with population and the number of hospitals. The notable exception to this was LaCrosse, which had the smallest population and the fewest hospitals, but the highest ratio of staff to hospital. This latter ratio probably reflects the fact that there are only two hospitals in LaCrosse and both have high staff ratios. The range of facilities is also of interest since it reflects the relative evenness of the distribution of resources among the areas where the network was implemented. Although in Milwaukee every facility listed by the American Hospital Association could be found, the range in the rest of the counties varied between 31 in LaCrosse to 39 in Dane County. The percentage of duplication of facilities reflects the varying depth of resources among the hospitals in each county. In Milwaukee and Dane Counties the extent of duplication is quite high, but it is much lower in the other counties.

Resources of the Network Institutions

Staff Resources. The staff resources at the headquarters were extensive and included all of the major specialty areas that would be required to manage head and neck cancer. The principal investigator was an otolaryngologist, and although he was head of the department, he was the only representative of his department in the program. In addition, a pathologist, a radiation therapist, a chemosurgeon, a plastic surgeon, a medical oncologist, and the director of cancer control at WCCC were participants. A head and neck nurse, a maxillofacial prosthodontist, a health educator, a tumor registrar, and an administrator were also on the headquarters staff. The participants in the network hospitals were all otolaryngologists except at Gunderson Clinic, where, in addition to the otolaryngologists, a pathologist and a radiation therapist also participated.

Beds and Clinical Facilities. The headquarters hospital at the University of Wisconsin had 626 beds, 36 of which were reserved for otolaryngology and 57 for oncology. In addition, the Department of Otolaryngology had extensive outpatient clinic facilities. This hospital had the broadest range of facilities of the network hospitals, and except for dental services (for which it contracted), it had all facilities for managing head and neck cancer.

Two points should be made about the Wisconsin network facilities. First, there were many hospitals that were well equipped to manage head and neck cancer patients. Second, some hospitals, such as Appleton Memorial, Methodist, Madison General, and St. Francis, were actually satellite hospitals to other participants that were more completely equipped to manage these patients. Thus, all participating units had access to facilities necessary to implement the treatment procedures that were the focus of the network program.

Patients. During the first year of the network program 245 head and neck cancer patients were seen at the Wisconsin network hospitals. Most of these were seen at the University of Wisconsin and at Milwaukee County General Hospital. However, the Veterans Administration Hospital and several other community hospitals representing most of the network regions contributed significant numbers of patients, again reflecting the evenness of the patient distribution throughout the network.

Preexisting Linkages

The WHNCCN was organized during a period when the WCCC was beginning to initiate a number of cancer control programs in the state. One of the primary links was between the Medical College of Wisconsin and the University of Wisconsin, which brought together more than 100 physicians and scientists throughout the state. The projects initiated by these investigators involved collaboration with many of the same hospitals that were ultimately included in the head and neck cancer network. The clinical program at the WCCC was also developing a clinical outreach program aimed at bringing patients from community hospitals into the large national clinical trials that were being initiated by the NCI. Two such networks in place were the Wisconsin Solid Tumor Group and the Wisconsin Hematology Study Group. Both of these involved community hospitals and were funded by the NCI.

A third cooperative program that involved several of the hospitals in the network was the tumor registry program being initiated by the biometry staff at WCCC. At the time of the organization of WHNCCN this program involved three of the network hospitals.

There were, however, no formal links specifically related to head and neck cancer. The principal investigator was active in the state otolaryngological society and through these activities knew most of the physicians treating head and neck cancers and the quality of their work. Thus, he activated these informal associations to obtain physician participation. Similarly, the director of cancer control at WCCC was also well connected throughout the state and could use his informal contacts to aid in formation of the head and neck cancer network. The sole formal tie existed between the principal investigator and the otolaryngologists in Appleton. They had been trained at the University of Wisconsin and maintained clinical appointments with the department.

Another point of interest in the various linkages is that the relevant links were not entirely with the University of Wisconsin. Appleton Memorial entered the program because of its relationship to St. Elizabeth Hospital, and St. Francis Hospital entered because of its relationship to Gunderson Clinic. Finally, the Milwaukee hospitals entered the program because of their ties to the Medical College of Wisconsin, not to the university.

Greater Delaware Valley Head and Neck Cancer Control Network (GDVHNCCN)

General Purpose and Objectives

The Greater Delaware Valley Head and Neck Cancer Control network was initiated as part of a larger radiation therapy network of 26 hospitals associated with the Hahnemann Medical College and Hospital in Philadelphia. The Hahnemann Radiation Therapy Treatment Planning Center (HRTTPC) was designed to develop treatment plans for radiation therapy (including the radiation dose distribution for each patient), to fashion devices needed for therapy, and to calibrate equipment and assure proper functioning of the equipment. The initial goals of the GDVHNCCN were an extension of these objectives to the management of head and neck cancer.

There were three ways in which the goals of the two networks were closely related. Both networks sought to (1) improve the overall quality of care received by network patients in their nearby community hospitals, (2) expedite the flow of information about patient management from the medical center (Hahnemann) to the community hospitals, and (3) strengthen the corps of physicians and related medical personnel available to a broad segment of the general population.

One program area of the network would focus on early detection by training dental hygienists, offering refresher courses to dentists and oral surgeons in diagnosis and treatment of these cancers, establishing screening programs in participating hospitals, and training house staff to perform head and neck examinations. A second program area would emphasize patient management and include educational programs on case management principles for professionals and lay persons, a maxillofacial prosthodontist training program, training for mental health professionals to cope with the psychosocial aspects of head and neck cancers, training oncology nurses in managing head and neck patients, and providing outreach services in speech rehabilitation. Finally, the third focus would be treatment, particularly radiation therapy, and would include consultation for radiation therapy treatment and cooperative trials for specific tumor sites.

The GDVHNCCN was expected to strengthen the capability within HRTTPC to manage head and neck cancer patients in two ways. First, resources from the contract would be used to hire support in epidemiology and biometry to collect and analyze relevant data on the impact of network care on patients. Second, there was a need to improve the rehabilitation capability within the region. A multidisciplinary approach to patient management was considered essential. There was an immediate need to attract and hire a maxillofacial prosthodontist. Also, in the area of rehabilitation, a psychosocial program for head and neck patients was to be initiated.

Environment

Although the GDVHNCCN was a program in a larger network, not all the hospitals in the larger program participated in it. The head and neck demonstration program was initiated mainly in the area immediately surrounding Philadelphia and southern New Jersey. This area included Bucks, Lehigh, Montgomery, and Philadelphia counties.

Sociodemographic Characteristics

The median age in the four-county area served by the GDVHNCCN was 31.2 years in 1970. Across counties it ranged from 26.1 to 32.6 years. The median percentage of the population over age 65 was 10.4% and ranged from 6.2% to 11.7%.

The region was predominantly urban. The median level of urban residence over all counties was 80.6% and ranged from 76.2% in Bucks County to 100% in Philadelphia County. The region was predominantly Caucasian; the median percentage white was 96.9%. Philadelphia, however, was only 65.8% white.

Although the median education level was 12.1 years, the median years of education in Philadelphia was 10.9, and in Lehigh County 11.9. Median income showed a similar pattern. The median income across all counties was $9744 in 1970, but it ranged from $7206 in Philadelphia to $11,061 in Montgomery County.

General Health Needs

The mean crude death rate in this network region was 9.5 per thousand, with a 1.8 standard deviation. However, in Philadelphia the death rate per thousand was

12, a rate consistent with the age and sociodemographic character of the city. The mean crude cancer death rate for the region was 1.9 per thousand. The rate per thousand in Philadelphia was highest at 2.3 per thousand. Overall, the ratio of cancer deaths to total deaths was 0.20; in Philadelphia the ratio was similar at 0.19 per thousand.

Professional Resources

To an extent, the medical personnel in the region were concentrated in Philadelphia. However, it is also clear that Montgomery County, and to a lesser extent Lehigh and Bucks counties, had local access to specialized personnel. There were not the wide gaps between the central urban center and the outlying counties observed in some of the other regional networks. Moreover, the concentration of specialists in Philadelphia, to the extent that it existed, reflected the distribution of cancer mortality and risk at that time.

Hospital Resources

The hospital resource distribution in the Greater Delaware Valley region followed a pattern similar to that found for the distribution of professional resources. Of the four counties, Philadelphia had a substantially larger number of hospitals, but this reflects the larger population of that county. The ratio of personnel to hospital was also highest in Philadelphia, followed by Lehigh. The level of staffing seems associated with the number of admissions and beds per thousand population. Finally, with the exception of Bucks County, which is actually a Philadelphia suburb with a young population, the four counties all seem to have had most of the resources listed in the 1974 American Hospital Association Guide to the Health Care Field (1974). Of the 46 facilities listed, Philadelphia had 45, Montgomery 43, and Lehigh County 44. The extent of facility duplication averaged about 0.81, with a small standard deviation, implying that facilities were fairly plentiful and relatively evenly distributed among hospitals in these counties.

Resources of Network Institutions

Staff Resources. The proposed network was grafted directly onto the existing radiation therapy network. The six hospitals that joined the network were already participating in joint programs. Thus, they had at least minimal staff to support the programs. All had at least one radiotherapist, oral surgeon, otolaryngologist, chemotherapist, and oncology nurse. In addition, a speech therapist was available at three centers, an audiologist at four, a social worker and home care coordinator at three hospitals. Services of a dietician, dentist, physical therapist, and tumor board coordinator were available at two hospitals. Hahnemann, the headquarters, had all the personnel that have been listed, as did Pennsylvania Hospital. The other hospitals lacked several of the support services but had the major medical staff. There was no maxillofacial prosthodontist available to the network when the program was initiated.

Beds and Clinical Facilities. By the conclusion of the first year, the number of hospitals in the network had grown to eight. For the most part, these participating hospitals were all equipped with a minimal level of facilities required for the management of head and neck cancer (usually at least 8 or 9 of the 11 relevant facilities). This level of resources is consistent with their participation in the larger radiation therapy network.

All but one hospital (Grand View) had X-ray therapy equipment, and all but two (Hahnemann Medical College and Metropolitan Hospital) had facilities for cobalt therapy. All but two hospitals (Grand View and Metropolitan) had approved cancer programs. Moreover, most participating hospitals had a substantial number of the facilities listed by the American Hospital Association. In general, the institutional resources for the network were strong and included a variety of hospital sizes and types.

Patients. During the first year of the network program the patient loads at the participating hospitals varied considerably. Hahnemann and Mercy Catholic Medical Center contributed the largest number of head and neck cancer patients: 65 and 51, respectively, out of a total of 199 for the year. Pennsylvania Hospital contributed 37 patients, and the other hospitals each contributed fewer than 20.

Preexisting Linkages

As we have noted, the principal linkage that preceded formation of the GDVHNCCN was the radiation therapy network centered at Hahnemann. This network by itself was insufficient to conduct all the activities required of the head and neck demonstration project. Initially, there were five affiliates. Of these, Grand View Hospital was a rural hospital located 40 miles outside of Philadelphia, and St. Luke's was located in another city 50 miles away. Of the other participants, one was affiliated with the University of Pennsylvania (Pennsylvania Hospital), one was with Jefferson University (Lankenau Hospital), and a third was a large osteopathic hospital. These were all located in the city or its suburbs. Two additional hospitals (Allentown and Mercy) joined later. These were both located outside Philadelphia.

Prior to the initiation of the head and neck cancer network, treatment programs for various head and neck cancers had been developed by the original six hospitals. Moreover, some of these hospitals shared facilities with the Hahnemann Medical College and Hospital. For example, radiation therapy conferences at Hahnemann provided the input for treatment planning and review of all patients receiving radiation therapy at Lankenau Hospital. Metropolitan Hospital and Hahnemann had a cooperative program in oncology, and there were staff affiliations in both radiation therapy and medical oncology. Grand View and Hahnemann also shared formal staff appointments, and fixed, prearranged referral links existed between these two hospitals. A similar preexisting referral system existed between Hahnemann and Metropolitan Hospital. There also existed a computer network that linked all the hospitals participating in the radiation therapy network.

Illinois Head and Neck Cancer Control Network (IHNCCN)

General Purpose and Objectives

The Illinois Head and Neck Cancer Control Network was organized by an otolaryngologist at Northwestern University Medical Center and a radiotherapist at

Rush-Presbyterian-St. Luke's Medical Center. The effort grew out of seven years of collaboration on head and neck cancer research. When the network was established the official goals were (1) to promote multidisciplinary management of head and neck cancer patients within the Chicago area, (2) to collect data that would provide information about the effects of multidisciplinary interventions, and that would permit epidemiologic research, (3) to conduct continuing education programs that promote multidisciplinary management, and (4) to enhance rehabilitation of head and neck patients.

At another level, however, the IHNCCN had the purpose of establishing a comprehensive cancer center in Illinois that would be formed from a consortium of the eight medical schools in the state. The objective at this level was to establish a model that would enable the development of cooperative research and service in the region addressed to a broad range of cancers. As part of the project, consortial agreements were developed and procedures for implementing and managing multi-institutional programs were established. The project also tested the capability of developing research and demonstration projects that allowed participation by community hospitals.

Environment

The area served by the IHNCCN was defined as the larger Chicago metropolitan area, a six-county region that included Cook County and all of the five collar counties: DuPage, Kane, Lake, McHenry, and Will counties.

Sociodemographic Characteristics

The sociodemographic characteristics of the region very much reflected the dominant urban environment of the city of Chicago. The median age for the six counties was 26.5 years, but it ranged from 24.2 to 29.5 years. The population over 65 ranged from 5.7% to 9.4% across the six counties, and the overall median was 8.1%. Cook County with Chicago had the highest median age and the highest percentage of residents over age 65.

As with most urban areas, the predominant race in 1970 was Caucasian: 95% over the six counties. In Cook County, however, the population was 77.5% white. Eighty-four percent of the six county region was urban, and the range was 99.7% in Cook County to 51.6% in McHenry County, which was also the least populated county.

The socioeconomic level of the service area was high relative to others that have been described. The median years of education was 12.2, and in no county was the median less than 12 years. Median income ranged from $9522 in Cook County to $13,297 in DuPage County. The median for the entire region in 1970 was $10,658.

General Health Needs

The mean crude death rate was 7.8 per thousand population in 1970, and it ranged from 5.7 to 10.3. The highest rate was in Cook County. The mean crude cancer rate was 1.4 per thousand, and it ranged from 1.2 to 1.9 across the six counties. Again, the highest rate was in Cook County. The ratio of cancer deaths to total deaths was 0.19 for the six counties, and there was very little variation in this ratio by county.

Professional Resources

Although Cook County had the most physicians per hundred thousand population in 1973 (210, with an average overall of 123), it did not stand out particularly on other medical manpower indicators. For example, the number of otolaryngologists per hundred thousand in Cook County equaled the average for the region (about 2), and there was very little variation across the six counties. More variation was evident in the number of radiologists per hundred thousand. Although Cook County was at the high end of the range, it did not have the highest ratio (5 per hundred thousand, compared to 6 in Lake County). Similarly, the ratio of specialists to generalists places Cook County slightly higher than the mean for the region. Thus, although Cook County had seven medical schools and 107 hospitals in 1973, the size of its population tended to place it near the mean for most of these measures.

Hospital Resources

In 1973 Cook County clearly dominated the six-county region in hospital resources, with 107 hospitals. The average number of hospitals in the other counties was about 5. The ratio of personnel to hospital was also highest in Cook County. Finally, of the 46 facilities listed in the AHA Guide, 45 were to be found in Cook County. In one county (McHenry) there were as few as 14 facilities, and in the other four counties this number was between 29 and 39. Facility duplication was very high in Cook County (0.98), indicating a large number of well-equipped hospitals. The extent of duplication in the other counties was considerably less, although it varied from 0.73 in Lake County to 0.44 in McHenry County, which had in general the lowest levels of health manpower and facilities.

Resources of Network Institutions

Staff Resources. The key staff of the IHNCCN were the group of otolaryngologists and radiation therapists at the four participating university hospitals. These key staff were in place at each of the four university hospitals that constituted the headquarters group at the Illinois Cancer Council. Each of the university centers had dental staff that were involved in the management of head and neck patients. At each center there was an oncology nurse. During the project all four university hospitals added rehabilitation teams, which included a speech pathologist, dentist/maxillofacial prosthodontist, social worker, dietician, and physicians.

The staff at the 12 community hospitals was more variable. In each instance there was an otolaryngologist or a head and neck surgeon. However, not all of these hospitals had adequate radiation facilities, and in some cases patients with this need were referred to the university center that served as that community hospital's headquarters. As will be noted below, many of these hospitals were satellites of the university centers for radiation and other services that they could not provide for themselves. The rehabilitation team concept was adopted at some level by eight of the community hospitals participating in the program. However, beyond the actual incorporation of teams, a high percentage of hospitals referred patients for rehabilitation to a university center.

Beds and Clinical Facilities. The hospitals in the network varied in size and in the extent of facilities. However, most were sufficiently well equipped to deliver the primary care required to treat these cancers. Where these facilities were absent, as we have noted, referral relationships were in place to deliver the service.

All but three of the network hospitals had facilities for X-ray therapy, and only five were unable to provide cobalt therapy, which was the other major type of radiation therapy used for head and neck tumors. Nine hospitals had no inpatient rehabilitation services, although this service was upgraded as part of the network activity. Only four hospitals had outpatient rehabilitation services, but social work services were available at all but three. All but four hospitals had dental services, and only three lacked speech pathology services. Thus, these hospitals had the capability of delivering multidisciplinary care either on the premises or through referral to another nearby facility.

Patients. In the first year, 519 patients were entered into the network data system by the 16 hospitals in the project. About 54% of these came from Northwestern, Rush, and the University of Illinois hospitals (the University of Chicago had not yet entered the network). The rest came from community hospitals. These hospitals contributed patients unevenly, suggesting that the delivery of services to head and neck cancer patients across hospitals was variable.

Preexisting Linkages

There were long-standing linkages in head and neck cancer therapy between the University of Illinois, Rush Medical Center, and Northwestern University. At one time Rush was part of the University of Illinois, and Cook County Hospital (which was linked to the University of Illinois for many types of cancer therapy, and shares the same "West-Side Medical Complex" location with Illinois and Rush) had a long-standing relationship with Northwestern University for otolaryngology.

In Chicago each of the seven medical schools had established relationships with networks of community hospitals that were used for medical education. However, these relationships were not exclusive, and community hospitals frequently related to different universities for different diseases or treatment modalities. These network links were activated by the various participants when the head and neck demonstration project was initiated and provided the basis for the program.

At the same time that the IHNCCN was being established, efforts were under way by the deans of the eight medical schools in Illinois to establish a consortium that would apply to become a comprehensive cancer center. As we have already noted, the IHNCCN became the first tangible evidence that the consortium could initiate collaborative research in the area. The contracts managed by the Illinois Cancer Council (ICC), which became the network headquarters, made the IHNCCN the first program of the center.

The possibility of collaboration was thus demonstrated by the implementation of the head and neck demonstration project. The fact that the ICC became the headquarters established the principle that the ICC would be "neutral ground" on which all universities could cooperate in areas where none could be successful alone.

Northern California Cancer Program Head and Neck Cancer Network (NCCPHNCN)

General Purpose and Objectives

The explicit, formal goal of the Northern California Cancer Program Head and Neck Cancer Network was to improve the management and control of head and neck cancer in the region. But, like the Illinois and Wisconsin projects, the network had the implicit and more fundamental objective of spearheading the establishment of the Northern California Cancer Program (NCCP) as a consortium cancer center for northern California and northwestern Nevada.

Environment

The geographic extent and diversity of the population in northern California and northwestern Nevada influenced the development of the NCCPHNCN. From the outset, the NCCP planned to implement a cancer control program throughout the entire region. In the developmental stages, however, efforts were limited to six Bay Area counties, plus Sacramento and Placer counties in California and Washoe County (Reno), Nevada. The description of the environment will be limited to these nine counties in which the planning efforts were initiated.

Sociodemographic Characteristics

The median age in these nine counties in 1970 was 30 years, and the range was 8.8. In San Francisco 14% of the population was over age 65, and in Santa Clara County 6% was above that age; the median for all nine counties was 7.8%.

San Francisco and Alameda counties were the only counties where the white population was less than 90%, and although the range on this measure was 25.5%, the median was 91.5%. Similarly, the region was predominantly urban. Over the nine counties the median was 95.1% urban.

The level of education in the region was quite high in 1970. The nine county median was 12.5 years of education, and there was a range of .5 years. Greater variability was evident in the income levels of these counties. Median income ranged from a low of $6765 in San Francisco to a high of $11,194 in San Mateo. The median income for the area was $8710.

General Health Needs

The crude death rate in the region varied from 12.5 per thousand in San Francisco to 5.9 per thousand in Santa Clara County. The mean was 8 per thousand for all counties. The cancer death rate followed the same pattern: 2.7 per thousand in San Francisco and 1.2 in Santa Clara. The overall mean was 1.7 per thousand.

The ratio of cancer deaths to total deaths for the nine counties was 0.21 and ranged from 0.24 in Marin County to 0.19 in Washoe and Placer counties.

Professional Resources

This was an area rich in medical specialists in 1974. The average number of physicians per hundred thousand population was 254 and ranged from 150 in Placer County to 570 in San Francisco. San Francisco also had the greatest number of otolaryngologists (7) and of radiologists (9) per hundred thousand population, while Placer County had the smallest number of these specialty groups (1 and 4 per hundred thousand, respectively). Finally, overall the ratio of specialists to general practitioners was highest in San Francisco (7.6) and lowest in Placer County (1.4).

Hospital Resources

Alameda County had the most abundant hospital resources of the nine counties, and Placer County had the sparsest resources. However, with the possible exception of Placer County, these counties were as rich in hospital resources as they were in specialized personnel relevant to head and neck cancer. The average number of personnel per hospital was 533.8. Of the 46 facilities listed by the American Hospital Association Guide in 1974, the average over the nine counties was 38.2. San Francisco County hospitals had all 46, and the hospitals in four other counties had more than 40 of the listed facilities. Facility duplication was quite high, with a mean for the region of 0.7. In San Francisco, Alameda, and Santa Clara counties the duplication rate was even higher (0.91, 0.89, and 0.85, respectively). The sparsest distribution of facilities was in Placer, Marin, and Washoe counties (0.35, 0.51, 0.54, respectively).

Resources of Network Institutions

Before the resources of the network institutions in the NCCPHNCN can be described, the membership of the network needs to be described. Just as the environmental context was quite diverse, so were the types of organizations to join the network. This breadth in membership was necessitated by the way in which medical care delivery was organized in this region.

The variety of institutions that participated in this network included four universities: the University of California at San Francisco (UCSF), University of California at Davis (UCD), University of the Pacific (UOP), and Stanford University Medical Center (SUMC). In addition, three private foundations, which were headed by physicians, were members and subcontracted to perform specific services for the network, including its day-to-day management. A planning council in Sacramento organized much of the activity in that area. Finally, the California State Department of Health provided the network data system. Thus, the institutional membership of the network was quite complex. Unlike the other programs, there was no single headquarters that provided the direction for the network and served as the primary source of the innovation. Rather, the network was directed by a consortium composed of the four participating universities, the participating foundations, and the

State Department of Health. The resulting diffusion strategy differed substantially from all other programs in form, although in philosophy it was similar.

Staff at the Medical Centers. The staff at the university medical centers and participating foundations provided the major services to the physicians in the community hospitals to whom the program was directed. These services were provided through pretreatment conferences that were established in the various regions of the network area, and to which physicians at participating hospitals were invited and encouraged to present their cases.

Both Stanford and UCSF had specialists in otolaryngology, general surgery, plastic and reconstructive surgery, and medical oncology. Radiation therapy was also available from SUMC and UCSF and from the West Coast Cancer Foundation (WCCF). Staff at SUMC included eight faculty, three physicists, and two dosimeterists. Five full-time radiotherapists were available from UCSF. Other support staff available through these two universities were audiology, nutrition and dietetics, dental hygiene, physical and vocational therapy, social work, and psychotherapy.

The Chair of the Division of Oral Biology in the School of Dentistry at UCSF was the principal investigator for the network project. The division included three units that served head and neck cancer patients: Oral Medicine, Maxillofacial Rehabilitation, and Oral Pathology. The University of the Pacific provided dental support for the hygienist screening programs. The UCD School of Medicine had staff in surgery experienced in treating head and neck cancer patients.

Beds and Clinical Facilities. Radiotherapy was provided in Sacramento through a private Radiation Oncology Center at Sutter Community Hospitals and Clinics. These hospitals had an average of 570 beds and an average of 1953.2 personnel. Of the 46 facilities listed by the AHA, they average 34. UCSF Hospitals and Clinics and Sacramento Medical Center had all the facilities relevant to the management of head and neck cancers. Stanford University Hospital lacked cobalt therapy, rehabilitation, and dental services, and Sutter Community lacked rehabilitation services. Thus, overall these centers were well equipped to deliver head and neck cancer care.

These four centers had a history of providing multidisciplinary clinics and/or conferences. At UCSF a specific conference dealing with head and neck cancer had been in place for 30 years and was attended by all relevant divisions. Particular note should be made of the Maxillofacial Rehabilitation Unit in the Division of Oral Biology at UCSF. This unit became the rehabilitation unit for the program, and the three maxillofacial prosthodontists provided services to the entire network. Eventually one member of this unit moved to Sacramento and established a program there as part of the network.

Community Hospital Beds and Resources

The remaining hospitals participated in the network through their attendance at one of the multidisciplinary treatment confernces held in various locations in the network service area. These hospitals were generally smaller than the university hospitals. All but one had fewer than 400 beds. They averaged 317 beds, compared with the 570 average in the university hospitals. The number of personnel ranged from 436 to 1992. One had nearly 2000, six had between 600 and 1000 personnel, and three had between 400 and 500 staff.

Facilities at these hospitals ranged from 11 to 34 of the AHA list in 1974. Generally, they had fewer facilities than the university hospitals, and the distribution across hospitals was less uniform. They average 22 facilities, compared with 34 at the university hospitals. Of the facilities associated with treating head and neck cancers, these hospitals most often had histopathology laboratories, therapeutic and diagnostic radioisotopes, radium, cobalt and X-ray therapy, and social work services. They were least likely to have rehabilitation services and dental and speech therapy.

Patients. The NCCPHNCN did not collect data from individual hospitals in the form used by the other network programs. Patient data for hospitals in five of the six Bay Area counties were obtained from the regional tumor registry. Supplemental data collection strategies were implmented for Sacramento, Placer, and Santa Clara counties. No data were obtained in Washoe County. For the first year of data collection, a total of 907 cases of head and neck cancer were entered. Forty-two percent of these were seen in the major network hospitals only (hospitals that treated more than 2.5% of the head and neck cancer patient population); 23% were referred to the major hospitals. The remaining 35% were seen in the minor hospitals (those treating less than 2.5% of the head and neck cancer population).

Preexisting Links

The links that enabled the establishment of the NCCPHNCN were the same links that had been employed in the formation of the NCCP. In addition, the core of physicians who established the NCCPHNCN had been practicing together before its formation.

The institutional links were of two sorts. There were collegial exchanges among professionals with common clinical and research interests in the region, including patient referrals. In addition, there were long-standing clinical appointments between institutions. Another link was between the universities and the community hospitals in residency programs at the medical schools. Thus, some of the faculty had clinical appointments at these hospitals, and in some instances house staff had appointments at the universities.

As was evident in other networks, one link of particular importance was implemented through the relationships established in the region for the delivery of radiation therapy. There were a number of such links because it was often more economical for community hospitals to refer patients for radiation therapy than to provide it themselves. Stanford, UCD, and UCSF each had such networks. In addition to the medical schools, the West Coast Cancer Foundation provided radiation therapy services to several of the participating hospitals. Finally, there was one group of community hospitals that also operated a shared radiation therapy facility.

Another set of preexisting links were organized with dentistry and maxillofacial prosthodontics. These links included UCSF and the College of the Pacific.

Finally, the private foundations were often used as a common neutral ground where area investigators met and could collaborate without concern for institutional barriers. Thus, the basis for interaction through these foundations was in place in the region and could be used to implement both the NCCP and the NCCPHNCN.

Network Environment and Response to Uncertainty

Performance Gaps and Definition of the Innovation

INTRODUCTION

Early in Chapter 1 we argued that organizational networks develop in social environments or communities, and network forms reflect the characteristics of these environments. In other words, the ecology into which the diffusion process is introduced influences how the need for the innovation is defined, the form the innovation must take if it is to be accepted, the type of channel through which it is diffused, and how the innovation is introduced through these channels.

This chapter and the next four will explore how the components of the innovation diffusion process are related to the environmental character of the social system into which the innovation is introduced. Following contingency theory, organizational performance depends upon meshing, or the contingent nature of environmental and technological constraints. Organizational structures develop to match those contingencies. This chapter will consider the fundamental premise from contingency theory that the environment limits and enhances organizational responses to uncertainty, defined here as a performance gap that threatens the organization's ability to perform its core functions. Also following contingency theory, we will examine the question of how innovations address uncertainty and yet create more uncertainty. Our analysis in this chapter will therefore focus on research questions 1 and 2 from Chapter 1:

1. How does the nature of the environment affect the perceptions and definition of a performance gap that could lead to the consideration of an innovation? What factors stimulate initial interest in an innovation among the target audience?

2. How are performance gap perceptions related to agenda setting within the networks?

The sequence of events that unfolded in these network projects is important background to keep in mind. Interest was stimulated primarily by an outside change agent, the National Cancer Institute (NCI). The request for proposals initiated the development of various network structures that were established at least superficially in the initial phase of the projects prior to implementation. Once in place, the networks defined the content of the innovation and the ways in which this content was introduced in each of the seven regions. Such a sequence reflects Weick's concept of "loose coupling" (1976) and the model of decision making within "organized anarchies" introduced by Cohen *et al.* (1972). Following Cohen *et al.*, organizational activities and decisions may be only loosely coupled to formal structures, structures determine strategies (rather than the reverse), and structures provide sets of procedures through which participants arrive at an interpretation of what they are doing and what they have done while they are in the process of doing it (1972, p. 2).

DIFFUSION AND UNCERTAINTY

Diffusion occurs when "an innovation is communicated through certain channels over time among members of a social system" (Rogers, 1983, p. 14). Thus, diffusion has several components. It is a *communication process* that takes place through *channels*. It occurs *over time*. It is *directed to specific members* of a social system. Finally, it *introduces something new* into the system in the form of a technology that reduces uncertainty about some key activity within the social system (Rogers, 1983). However, Rogers also notes that when first introduced, innovations create uncertainty until it is determined whether they are better than the things they replace. As experience with the innovation increases, this uncertainty decreases.

Rogers identified two kinds of information that reduce uncertainty. Software information contains guidance about how the innovation works and is embedded in the technology. Again, as experience with the innovation increases, questions about how the innovation works tend to be reduced. The other kind of information is innovation-evaluation information, which concerns the assessment of outcomes. As evaluation information is acquired, uncertainty about the potential costs, outcomes, and relative merits of the innovation is reduced.

Innovation diffusion is not a single concept. It has two principal dimensions: the innovation itself, which may be a new idea or technology, and the diffusion process by which that idea or technology is transmitted. Furthermore, following Rogers (1983), the innovation includes the technology itself, or hardware, the software or information base that defines how the technology is to be implemented, and the rationale for its application in various contexts. In some instances the technology and software are distinct; in others they are integrated to the point that it is hard to distinguish one from the other. Frequently, the technological component of the innovation is actually a set of technologies, or a technology cluster (Rogers, 1983), which is developed in response to major changes in the knowledge software or in the information base associated with the field into which the innovation is introduced. It is usually a response to a performance deficit. In other words, innovative technology is often an instrumental reaction to uncertainty, or it results from a perceived performance gap created by changes in the information base of the organization's core technology (Rogers, 1983; Zaltman et al., 1973).

In this particular instance, the pressure for innovation was a response to changes in the information base that had for years governed how cancer was managed. At the time the networks were being organized there was a growing awareness that some cancers would respond to chemotherapy as an adjuvant therapy, or even as an alternative to traditional treatment by surgery and radiation. A relatively new subspecialty, medical oncology, was being recognized, and board certification in this subspecialty of internal medicine was being considered. There was also an associated recognition that multidisciplinary management would benefit even the terminal patient by enhancing the quality of the survival period. Thus, in addition to new treatment strategies, there was a growing recognition that more could be done for the cancer patient.

As we indicated in Chapter 1, the staff at the NCI and many leaders in oncology were increasingly convinced that a performance gap existed, particularly in community hospitals. In their view these new ideas about patient management needed to be diffused into community settings where the existing technology could be reorganized to deliver the new form of multidisciplinary care. Head and neck cancers were identified by these groups as one type of cancer that would respond to such a multidisciplinary approach. To introduce it, however, required a reconceptualization of the existing knowledge base and treatment rationale. It also required convincing practitioners that new forms of patient management would in fact improve either survival or the quality of life of terminal patients. Thus, the innovation was formulated into a set of guidelines that incorporated these new ideas and treatment concepts.

These seven networks were formed in a context characterized by several sources of uncertainty. First, there were the questions of the NCI and among some in the academic medical community about whether state-of-the-art treatment was available in community hospitals where considerable numbers of cancer patients were being treated. Second, from the standpoint of the academic medical centers, there was the related concern that an increasing number of patients were being treated in community hospitals. As a result, there were fewer patients available to the university hospitals for research and training. Third, the community hospitals were able to attract better-trained physicians with specialization in oncology. These physicians expected modern treatment facilities and access to the experimental drugs that had been available to them in their residencies. The community hospitals had to deliver or face the threat of losing these young physicians to other places willing to provide such access. Fourth, Congress had mandated implementation of a cancer control program as part of the newly passed National Cancer Act of 1971. Although there was no clear definition of what such a program would entail, it was clear that Congress wanted the results of scientific research disseminated to the community.

In addition to the above concerns, part of the mandate in the National Cancer Act established comprehensive cancer centers. These centers were to provide stable and continuing support for both cancer research and cancer control. Cancer control was to be implemented through programs that reached out into the community and ensured delivery of state-of-the-art care to the public at large. However, these new programs were threatening to the research-funding relationships established between academic medicine and the NCI, since cancer control programs could potentially compete for the research funding that had traditionally gone to the universities. It became clear that unless the universities participated in these new programs, their access to these new resources might be limited.

Some universities elected not to participate. Those that did choose to participate had to reallocate internal resources and consider the impact of this participation on what they defined as their core activities. Frequently, they did not have the staff or resources to develop new cancer control programs. Moreover, there were no clear precedents or guidelines for establishing such outreach programs. The one network program that had been attempted by the NCI met resistance from organized medicine, especially the American Medical Association and some community hospitals that resisted any form of federal support (Breslow, 1977). Thus, there was considerable uncertainty in these environments about whether the cancer control programs that incorporated the network concept would be accepted by the community hospitals to which they were addressed. So the changing environment was a source of uncertainty for the change agent, for the NCI, and for the university hospitals. The new programs represented innovations that might resolve the uncertainty about the level of care given to patients treated in the community, but they created uncertainty about the continued availability of both research and cancer control resources.

The participants in this program interpreted these environmental uncertainties in different ways, depending upon their own situations, but overall the response was consistent with the Cohen *et al.* (1972) model. They uniformly saw the network demonstration program as an opportunity to obtain resources that could be used to reduce uncertainty in the supply of research funds. By reorganizing their environments into "networks" they could obtain predictable access to the resources being reallocated by the NCI to cancer control as a result of the 1971 National Cancer Act.

Three of the networks formulated agendas that specifically focused their network activities on the development of comprehensive cancer programs for their regions. Wisconsin planned its program with the university as the center and community hospitals as participants. Illinois and Northern California saw the network program as a chance to capitalize on existing linkages and develop regional consortia that would provide the basis for a variety of cancer programs. Each of these programs had participating units that were heavily involved in a variety of clinical trials programs. Thus, the network also provided a base for developing links with community hospitals that would be participating in clinical trials.

Greater Delaware Valley was primarily oriented to one clinical modality, radiation therapy. Its network was already committed to a cooperative radiation therapy program and the head and neck demonstration program enhanced this cooperative link. The Eastern Great Lakes, Mississippi, and Arkansas programs were more specifically oriented to head and neck cancer and each sought to establish the headquarters as a center for the management of such patients. There did not seem to be any larger objective behind collaboration with the community hospitals for these programs.

A second source of uncertainty was the concept of multidisciplinary care incorporated into the innovation. Some clinical research had established the benefits of multidisciplinary management of patients with cancers of several sites, most notably breast cancer, where adjuvant or combined therapy had recently been found to be a promising new breakthrough in several large-scale clinical trials. Chemotherapy had also been demonstrated to be beneficial in treating childhood cancers and adult leukemia and lymphomas, including Hodgkin's disease. However, there was no compelling clinical evidence that either chemotherapy or multidisciplinary management would be effective in treating head and neck cancer patients. At the time of the network programs this disease was primarily treated by surgery alone or with radiation therapy. Even among the two surgical groups that treated it, otolaryngologists and head and neck surgeons, there were differences as to which group was most qualified to manage these patients. Although new research was showing that rehabilitation and presurgical planning could impact favorably on the quality of survival, there were no data from large-scale clinical trials to support these clinical impressions, and no data to indicate the benefits from chemotherapy.

The uncertainty regarding the potential benefit of the proposed innovation was not specifically directed at the actual technology. Surgery and radiation therapy were the treatments of choice for these cancers, and the treatment strategies suggested by the NCI did not propose any basic change in the use of these treatments. The uncertainty was really more related to how the treatment strategies that were advocated were to be introduced. It was the software, then, rather than the hardware, that was problematic. The innovation of multidisciplinary treatment called for involvement of nonphysicians such as speech therapists, oncology nurses, nutritionists, and social workers in the treatment planning. This approach interfered with the authority of the physician. Moreover, it required pretreatment planning, which put constraint on the surgeon to commit to a surgical strategy involving nonphysicians before treatment was administered. These were new ideas for surgeons who were used to complete autonomy. Because the treatment plans incorporated rehabilitation, which was not part of the surgeon's specialty, there was an implicit threat of evaluation of his work in the posttreatment phase when the rehabilitation specialists began their work with the patients. Thus, new relationships had to be formulated that left room for a potential, albeit small, challenge to the authority of the surgeon. And, as we have noted, there was no clear scientific rationale that could be derived from large-scale clinical research that the proposed strategies were in fact more effective than the existing management techniques.

TYPES AND CHARACTERISTICS OF INNOVATIONS

Considerable work has focused on the problem of developing innovation classification schemes and lists of variables that characterize various innovations (Beyer and Trice, 1978; Downs and Mohr, 1976; Rogers, 1983; Zaltman et al., 1973). Early work by Becker (1970), Kaluzny (1974), and Mohr (1969) focused on characteristics of the innovation and perceptions about the innovation's compatibility with the institution or environment into which it is introduced. In examining some of these studies Downs and Mohr (1976) point out that for all of the voluminous research that has accumulated on organizational change and innovation, no general theory incorporating characteristics of innovations and their adoptability has emerged. Characteristics that seem positively related to diffusion in one study are negatively related in a second, and unrelated in still another. Some authors (Moch and Morse, 1977; Rowe and Boise, 1974) have concluded that it may be impossible to develop a general theory of innovation because of the diversity of forms that innovations take.

However, Kaluzny (1974) found characteristics of the innovation and those of the organization to be correlated, particularly when the innovation has high adoption potential, defined as compatibility with existing values and institutional norms. Thus, characteristics of adoptable innovations were different for hospitals than they were for health departments, reflecting differences in the goals of the two institutions. Downs and Mohr (1976) generalized this observation in their summary of conceptual problems that have led to disparate results in innovation diffusion studies. They concluded that characteristics of the innovation and the adopting agency cannot be studied separately. The characteristics of the innovation must be compatible with those of the organization. This approach ties innovation diffusion into the contingency framework, where the organization and its environment are linked with the innovation's form and character.

Many studies have focused on the characteristics of the innovation. Within the organizational literature at least three dimensions have been identified as important in any study of innovation. These are (1) whether the innovation affects the administrative activities of the organization or its technical core (Daft, 1978; Evan, 1966; Kimberly, 1978; Kimberly and Evanisko, 1981; Teece, 1980), (2) whether the innovation is internally or externally generated (Beyer and Trice, 1978; Daft, 1978; Mohr, 1969; Rogers and Shoemaker, 1971; Roman, 1980), and (3) whether the change is mandated or voluntary (Aldrich, 1979; Beyer and Trice, 1978). These factors relate to how the innovation is initiated and where its impact will be felt in the organization. The nature of the innovation, for example, will determine which actors in the organization will have most voice in the adoption of the innovation, other things being equal. However, as noted in Chapter 1, the medical care industry is changing rapidly, and some have observed that even technical innovations that were formerly the province of the physician may be adopted by administrative authorities who then hire the professionals to implement them (Greer, 1986). In such instances the innovation may represent an aspect of organizational efforts to retain or enhance scarce resources, such as a share of the patients in the region. As we will see in the discussion of the diffusion process, core resource acquisition played a key role in the way the diffusion process was initiated in these head and neck cancer demonstration programs.

From a contingency standpoint, whether the innovation is introduced internally or externally is less significant than whether it is compatible with the organization's objectives and structure. Rogers has introduced the concept of "reinvention," which he defines as "the degree to which an innovation is changed or modified by a user in the process of its adoption and implementation" (1983, pp. 175–182). This concept is important in the study of medical diffusion networks because it draws attention to how the basic idea of an innovation, found in its software, may be adopted and then the hardware and hardware-related software modified to meet specific organizational or environmental objectives, such as perceived performance deficits. Chapter 7 will describe in detail how reinvention took place as these cancer networks confronted the major areas of uncertainty and attempted to implement the objectives of the contracts in their regions.

Whether the change is mandated or voluntary raises other important questions. The first issue is where in the diffusion process the mandate is issued or the voluntary adoption occurs. A decision to implement new technology may be made by administrators or by the relevant professionals. If it is made administratively, then it is a mandated change. The decision to participate in the head and neck demonstration project and adopt the innovations that were part of that program was voluntarily implemented through a contractual arrangement entered into by the principal investigators. Moreover, the form of the innovation adopted, and the procedures for defining its content, were left to the contractors to resolve.

The timing and clustering of innovations is also important and may reflect change in the underlying knowledge base or paradigm (Kuhn, 1962; Rogers, 1983) into which the technology of the innovation fits. We have already indicated that the networks were initiated in response to such changes in the understanding of the natural history and course of cancer as a disease, and in the kinds of treatment and management that could potentially be applied.

When such changes in the underlying knowledge base occur, they are frequently followed by clusters of innovations that reflect the alteration in the knowledge base. Then, as new innovations develop, they are often in competition for scarce resources with parallel or competing innovations. More frequently, innovations occur synergistically and one innovation opens a path for the adoption of subsequent modifications or enhancements. Thus, adoption may be sequentially ordered (Fennell, 1984). Change agents may introduce a cluster or package of innovations representing a complex change in the knowledge base, which then produces an innovative software that requires a cluster of technology to be implemented. This was the case with the changes in the management of head and neck cancer. The proposed changes in patient management followed changes that had occurred in the overall concept of how cancer developed and could be treated, and they signaled the introduction of systemic treatments such as chemotherapy to be used in conjunction with the standard surgery and radiation.

Rogers has reviewed most of the literature about innovation diffusion and has produced the most parsimonious set of characteristics of innovations that specifically draw attention to the link between characteristics of both the innovation and the adopter (1983). These characteristics help explain why some innovations spread rapidly and others more slowly. Following Rogers, five characteristics are most important:

1. *Relative advantage* refers to the degree of uncertainty that surrounds the innovation. It is the degree to which the innovation is perceived by the target audience as better than the idea it is intended to supersede.

2. *Compatibility* also affects uncertainty. It is the degree to which the innovation is perceived by the target audience as consistent with existing practice, central values, past experience, and the current needs.

3. *Complexity* is the degree to which the innovation is perceived by the target audience to be difficult to understand or to use. Note that complexity refers to both the software and the hardware.

4. *Trialability* describes the extent to which one can reduce uncertainty before making a final decision to adopt. It is the degree to which an innovation can be adopted or tried on an experimental or limited basis before a final decision and commitment of resources are made.

5. *Observability* is the degree to which the results of others' use of the innovation are visible to the target audience.

Very often these five characteristics can interact in their effects on adoption decisions. For example, if an innovative technology is introduced and requires significant investment in facilities or complex staffing to implement, uncertainty about the potential impact of such an innovation will have a decided effect on the adoption decision. Given the type of organizational commitment required, it is unlikely that the innovation will be adoptable on a trial or experimental basis before substantial resources are committed. In such a situation the relative advantage will have to be quite high and clearly observable from reliable sources within the organization who are in a position to influence the decision. Such innovations are more likely to be adopted if they are compatible with organizational goals and objectives. Thus, one would expect organizations that adopt complex and costly innovations to have an agenda in which such technology plays a critical role.

THE INNOVATION IN HEAD AND NECK CANCER TREATMENT

At this point in the discussion, it is worthwhile to look at the innovation and attempt to characterize it according to some of the criteria that have been described. This characterization will have to be quite general because the innovation as introduced by the National Cancer Institute, acting as a change agent, was quite general. However, as will be discussed in Chapter 7, the individual contractors reinvented the innovation in accordance with their agendas to meet specific performance gaps in their regions.

The Head and Neck Network Demonstration projects were introduced by the NCI as part of the newly organized cancer control program. They were to disseminate state-of-the-art treatment from the academic medical center into the community. Thus, at one level the innovation to be diffused was multidisciplinary state-of-the-art medical management of head and neck cancers. As a result of the clinical trials program that had been in effect prior to the implementation of cancer control programs, it was becoming apparent that cancer management was changing. In particular, two related concepts were emerging. First, care for some tumors was found to be most effective when it was multidisciplinary and the treatment team included a surgeon, a radiologist, and a medical oncologist. This last member of the team was added when it became increasingly apparent that many cancers responded to chemotherapy as a curative measure and that adjuvant chemotherapy could even enhance the effects of surgery and/or radiation. The second and related concept was that even in the absence of cure, survival with some cancers was enhanced when posttreatment care was planned before the primary treatment intervention. Survival rates for head and neck cancer patients improved when planning for speech therapy and swallowing and dietary management took place before the primary treatment. In particular, performance of speech and swallowing following surgery could be dramatically enhanced by such planning. The concept of pretreatment planning by a multidisciplinary team was an innovation in the software associated with the technical management of head and neck cancer patients.

In summary, the technology being introduced involved an alteration in the paradigm or knowledge base of cancer treatment because it called for acceptance of a new concept of the disease as systemic, a concept that allowed for multidisciplinary interventions and shared decision making regarding the status of the patient. In addition, the implementation of this multidisciplinary approach required access to sophisticated hardware in the form of complex and costly radiological apparatus and the addition of staff in speech therapy, nutrition, oncology nursing, and medical oncology. Thus, the innovation of multidisciplinary management of head and neck cancer was complex and trialable only in an environment with appropriate hardware and personnel. It would be compatible in settings where these facilities were available and head and neck cancer was treated in sufficient numbers to warrant investment in the hardware and personnel.

However, the scientific rationale for the proposed innovation was shaky. Although clinical trials had been conducted and had demonstrated the effectiveness of multidisciplinary management of cancers of other sites, there had never been extensive clinical research demonstrating the effectiveness of chemotherapy in treating head and neck cancer. Nor had the rehabilitation efforts that were included in the concept of multidisciplinary treatment planning, the basis for the Head and Neck Demonstration Network program, ever been systematically evaluated. Thus, the observability and relative advantage of this innovation was not documented in the research literature, although clinical and other experience suggested that it would be beneficial. The participants accepted the innovation primarily on the basis of their own experience with management of these cancers.

A second innovation was also introduced as part of this program. It was more organizational or administrative than technical, following the distinction made in the literature (Daft, 1978; Evan, 1966; Kimberly, 1978; Kimberly and Evanisko, 1981; Teece, 1980). This innovation was the effort to link community hospitals and primary care physicians with research medicine in some systematic way. The Head and Neck Demonstration Networks provided slack resources to the participating universities and treatment centers in a way that would facilitate their development of these linkages, and to promote the formulation of strategies that would facilitate technology transfer.

This second innovation was primarily software-related. "Linkage," as conceived in this program, did not require adoption of any hardware. However, it was a unique idea that had not been tried by the National Institutes of Health except on a very minimal basis. The resources of the program made the concept trialable. The uncertainty associated with the implementation primarily involved the extent to which the resulting exchange relationships would give the university-based headquarters some unfair advantage over the community hospital by taking their patients. In one instance, this fear on the part of community hospitals limited the capability of the headquarters to form a network. However, for the most part, as we will show in Chapter 5, the formal, contractual relationships between the headquarters and the participating hospitals limited this risk. This component of the innovation was not observable to the medical community, and no data existed on the possible relative advantages of implementing the network principle as a means of promoting diffusion. The concept was compatible with existing interorganizational relationships in some areas, if the networks built on those relationships. In other regions it represented a change in the preexisting relationships, which caused some concern. The concept was not complex, although it required a certain amount of bureaucracy to manage it.

PERFORMANCE GAPS, AGENDA SETTING, AND THE NETWORK PROGRAMS

We are interested in innovation diffusion in and between organizations. As we will show in the next chapter, not all the networks were based on links between organizations. How the networks were formed was constrained by the environment and the ability of the organizations in the environment to adopt the multidisciplinary approach to head and neck cancer patient care. However, all the headquarters saw adoption of both multidisciplinary patient management and the network concept as innovations that would improve some aspect of their performances or protect some aspect of their core activities.

Rogers (1983) has characterized the process of organizational adoption of innovations as occurring in five sequential stages: *agenda setting* or targeting performance gaps in which problems or areas for potential development are established; *matching* performance problems with proposed innovations; *redefining* or restructuring the innovation to fit the organization's structure (or reinvention); *clarifying* the meaning of the innovation; and *routinizing* it as part of the organization's regular activities. In the remainder of this chapter we are primarily interested in the earliest stages of this process: agenda setting and matching. We will show how agenda setting followed the identification of performance gaps at the national level, in the academic medical centers, and in the community. Thus, we will begin by considering the nature of a performance gap.

Following Zaltman *et al.* (1973), a performance gap is a discrepancy between what the organization can do in response to a goal-related opportunity in its environment and what it actually does in exploiting that opportunity. It is recognized as a discrepancy between what an organization does and what those in decision-making positions within the organization believe it ought to be doing. Thus, it is acted upon only when recognized. Such recognition may occur in many ways, as March and Simon (1958) note. Usually there is impatience with the *status quo*. This definition of performance gap is consistent with the assumptions of contingency theory because the performance gap is ultimately recognized when changes in the environment constrain the performance of the organization and are perceived as impeding effectiveness.

The recognition of a performance deficit frequently leads to interest in innovation. However, recognition of the innovation as a possible solution may not be an immediate consequence of recognizing performance deficits within the organization (Zaltman *et al.*, 1973). The potentially relevant innovation may have to be introduced by an external source. This is especially likely if the innovation is not clearly articulated or if its relevance is not immediately obvious. It is also likely if the organization does not have access to resources necessary to implement the innovation. Finally, external introduction is likely if the organization's leaders do not have access to sources of information that would enable them to recognize the relevance of the technology.

Recognition of performance deficits and matching these needs with innovations is most likely when the organization is prepared. Agenda setting is the first stage in the Rogers (1983) model of organizational diffusion and is one way in which the organization becomes prepared to recognize an innovation. Organizational agendas serve to identify general organizational needs, problems, and long-term goals. As these agendas are formulated, performance gaps may be identified and strategies devised to address them. Agenda setting defines the organization's goals and identifies the potential problems that need resolution if these goals are to be achieved. Organizations or individuals that engage in agenda setting are likely to be leaders in their fields and among the earliest adopters of innovations once they have shown some effectiveness.

Although organizations may set agendas, innovations may also be adopted opportunistically. According to March (1981), the most successful organizations continuously monitor their environments for potentially beneficial ideas. As March further observes, there are so many problems in most organizations that any quality innovation that addresses any of the organization's functions is likely to be compatible with one or more aspects of an organization's agenda.

Even those organizations with established agendas may fail to recognize a particular performance gap, or the agenda may contain higher priorities. In such instances an innovation may be unnoticed by the organization's leadership, and its relevance may depend upon recognition by someone external to the organization who them stimulates initial interest within the organization. Or, recognition may come from someone in the organization who is not directly connected with agenda-setting activities. In either case, frequently the relevance of particular innovations may be recognized by others who then stimulate the interest of the organizational leadership by calling attention to the match between the innovation and the organization's agenda. Thus, finding a potentially beneficial innovation requires a certain degree of serendipity, which is most likely when the discoverer is prepared to recognize the relevance of the innovation.

We have adopted a contingency model to explain how the participating network organizations were recruited to address a performance gap perceived at the national level. These organizations were given a general set of guidelines and told to develop their networks, through which they would disseminate the information on state-of-the-art care for head and neck cancers. As Scott (1977) notes, following contingency theory, what constitutes a "good" organizational arrangement depends upon the organization's goals. Hence, the major question in assessing the potential relevance or benefit of the innovation to these networks is its match with those goals. Thus, as we consider these networks and their various approaches to diffusing the innovation of multidisciplinary patient management, we must look at how both the content of multidisciplinary care and the network principle of organization matched with the agenda that each of the seven established.

As we have indicated, there were three key actors or actor groups involved in this program. These were the federal government, the academic medical centers, and the community hospitals. The federal government included the president, who had set finding a cure for cancer as a major objective of his administration, Congress, and the staff at the National Cancer Institute and its advisory panels. Academic medicine included the headquarters institutions, the members of the advisory panels to the National Cancer Institute, and others who participated in the research programs sponsored by the National Cancer Institute. The community hospitals were of varying size and degree of sophistication, as we will show later. In most cases, however, there was some commitment to participate in the program prior to the award of the contracts.

Recall that there was uncertainty within the federal government regarding the extent of dissemination of state-of-the-art cancer treatment. Congress acted on the president's agenda for cancer by passing the National Cancer Act, which mandated that the NCI take action to ensure that the state of the art in cancer management was made available to anyone, wherever he/she was treated. State of the art was to be defined by the results of the clinical research programs that were ongoing under NCI sponsorship. Hospitals with magnificent treatment facilities and highest quality staff existed in the same environment as hospitals with limited facilities and limited access to qualified staff, and both sorts of institutions treated cancer patients (Jesse, 1981). Thus, there was pressure to encourage both referral and upgrading of community facilities to enhance the level of care available.

It was also becoming apparent to the academic medical centers that patients with cancer, who in the past would have been referred to the university or tertiary treatment center, were now being treated in community hospitals (Carbone et al., 1978; McCusker et al., 1982; Murphy, 1981; Smart, 1981). The community hospitals were increasingly sensitive to the fact that the shift in patient distribution was due in part to the influx of young, newly trained medical oncologists who expected to treat cancer patients in community settings. These young oncologists were not interested in entering academic medicine. They could attract patients to the community hospital, but they would also increasingly expect the community hospitals to provide the facilities needed to treat patients with the up-to-date methods they had been taught in medical school. The community hospitals, therefore, had some incentive to upgrade their facilities. The networks could provide the funds to make this possible.

In part to meet the demands of these newly trained oncologists and to attract patients, the facilities improved at the community hospitals. As the newly trained oncologists began to treat their patients in these hospitals, there was increased competition for patients. This competition resulted in decreasing numbers of patients available at the medical centers. This meant fewer patients available through these major centers for research and for training new students. The medical schools needed to establish new relationships with the community hospitals that would provide training for their students and patients for their research protocols. One outcome of this need was the development of residency programs in these community hospitals, often based on relationships between medical school alumni and the departments where they trained. These relationships formed the basis for the network programs that were being introduced by the National Cancer Institute in several of the network demonstration regions, particularly Illinois, Wisconsin, the Greater Delaware Valley, and Arkansas.

By the end of the 1970s more than half of all patients enrolled in the protocols developed by the large national cooperative research groups would come from these community hospitals (Begg et al., 1982; McCusker et al., 1982; Murphy, 1981). The quality of the data from these programs indicates that quality care was frequently available. Thus, for some medical centers these early cancer control initiatives by the NCI provided the necessary resources to link them with community hospitals. As we noted earlier, the linkages to community hospitals in support of clinical trials was an apparent component of the agendas for Illinois, Wisconsin, Northern California, and the Greater Delaware Valley. It was less obviously the case for Arkansas, the Eastern Great Lakes, and Mississippi. These linkages would later be expanded to other forms of collaboration, or they would provide the basis for comprehensive cancer programs in their regions.

As part of the National Cancer Act, Congress mandated funds for the establishment of comprehensive cancer centers. These funds were to be used to provide secure and continuous funding to advance the basic and clinical research activities at established research centers across the United States. However, the funding criteria stipulated that to be "comprehensive" these centers would have to incorporate epidemiology and cancer control as well as clinical and basic research. Cancer control activity at that time did not include research but emphasized demonstration programs and outreach designed to disseminate the results of research to community treatment centers. Congress's cancer control mandate was to be implemented with funds incorporated into the NCI budget as a line item. These funds were a significant portion of the budget of the National Cancer Institute, and programs were designed to encourage links between the research centers and community hospitals. Developing a comprehensive cancer center was part of the agenda of at least three of the networks: Illinois, Wisconsin, and Northern California.

However, as we will describe in more detail in the following chapter, not all the network regions had the resources to support cancer centers or even multihospital networks. Some of these programs had identified performance gaps in the ability of hospitals in their service regions to deliver care to head and neck patients. Thus, their agenda included the need to attract specialized personnel or equipment that would enhance treatment opportunities. Networks with this agenda included Arkansas, the Greater Delaware Valley, and Northern California. Several networks recognized the need for coordination of care around certain shared facilities, such as expensive radiation therapy facilities, and sought to become tertiary referral centers, using resources from the network for this purpose. These networks were Arkansas, Mississippi, and the Greater Delaware Valley.

Not only was there no prior experience or precedent for cancer control in the academic medical centers, there were also no program staff at the NCI with experience in managing such programs. Thus, another performance gap was the ability to initiate these programs. On a more general basis, the agenda of the NCI had to include developing an infrastructure for cancer control.

Moreover, the National Cancer Institute generally operated with a peer review system in which scientists who were established experts in a given area reviewed the proposals of other scientists with similar credentials. This system worked well in the basic and clinical sciences where there were well-established cadres of investigators and where the knowledge base was well established. All these things were lacking in cancer control for the historic reasons described earlier in Chapter 1. There was no obvious investigator clientele and no identifiable set of peers to review research programs in the field of cancer control. Much of the initial activity initiated in cancer control was contractual and directed by staff who were inclined to let the investigators exercise their expertise. The leadership of these efforts both within the National Cancer Institute and in the academic centers typically came from physicians, supported sometimes by statisticians and epidemiologists, and sometimes by other personnel who were not even trained for research. Skills were lacking in health services research, health care planning, and the basic social sciences needed to formulate a realistic and evaluable implementation plan for this agenda.

Finally, many were convinced that there were new clinical findings that should be quickly transmitted to the community physician. These groups believed that once available, this new technology would genuinely improve the quality of cancer care in the community. New ideas were not available for every cancer site. Thus, to build a sophisticated network of hospitals that would support cancer control programs developed by the universities, the medical centers had to provide access to modern treatment facilities and methods and new treatment procedures to be transmitted. Although they were not always new, there were prevailing standards for treating most forms of cancer. But they did not always call for multidisciplinary treatment. Both within the NCI and in the academic medical community there were those who believed that these standards could and should be transformed into guidelines that would be less rigorous than research protocols, but nevertheless useful in guiding the management of certain cancers in community treatment centers. These guidelines would then be the vehicles by which modern treatment methods could be made available to all patients wherever they received treatment.

As we shall see in Chapter 7, however, patient guidelines were not uniformly accepted either in the community or by the academic medical centers at which they were supposed to be developed. Nor, as it turned out, were treatment procedures as commonly accepted as it was believed.

In summary, each of the three interest groups had an agenda. The federal government's agenda was defined by the president's priority to find a cure for cancer. One aspect of this was to establish an infrastructure that would support the cancer control programs mandated by Congress. Academic medicine's agenda was to establish new sources of patients for training and research, to secure access to new funds for cancer control activities, and to be eligible to become comprehensive cancer centers or establish themselves as regional referral centers. The community hospitals' agenda was to attract young physicians and their patients who could provide revenue to further build their facilities and patient base.

In Chapter 2 thumbnail descriptions of the seven network programs were presented. Included were descriptions of the goals and objectives of each network as stated in the proposals prepared by the headquarters institutions. Since these proposals were written in response to a "Request for Proposals" prepared by staff at the National Cancer Institute, they had to be responsive to the specific objectives outlined in that document. They constituted, then, the manifest or formally stated organizational agenda for each network. They appear, therefore, to be consistent with the agenda as set forth by the NCI. For purposes of this analysis, one level of definition of organizational goal is the formal statement of measures by which each of the seven networks would address the problem of disseminating state-of-the-art treatment strategies to community hospitals as mandated by the NCI program.

The top portion of Table 3.1 summarizes these formally stated objectives, as distilled from the network proposals. Clearly, the general goal of dissemination of multidisciplinary care was translated by the network principal investigators in a variety of ways, but these stated objectives are classifiable into three broad categories: patient care, network building, and education.

As Perrow (1961) and others have noted, stated goals may or may not reflect the organization's activity or operant goals. Otherwise put, the networks had latent agendas that were stimulated by the performance gaps described earlier, and by the overall perception that the environment of support for clinical and basic research was changing. However, the individual agenda developed by each network tended to closely reflect the political and social climates in which the networks were to be developed. These latent agendas reflected alternative motivations of the headquar-

Table 3.1. Stated Network Objectives and Latent Agendas[a]

	Arkansas	Eastern Great Lakes	Mississippi	Wisconsin	Greater Delaware Valley	Illinois	Northern California
Stated objectives							
Improved patient care							
Generally improve management					X		X
Provide multidisciplinary treatment		X	X		X		
Evaluate multidisciplinary treatment through data collection and analysis		X	X		X		
Develop patient management protocols		X	X				
Increase access to needed care					X		
Specifically enhance rehabilitation							X
Network enhancement							
Develop referral links between MDs	X						
Develop linkages between hospitals	X						
Evaluate effectiveness of network	X						
Education							
Educate health professionals	X	X		X	X	X	
Educate public	X			X			
Train dental hygienists	X		X		X		
Domain enhancement							
Establish HQ as principal regional treatment center			X				
Latent agendas							
Establish HQ or PI as regional treatment center	X	X	X		X		
Enhance research in area through establishment of consortium cancer center				X		X	X
Hire needed specialists for region	X				X		X

[a]Source: Network case materials.

ters for pursuing the development of network demonstration projects as an appropriate solution to performance gaps in patient treatment and knowledge dissemination.

The bottom half of Table 3.1 summarizes what we observed as the latent agendas or operant goals of each network. Two themes emerge here, dictated in large measure by environmental constraints. In one theme the emphasis was placed on establishing the institution or principal investigator as the center for head and neck treatment in the region. This strategy was adopted by four of the networks: Arkansas, Eastern Great Lakes, Mississippi, and Greater Delaware Valley. The other theme, adopted by Wisconsin, Northern California, and Illinois, was to enhance the regional capability for cancer research and improvement of treatment by implementing an interinstitutional network linking university and community hospitals and sharing data management resources, technical expertise, and patient information. In addition to these two general approaches, the Greater Delaware

Valley, Arkansas, and Northern California programs used some of the resources to add personnel to their programs that would serve the region. In each case the resource was a key rehabilitation person, and so the addition was consistent with the program. In Arkansas, a person who specialized in developing facial prostheses was added. In the Greater Delaware Valley and Northern California, maxillofacial prosthodontists were brought into the service region.

Of the seven networks that were established under this program, six survived and completed the program. The Mississippi Head and Neck Demonstration Network was unable to advance from the planning to the implementation phase. It is of considerable interest to note in Table 3.1 that manifest and latent agendas in Mississippi both emphasized domain enhancement as a primary objective. The Mississippi proposal specifically indicated the intention by the university of establishing a tertiary treatment center for the managing of head and neck cancer in Mississippi. Although there is no direct evidence that this direct statement contributed to the failure of the Mississippi network, the investigators in their report indicated that they were unable to obtain the necessary cooperation either from within the network or from the hospitals that were originally proposed to be in the network program.

These two themes also affected how the network concept was implemented in each network region and the form of diffusion that occurred. In the following chapter we will argue that three factors in the environment (resources, diversity of organizational form, and preexisting linkages) influenced how the innovation process proceeded. These environmental constraints also influenced which of the two themes were adopted to resolve the performance gap in a particular network. The themes reflect two strategies for dealing with both the need to establish linkages with community hospitals and the requirement of disseminating state-of-the-art treatment into community settings. These were the formal objectives. However, the latent or operant objectives reflected some desire to establish the centrality of the headquarters institution as the center for research and treatment of cancer in the region. In this sense the headquarters institution used head and neck cancer care and the interests of the principal investigator for broader objectives aimed at positioning the institution to compete for other funding becoming available through the NCI. Through this effort the headquarters was also attempting to acquire greater access to important patient resources in the region.

To summarize, it appears as if agenda setting, both manifest and latent, occurred in all networks. With one exception, there were discernable differences between the manifest and latent components of the agenda at each network. Stated objectives tended to be quite consistent with the agenda established by the federal government and explicitly outlined in the "Request for Proposals." They stressed the need to improve patient care and to devise strategies to enhance cancer knowledge among both lay and professional publics. The latent agendas more often were explicit in their domain enhancement objectives. Two forms of domain enhancement strategy were implemented. As we will see in Chapter 4, the adoption of these various strategies was very much influenced by the context into which the network was introduced.

4

Considering the Environment
Environmental Context and Network Form

INTRODUCTION

The preceding chapter considered uncertainty in the ability of organizations to perform their key functions, and the relationship of uncertainty to innovation diffusion. We applied contingency theory to help explain how organizational leaders deal with uncertainty by first identifying performance gaps and then by developing agendas to address these performance deficits. These basic concepts were then used to analyze how the key actors—the National Cancer Institute, the academic medical centers, and the community hospitals—in the head and neck demonstration projects defined the innovation and set agendas that addressed specific performance gaps related to their core activities. The agendas that emerged from the networks were constrained by the environments in which the programs were established.

Following up on the questions we posed at the end of Chapter 1, our focus here is on question 3: How does the environment influence the formation of channels through which the innovation is diffused? Specifically, under what circumstances will diffusion occur through interpersonal or interorganizational channels? Chapter 5 will continue our examination of environmental influences on network formation, considering the structure of the networks in finer detail.

We will also continue the themes introduced in Chapter 3. In that chapter we focused on agenda setting within individual organizations and did not consider the interaction that developed across organizations as the headquarters organizations began planning to implement their agendas. As we described in Chapter 3, the innovation had three components: the concept of multidisciplinary care, developing a standard definition of multidisciplinary state-of-the-art care in a common format for dissemination (the guidelines), and the development of networks through which to communicate the content of the guidelines. Since these innovations were developed to address the performance gap of uneven care in community hospitals in each network service area, the objective of the program was to disseminate the concepts to all hospitals in the region. The diffusion effort required the creation of some form of linkage or communication channel among health care delivery units within the region. However, the establishment of these channels proved to be a multilevel problem, defined in part by characteristics of the regions in which the programs were introduced. How these channels were formed was related to the interpersonal interaction between the leadership in the network headquarters and the community physicians, the decision makers in the hospitals, and the characteristics of the hospitals in the region.

BOUNDARY SPANNERS AND INTERORGANIZATIONAL LINKAGE

At the most basic level, innovation diffusion across organizations involves two factors: the organizational capability in the region and the individuals in the organizations who make decisions. Ultimately, however, the diffusion process takes place between individuals who represent both their own interests and the interests of the organization to which they belong. Thus, innovation diffusion is a boundary-spanning activity. As such, the basic linkage is between individuals who form a communication network through which information about the innovation is disseminated, and who influence perceptions of its applicability.

The individuals who form these linkages are called "gatekeepers" or opinion leaders (Rogers, 1983). Opinion leaders exercise leadership that is informal rather than formal. Their leadership position is based on the recognition by others in their group or organization that they have special competence in a particular area of central interest to the group. In addition to their technical competence, they are usually accessible to the other group members and conform with the central norms of the group. Thus, above all they tend to be compatible with the group on its central characteristics, yet at the high end in terms of competence and success as defined by the norms of the group.

In addition to their special place within the group, opinion leaders have linkages outside the group to sources of information regarded as important to the group's activities. Although locally influential, they have access to "cosmopolitans" who are leading figures in their areas of influence. These individuals have higher social status and are more open to new ideas than other members of their groups (Coleman *et al.*, 1966; Katz and Lazarsfeld, 1955; Rogers and Shoemaker, 1971; Warnecke *et al.*, 1976).

The central role of the opinion leader is to mediate the flow of information about innovations within the group. The opinion leader interprets its meaning and often makes a preliminary assessment about its potential utility for the main activities of the group. Their centrality in the group stems from their knowledge about the group's agenda. These individuals will most likely influence the attitudes of the group members about the innovation and their willingness to try it.

The opinion leader is generally found in communities or informal groups. It is an informal role which is recognized but which has no defined status within an organization. When the role is formalized within an organization, its occupant is often described as a boundary spanner. As discussed by Aldrich (1979), Kaluzny

(1974), Rogers (1983), and Scott (1977), boundary spanners influence the internal decisions within the organization and also represent the organization to the external environment. Although these roles often contain both formal and informal elements, occupants are usually recognizable because of the central relevance of their activities to the main or core functions of the organization. For example, in Greer's recent (1986) study of technology diffusion in hospitals, she found that key boundary-spanning roles were played by hospital-based specialists, such as radiologists or pathologists, who performed key services for others who were more dependent upon the community, such as internists and surgeons, and who depended upon their ability to manipulate both the hospital bureaucracy and these community-based physicians to maintain their status. These actors are particularly influential in decisions to acquire technology because much of their activity is dependent upon the availability of powerful technology.

As information processors, boundary spanners receive, filter, and control the flow of information from the environment into the organization. The organization is dependent upon them for information about the environment, including those aspects most critical to the organization's survival and growth. As the external representatives of the organization, they may acquire and dispose of organizational resources, ensure the organization's political and social legitimacy, and manage the public image of the organization. When the role combines external representation and resource management, the boundary-spanner role becomes very powerful, and whoever performs it must exercise discretion and sensitivity.

The power of the boundary spanner depends upon the authority of the individual playing the role, especially in organizations with dual lines of authority. In organizations such as hospitals, the administrator manages the organization through acquisition of resources and maintenance of institutional boundaries, but the administrator also has to coordinate nonroutine hospital events in which the autonomy of the professional takes precedence over bureaucratic authority (Perrow, 1965). Kaluzny (1974) noted that within such organizations administrators must negotiate with the physicians, especially when the administrators need to make technical decisions beyond their levels of competence and must simultaneously respond to the demands of their lay constituents to limit costs and operate within the institutional budget. However, Greer (1986) found that administrators frequently set hospital goals and then acquire technology and professional staff to accommodate these goals without consulting the professionals who may resist change. In such instances the administrator plays the powerful boundary-spanning role and may even bring in new professional staff to legitimate the decision to acquire technology.

When the boundary-spanning role is held by a senior professional, such as the chief of a service, its power is usually considerable. When a junior professional or administrator attempts to play the boundary-spanning role, its power is often constrained by the amount of authority that is specifically designated to the position. In such cases the relationship between the professional and senior professional and administrative staff is critical.

However, when a decision requires organizational commitment of major resources, the power relationships are likely to be altered. Any professional in a boundary-spanning role has the necessary expertise to make and legitimize major technical decisions relevant to the organization's central or core activities. But, unless the professional also controls the necessary organizational resources, his/her power to implement a decision requiring major resource commitment may be limited. A nonprofessional can never legitimize a decision that affects the central activity of a medical center, but, as we have noted, when the innovation requires major organizational resources and affects the external capability of the hospital to maintain its position within the environment, the administrator can make such decisions and then bring into the hospital professional staff that will legitimize the activity. The nonprofessional or administrator may thus represent the organization in the environment and may bring in resources and expend them, but the successful introduction of a technical innovation into the hospital must ultimately depend upon the availability of professionals to implement it.

Changes in the context and organization of the practice of medicine have effected a basic shift in the control of the adoption of medical innovations from the individual physician to the health care management system, which is often represented by the administrator. The result has been a decrease in the impact of the physician on major technological decisions within the hospital. More often now the decision to implement a new technology is influenced by cost, the impact of the acquisition on the market position of the hospital within the region, and its ability to attract staff that will increase the utilization of the facility. As discussed in Chapter 1, innovation diffusion within organizations that requires major technological or personnel expenditures tends to embody contingent decisions in which both adminstrative and professional criteria are applied. Although the target of innovation diffusion may continue to be the physician, the organizational milieu and the characteristics of the technology required to implement the innovation influence the potential for dissemination and how the dissemination can occur. The models of diffusion that might apply are thus our next consideration.

THE INNOVATION DIFFUSION MODEL

The original conception of innovation diffusion as developed by Rogers (1983) and others was that the individual was the adopter. Organizational variables were not considered, or if they were, they were not directly related to the diffusion process. When diffusion occurred in an organization, it was assumed that the adoption decision was made by a person in authority, and once a decision was made, it would be carried out within the organization.

The concept of individuals acting autonomously in the adoption process was quite appealing when the target of the innovation was a professional. The autonomous adopter was consistent with the image of the professional as having the license to act autonomously in professional matters. Indeed, when Abraham Flexner (1910) recommended reforms for professional medical education, the elements of that reform replicated the elements of the classic innovation diffusion model. It is clear in Flexner's recommendations that he viewed the physician as a free agent reviewing the medical literature and adopting treatment strategies based upon his/her evaluation of the research reported in the literature. The model used by Flexner was well grounded in direct experience since it reflected the way medicine was practiced at the time and how the practitioner behaved in assessing new treatment regimens.

The individual's decision to adopt an innovation usually is reached in a series of steps. In the first step (*knowledge*), targeted individuals become aware of the innovation and begin to associate it with needs or activities to which it is relevant, to an agenda, either personal or organizational. At each step in the adoption process certain characteristics (see Chapter 3) of the innovation are particularly relevant. At the knowledge step, the complexity of the innovation and information about how it can be used are important. Complexity influences the adopter's assessment of how easily it can be implemented. It also refers to the understandability of the underlying principles that govern how the innovation is used and under what circumstances. Clearly, professional judgment is required to assess whether the innovation is sufficiently advanced and tested to be considered for implementation.

For example, an innovative treatment may involve using a new member of a well-known family of drugs that has been in use to treat a disease. In such an instance, adopting the new drug may not require any change in the underlying software that governs how the disease is treated. On the other hand, the same drug may represent an entirely new approach to treating the disease based upon new insights into how the disease behaves. In this case, the software component is the most important aspect of the innovation and must be accepted before the technology can be implemented.

Another characteristic of the innovation that is important at the knowledge step is its compatibility or relevance to other activities that are part of the core tasks of the organization. When the software requires complex changes in orientation to the core tasks, compatibility and complexity become competing issues. If the software of the proposed innovation departs too radically from the conceptual framework of those to whom it is directed, more effort will have to be made to reconcile the underlying conceptual understanding of the principles on which the innovation is based with existing practices and principles. Thus, the more complex the software, the less likely the innovation will be perceived as compatible with existing technology or activity.

At the knowledge step, the important sources of information tend to be objective and impersonal. Magazines, technical journals, discourses by renowned authorities who occupy positions similar to that occupied by the target audience, and texts are often crucial sources of information. Often these sources of information play a critical role in reconciling the apparent conflicts between the new ideas embedded in the software of the innovation and existing practice. The opinion leaders at the local level are often those with direct contacts to these sources.

The second step in the process is *persuasion*. At this step other features of the innovation become significant, namely, its observability and technical advantage relative to standard practice. If the technology is complex and apparently varying from accepted ideas, its justification by significant individuals in the profession may resolve or reduce uncertainty. However, the motivation to implement such change will depend upon evidence that individuals such as those in the target audience have experienced success in implementing it. Such evidence, to the extent that it comes from informal or clinical evidence in contrast to formal reports of clinical trials, will be heavily dependent on collegial contact. Thus, at this stage the local influentials, opinion leaders in the local community who are well known and viewed as successful, are most likely to be able to persuade others to try the innovation (Coleman *et al.*, 1966; Downs and Mohr, 1976; Kaluzny, 1974).

Relative advantage is defined statistically and through clinical experience with the innovation. The effects of the innovation are assessed through tangible results. In the case of medical technology these are often reduced mortality or morbidity, improved access to critical resources, improved cost/benefit ratios, or, most likely, some combination of these outcomes. Evidence of such outcomes can be observed in the literature through reports from clinical trials or experiments set up to specifically evaluate the relative advantage of the innovation over existing practice. However, more than likely the innovation will not be adopted until local influentials report successful use of it through informal channels (Coleman *et al.*, 1966).

The trialability of the innovation is a major factor influencing the third step, the *decision* about whether the innovation will actually be implemented. Trialability is determined by whether the target audience has the resources to implement the innovation and by how permanent the initial decision has to be. Thus, if the innovation can be tried at no great risk to the adopter, and if there are slack resources available to the initiator or the organization to support trial use, it is more likely to be adopted on a trial basis than if such resources are scarce and/or the decision once made is difficult to reverse. Innovations that can be adopted on a trial basis are more likely to be adopted. Trialability of medical innovations is often enhanced by the availability of research funds or third-party payers who will reimburse the organization for any costs associated with the trial. Thus, the decision step is conditional on the availability of organizational resources to support a trial implementation, and on the possibility that the trial can be reversed at marginal cost to the innovator.

Since the decision to adopt usually occurs over time, the adoption process includes a fourth step, *confirmation*. Because the adoption process never really ends, this step is never fully observable. However, its incorporation in the model serves to emphasize that adoption of an innovation is always conditional on the continued confirmation that the innovation makes a contribution to the core activities of the organization or individual making the decision to adopt. Thus, adoption implies an initial decision, which then must be confirmed by continued experience. There is always the possibility that the adopter will revert to earlier practice or replace the innovation with an even newer technology or software.

This traditional four-step model has been found unsatisfactory when applied to studies of organizational diffusion (Greer, 1977; Rogers, 1983). This dissatisfaction stems from the inability of the model to deal with factors in the organizational context that influence how the adoption decision is made, even when it is made by an individual.

As medicine and its organizational milieu have become more complex, the traditional model of innovation diffusion has been found particularly inadequate to explain the diffusion of medical technology. Although the physician is still the key boundary spanner in the diffusion of medical technology, the organization and its administrators play an increasingly larger role in the process. Hence, the appropriate model in some instances may be a contingency model in which innovations are adopted only after several key organizational actors are convinced that it will support the core activities of the adopting organization.

Historically, two major theoretical perspectives on organizational innovation adoption have been described by the literature. One takes the perspective that innovation adoption represents an outcome of political or interest group competition within organizations (Fennell, 1984; Greer, 1977; Kimberly, 1981; Moch and Morse, 1977; Pfeffer, 1981). A second argues that characteristics such as the size, complexity, centralization of decision making, interconnectedness, and urban location of the organization influence the adoption decision (Hage and Aiken, 1967; Kimberly, 1978).

In recent years, a third formulation has surfaced, which views innovation adoption as a response to institutional pressures in the organization's environment, rather than as the outcome of rational decision making based on expectations of the technical advantages afforded by an innovation (DiMaggio and Powell, 1983; Fennell, 1980; Meyer and Rowan, 1977). This neoinstitutional perspective argues that adoption will occur whether or not the technical merits of the innovation have been demonstrated, if the innovation has *already* been widely adopted by other organizations (Tolbert and Zucker, 1983). Late adopters, then, are influenced more by the normative expectations and pressures surrounding an innovation that has become popular than by whatever it is the innovation is purported actually to do. In the medical arena such a process may have been responsible for the spread of many high-cost technologies during the 1960s and the early 1970s while resources were still relatively plentiful. However, as slack resources have become increasingly rare, it is more likely that the political process model of negotiation between interested groups better fits reality in the hospital sector.

Using the political model, adoption is viewed as a process through which decisions are made to commit slack resources within the organization to new programs. From this perspective, the adoption process may itself influence who gains or maintains control of the organizational agenda. March and Simon (1958) and Pfeffer (1981) define slack resources as those resources that have not already been committed to other organizational participants or programs. Acquiring slack resources or influencing their allocation to new programs or technologies can become a significant means to gain or maintain power within the organization. As we have already noted, in modern medical organization this power may be in the hands of boundary spanners. Moreover, commitment of these resources for innovations is likely to require negotiation between the administrative and professional authorities within the organization. These negotiations can take place when the organization sets its agenda. Administrative authorities will probably be more concerned about the financial and bureaucratic implications of the innovation; professional authorities will be more concerned with the technical and software aspects of the innovation.

The necessity of these two groups within the organization to negotiate for the adoption of the innovation illustrates well the contingent nature of the process. In the organized medical setting an individual cannot always independently adopt an innovation. The decision requires legitimation through which the bureaucratic component commits the slack resources required for implementation and the professional authority concedes the technical merits of the innovation. The professional authority must secure consensus among other relevant professionals that the innovation will enhance patient care within the hospital. This consensus is especially important when the innovation involves these other professionals or the resources that they control (see Chapter 8 concerning the case of the Mississippi network). Without either of these commitments the innovators may experience resistance and the innovation will not be adopted.

How complex the adoption process becomes depends in large part on the innovation and its potential impact on the hospital's resources. If the innovation can be easily implemented within the existing hospital structure and resources, then the extent of political maneuvering is likely to be small or nonexistent. As the complexity of the innovation increases and more components within the organization are involved in its adoption and implementation, the political process becomes more complex.

Many studies of innovation adoption within organizations conducted during the 1960s and 1970s emphasized the importance of the software component, especially the importance of access to information about innovations, and integration of the organization into informational networks during the adoption process (Beyer and Trice, 1978; Crane, 1972; Hage and Aiken, 1967: Kimberly, 1978). From this perspective, structural and contextual characteristics of the organization such as size, complexity, centralization, interconnectedness, and urban location affect the likelihood that an innovation will be recognized and accepted by the organization, by affecting the amount of information about innovations that enters the organization. The more information about innovative technologies and/or programs that flows through the organization, and the more varied the sources of information, the more likely the organization will be innovative or adopt innovations. Thus, the political process model offers guidance about the contingent factors that influence the decision and confirmation steps of the classical model. The second perspective suggests that the likelihood of linking organizational agendas to particular innovations is increased as information-flows into the organization increase.

Both of these perspectives have generated an impressive amount of empirical work on innovation in organizations. However, as Rogers (1983) and others (Kimberly, 1981; Kimberly and Evanisko, 1981) have noted, most of the work has produced disappointingly low correlations between the supposed predictors of innovativeness and actual adoption of innovations. One reason is the failure of much of the organizational research to study the adoption/diffusion process over time and to consider the different effects that many of the independent variables may have on adoption at various steps in the process. As described in Chapter 3, these steps include agenda setting or targeting performance gaps, matching or connecting identified problems in performance with the proposed innovations, redefining or restructuring the innovation to fit the organizational setting (reinvention), clarifying the meaning of the innovation for the core activities of the organization, and routinizing the innovation as part of the organization's regular activities. In Chapter 3 we described agenda setting. In this chapter we will consider how matching the innovation with the organization and its context influences the adoption process.

CONSIDERING THE ENVIRONMENT

Throughout this book we are using contingency theory as the basic framework for examining the effects of context and structure on the emergence of the network demonstration projects. The complementary assumptions of resource dependence are incorporated into the analysis to help understand how and why organizations participate in cooperative ventures, i.e., establish linkages for the purpose of innovation diffusion. The fundamental assumption of resource dependence is that an organization can and does take action to increase its access to resources in the environment (Aldrich and Pfeffer, 1976; Jacobs, 1974; Mindlin and Aldrich, 1975; Yuchtman and Seashore, 1967). These resources are sought in light of their relevance to the organizational tasks or, as Jacobs (1974) notes, their "essentiality" to organizational goals.

The resource dependence approach assumes that when organizations are unable to generate these resources on their own, they must interact with other organizations in their environments to ensure resource availability. The availability and distribution of those resources in the environment determines the level of competition for them and the degree to which an organization will have to depend upon other organizations to obtain them. On the one hand, if the environment is rich in resources and they are available from several sources, dependence on any single source is reduced and, in fact, may be reversed to the point where the suppliers become dependent upon customers. On the other hand, where there are few providers of a valued resource, the supplier has control. Whichever is the case, organizational effectiveness, according to the resource dependence perspective, is contingent upon the organization's ability to maximize access to essential resources and to minimize dependence on other organizations (Yuchtman and Seashore, 1967).

In Chapter 1 we reviewed the fundamental assumptions of contingency theory, which led to the proposition that good matching between environmental constraints and organizational structures (strategic contingency) leads to good performance. We are interested here in explaining how these networks formed. Although all seven networks had the formally stated objective of disseminating state-of-the-art treatment to their target communities, they were not all based on interorganizational linkages. As we will show, the network structures to develop reflected the supply and distribution of resources in the network environment. In particular, we hypothesize that the form of diffusion channel that emerged in each environment was determined by the resources in the region, how they were distributed among various organizations, and the preexisting linkages between organizations in the environment. The significance of the concept of multidisciplinary management of head and neck cancer patients to the organizations in the environments, as well as their level of participation, depended upon the potential relevance of treating those kinds of patients to the organizations involved. It also depended on the compatibility of the other technical and software components of the innovation with the participating organization's manifest and latent agendas.

Environmental Context and the Form of the Diffusion Channel

Our basic argument, then, is that how the diffusion channels formed was constrained by the resources in the environment, the ability of the organizations in the environment to adopt the innovation, and the preexisting relationships among the organizations in the environment. A number of organizational theorists who have examined the influence of the environment on interorganizational dependence relationships have noted that, consistent with the contingency argument, different patterns emerge in different environments (Hall, 1963; Lawrence and Lorsch, 1967; Perrow, 1967; Pugh et al., 1968, 1969; Thompson, 1967). Following these theorists, we hypothesize that network form depends upon those environmental factors that influence the organization's ability to obtain the necessary resources for achieving its objectives. Thus, the different settings in which the head and neck cancer network demonstration projects were implemented nurtured various patterns of organizational linkage to implement programs.

A variety of studies have examined the effects of the environment on innovation diffusion strategies. Consistent with our hypotheses derived from resource dependence and contingency theory, three factors emerge as most relevant: (1) whether the organization or group to which the innovation is directed has access to the resources necessary to implement the innovation, (2) the compatibility between the innovation and established practices and technology available, and (3) the existence of prior channels of communication that may be used to transmit the current innovation (Aldrich, 1979; Downs and Mohr, 1976; Hage and Aiken, 1967; Kaluzny, 1974; Mansfield, 1973; Rogers, 1983; Warner, 1975; Zaltman et al., 1973).

Resource Capacity

If the purpose of the network is to disseminate complex treatment technology, the institutions in the network must have access to the resources needed to implement the innovation. Where the resources are limited or unevenly distributed, the number of institutions capable of implementing the innovation may be limited. Alternatively, the method of dissemination or adoption may be redefined.

Three types of resources are critical to the medical care delivery system. These are access to the relevant technology and facilities for delivery of the care, the availability of qualified medical staff and related professionals and technicians, and patients requiring the type of care offered by the institution and financially able to afford it. In general, the availability of patients is the most basic of these resources. Institutions are unlikely to invest in complex and costly equipment and high-quality professional staff if the prospect of attracting patients is limited. Similarly, those skilled in treating specific types of patients are not apt to accept an invitation to join the staff of a hospital with no patients in need of their specializations.*

Compatibility of Organizational Form

The availability of patients and other resources indicates the capacity of the environment to support innovative programs. The compatibility of the organizations participating in the programs affects the ease with which the innovative program can be diffused. Compatibility between channel members, or what has

---

*Although the number of patients is used more commonly by health economists to measure the demand for medical care, from an organizational perspective patients represent an essential resource dimension of the task environment. Patients neither choose their own hospital services nor directly pay for them, so their role as consumers (or the demand side) is debatable. Patients are used, however, as justification for the adoption of innovations deemed necessary by physicians (Greer, 1984). Thus, an ample supply of patients at risk of head and neck cancer represents an important resource in the environment of targeted hospitals within the network regions.

been called "homophily" (Rogers, 1983), includes similarities of size, level of specialization, functional differentiation, and agenda. An environment consisting of homophilous organizations is more conducive of interorganizational diffusion. This consideration has been well documented in the literature on innovation diffusion at both the individual and collective levels (Aiken and Hage, 1968; Downs and Mohr, 1976; Hage and Aiken, 1967; Mansfield, 1973; Rogers, 1983). The basic conclusion is that innovation diffusion is most likely to occur between organizations or individuals that are compatible and comparable on dimensions central to implementing the innovation.

The extent to which the organizations in the environment are structurally homogeneous will influence the degree and level of innovation that occurs. Homogeneity is particularly pertinent in characterizing those organizations defined as eligible network participants, or organizations toward which the innovation is directed. If the participating institutions are sufficiently similar to the institution that initiates the innovation, direct adoption of the innovation is possible, and interorganizational linkages for diffusion are likely.

The type of linkage through which the innovation is disseminated is then directly associated with the way in which the innovation is eventually adopted. The level and mode of diffusion depends upon existing practical conditions. The target organizations must have the necessary complement of characteristics to create a homogeneous environment for network development.

Preexisting Linkages

A third dimension of the environment that influences the development of diffusion linkages is the nature of the linkages already present. Three characteristics of these linkages are particularly relevant: density, stability, and domain consensus.

The concept of density was introduced by Barnes (1954) and Mitchell (1969) to characterize the level of connectedness within an organizational environment. Density is defined by the number and extent of relationships within an environment; high levels of density may indicate that the organizations in a network or set have had sufficient experience with each other to permit the creation of mutually beneficial relationships. In this case, density of linkages would create stability and provide a basis for establishing diffusion channels. On the other hand, density may also indicate an abundance of competitive relationships or a level of interdependence that is threatening to some organizations within the environment. A very dense environment is one in which all organizations interact directly. However, density is not synonymous with stability (Weick, 1976). As described by Aldrich (1979, p. 326), disturbing influences travel very quickly throughout very dense environments, thereby disrupting the whole network.

Stable, long-standing linkages between organizations may also support the *status quo*. The extent of such linkages will influence the possibility of new relationships forming. If diffusion channels can conform with these preexisting relationships, then their development and stability may be enhanced. If, on the other hand, new linkages threaten or compete with these relationships, they may not be very stable or likely to survive. Particularly at the persuasion and legitimation stages of the diffusion process (when local influence and observability of success are likely to be important factors), the stability of the relationships through which information about the innovation is communicated will influence acceptability (Rogers, 1983).

Although domain consensus is regarded as a secondary factor within the resource dependence perspective, in the context of innovation diffusion it is an important feature of the environment. Within an environment, consensus as to each organization's domain includes recognition and acceptance of the organizations' boundaries and appropriate tasks. If a particular target audience is within an organization's accepted boundaries, or if interacting with it is part of the organization's recognized tasks, involvement of that audience in the organization's attempt to diffuse the innovation will be considered legitimate. In a situation where several organizations attempt to effect innovation, domain consensus prevents volatile competition. In the establishment of the head and neck cancer networks, competition among multiple headquarters for target audiences or special roles in implementing programs could impede the diffusion of the innovation. However, the successful networks seemed to resolve this issue, as we will show. Consensus about the legitimacy of old and newly established domains facilitates diffusion.

Interorganizational versus Interpersonal Channels

Following the resource dependence perspective, we have assumed that patients are the primary resource for which competition or cooperation among medical institutions occurs. Access to patients fulfills differing needs according to the circumstances and nature of the organization. For example, a community hospital needs a large and sufficiently diverse patient pool to attract staff with the medical training to handle the ever-increasing complexity of modern medical care. Simultaneously, patient fees are necessary to support up-to-date treatment facilities demanded by a range of modern treatment strategies. To maintain itself as an adequate medical facility the community hospital must to some degree keep abreast of medical advances.

The assurance of a reliable patient pool fulfills different needs for the tertiary academic medical center. Access to patients who require complex treatment or who have rare diseases attracts high-quality students and faculty. The university medical center can then compete with other universities and research centers for federal and foundation financial support for specialized research programs, which further support the faculty and students. The perpetuation of the tertiary center depends upon those funds to conduct the research that contributes to its distinction as an academic medical research center.

Following this logic, we hypothesize that as long as cancer care, particularly head and neck cancer care, was relevant to the organizational goals of the two kinds of institutions that were targeted participants in the network programs, patient access was the immediate impetus to participate. Exchange relationships were formed in the establishment of a network to diffuse and implement the innovative patient care. The exchanges were set up to redistribute the patients to the mutual benefit of both types of organization.

This model assumes two possible motivations on the part of the tertiary facility. In environments where academic facilities compete for patients with large, well-equipped community hospitals, establishment of referral relationships in which community hospitals treat the common or routine cases and refer the complex ones to the tertiary center creates a larger market to support the more sophisticated services of the tertiary facility. As part of the exchange, the tertiary center may help the community hospital obtain access to experimental drugs or equipment. It may also establish residency and internship programs at these hospitals. In these ways, access to more patients is obtained but, in exchange, the community hospital gets to participate and enrich its own services. In return for the technology to treat some formerly referred cases, the community hospital provides access to patient information for research and refers the most complex and rare cases to the tertiary facility. In such cases, treating cancer patients is part of the agenda for both community and tertiary facilities.

Alternatively, if cancer care is not a significant component of the community hospital's agenda (specifically if treating head and neck cancer patients is not included in the hospital's agenda), then access to these patients will not motivate the hospital to participate in the program. These particular patients are not a resource upon which the organization depends. In such a region, establishment of interorganizational channels will probably not be possible since there will be no basis for their implementation. The hospitals in these environments will have limited treatment facilities, and those that are available will probably not be suitable for treating complex cancer patients. The technical facilities are likely to be concentrated and controlled by one or two academic medical centers, perhaps in conjunction with staff at one or two large community facilities. The innovation may be instituted at these tertiary facilities, but the less well-equipped community hospitals will not be willing to participate in programs designed to promote complex treatment in their hospitals.

The question for the tertiary center in such circumstances then becomes how to increase its access to the patients necessary to implement the innovation if the community hospital with patients has no motive to cooperate in an exchange relationship. The most obvious alternative is for the tertiary facility to establish liaisons with individual, primary care physicians, and to establish an interpersonal network. Detection and preliminary diagnosis within interpersonal networks would occur in the community, and then the patient is referred to the tertiary center for state-of-the-art primary treatment and is eventually returned to the care of the referring physician for follow-up management. The key to these relationships is that the referring physician retains control over the patient, and the tertiary facility delivers only the most complex treatment components. In such settings the community hospital does not have to locate and expend slack resources for new treatment facilities, and the tertiary care center has the patients to support their treatment facilities. Further, the community physician is capable of at least indirectly providing state-of-the-art care.

The differences between interpersonal and interorganizational networks in terms of boundary maintenance and resource allocation are significant. In the latter, the exchange is based on the distribution of patients within an organizational network in exchange for access to resources. In the interpersonal network, the tertiary headquarters facility seeks to attract all eligible patients to the headquarters for primary treatment of the tumor. The innovation is diffused by referral rather than by dispersal of the treatment capability to many centers. The appropriate management strategy is defined by the network headquarters and all resources are located there. In the interorganizational network, information and technology transfer is from headquarters to the community treatment centers, and use of the innovative treatment strategy is encouraged at the community hospital through manipulation of resources that will support the initial implementation.

In environments where interpersonal strategies are employed and the resources are clustered in more than one hospital, there may be competition for referrals. This is likely to be handled by establishing a multihospital headquarters. In environments where interorganizational networks are established, and there is competition, the competition among the tertiary facilities is more likely to be for domain. In such circumstances a multiinstitutional headquarters may be established where each tertiary facility has an established domain.

Resource capacity, the presence of compatible organizational forms, and preexisting linkages are the major environmental characteristics that influence the form of diffusion channels likely to emerge in a given environment. Of these three characteristics, the availability and distribution of technical facilities, skilled personnel, and patients are the factors most likely to influence the form of medical innovation diffusion that can occur and, hence, the type of channel, or network, that will form.

RELATING ENVIRONMENTAL CHARACTERISTICS TO DIFFUSION CHANNEL FORM

We now turn to a consideration of the form of diffusion channel to emerge in each of these seven network demonstration projects and the environmental characteristics of each region (resources, organizational homophily, and preexisting linkages). Both forms of network (interpersonal and interorganizational) emerged as diffusion channels. In the Arkansas and Eastern Great Lakes networks, interpersonal linkages were used to diffuse the innovation. In the Greater Delaware Valley, Wisconsin, Northern California, and Illinois networks, interorganizational channels developed. Mississippi withdrew from the program before any linkages were established. However, it is interesting to look at its characteristics since its objective was to establish interorganizational linkages. We will begin with an examination of the effects of the resource base in the region on the form of channel that emerged.

Resources

If the purpose of a network is to disseminate complex treatment technology, the institutions in the network must have access to at least the minimal level of resources necessary to implement the innovation. Thus, we hypothesize that the availability and distribution of important resources among the receiving organizations will limit the extent of that diffusion. Adoption of treatment innovations will be more readily accomplished among organizations where resources are plentiful than where they are scarce. However, this assumption must be qualified to allow for the demand for resources. Thus, in regions where the resources are scarce or lean, the demand for them by organizations and the distribution of organizations may influence the impact of scarcity on the form of diffusion channel. Moreover, the distribution of resources among the organizations must also be considered. In this section we have defined three types of resources as critical: patients requiring the types of care offered by participating institutions, the availability of qualified medical staff and related professionals and technicians, and sophisticated facilities for delivery of complex treatment. Of these resources, we have argued that patient availability may be most critical. It will be considered first.

Patients as Resources

The patient populations of each network area constitute a very important resource for the development of network projects. Patients in need of sophisticated treatment involving special equipment must be available before health institutions will invest in costly facilities and the staff to operate them. Since utilization of hospital facilities varies by certain demographic characteristics (Andersen and Anderson, 1979), this section will begin with a general cross-network comparison of patient demographics—specifically, age, race, average income and education of the population, and proportion of the population residing in urban areas. Then we will consider variation in the population of head and neck cancer patients by network area.

The median age in the seven network regions varied from 31.2 in the Greater Delaware Valley region to 25.9 in Wisconsin, placing the median age of all seven networks as young adult. Of particular interest is the percentage of the population

Table 4.1. Population Characteristics of Network Areas: Medians and Range (1970)[a]

Network demonstration project	N of counties in network area	Median age (years)	Percentage of population over 65	Percentage of population white	Median education (years)	Median income (dollars)
Arkansas	9	30.5	11.6	90.4	11.5	5,365
		(11.8)[b]	(9.0)	(40.5)	(1.2)	(2,382)
Eastern Great Lakes	9	28.3	10.9	96.7	12.1	8,195
		(6.1)	(3.1)	(9.0)	(0.8)	(3,746)
Greater Delaware Valley	4	31.2	10.4	96.9	12.1	9,744
		(6.5)	(5.5)	(33.1)	(1.5)	(3,855)
Illinois	6	26.5	8.1	95.2	12.2	10,650
		(5.3)	(3.7)	(22.3)	(0.5)	(3,775)
Mississippi	6	24.8	9.2	62.3	11.7	4,547
		(6.2)	(4.7)	(30.1)	(2.5)	(2,060)
Northern California	9	30.0	7.8	91.5	12.5	8,710
		(8.8)	(8.0)	(25.5)	(0.5)	(4,429)
Wisconsin	6	25.3	9.3	98.8	12.2	8,929
		(5.5)	(4.0)	(10.6)	(1.0)	(4,412)

[a]These data were compiled from the data utilized for the individual case studies.
[b]Numbers in parentheses are the range for each measure, based on county-level census data.

over age 65. This is the age group at greatest risk for head and neck cancer. As shown in Table 4.1, Northern California had the smallest percentage (7.8%) in this age range and Arkanasas had the highest (11.6%). In all regions but Mississippi, over 90% of the population was white. However, the range in percent white by county varied considerably across the network demonstration areas, as shown in Table 4.1. The Eastern Great Lakes and Wisconsin network service areas had the least variability. By contrast, the percent white in the Arkansas counties varied by 40%.

Highly educated people tend to use specialized health care facilities more often than those with less education (Andersen and Anderson, 1979). Higher income levels within a service region indicate a broader income base to support implementation of more sophisticated treatment than in areas with lower income levels. Median education varied by 1 year across the seven network service regions from a low of 11.5 years in Arkansas to a high of 12.5 in Northern California. Only Mississippi, besides Arkansas, had a median educational level below 12 years. Median income varied substantially from a high of $10,650 in Illinois to a low of $4547 in Mississippi. Within the regions the greatest range in income level occurred in Wisconsin and Northern California. Populations in Mississippi and Arkansas had the lowest income levels and there was very little internal variation across counties.

Of the seven regions, the populations of Northern California and Illinois were the most urbanized. Arkansas, the Eastern Great Lakes region, and Mississippi were most rural. Wisconsin and Greater Delaware Valley were urban with some very rural counties.

Table 4.2 presents data on the number of hospitals in each network area that participated in data collection during the first year of data entry, the number of head and neck cancer patients registered by each network, and the most common tumor site and stage of diagnosis at each cancer center. These data allow some comparison of the number of participating hospitals in each network, the size of the

Table 4.2. Distribution of Patients within Networks by Site and Stage, First Year of Data Entry[a]

Network demonstration project	N of hospitals contributing patient data	N of head and neck patients	Most common site	Most common stage
Arkansas	14	297	Oral cavity, larynx	I, unstaged
Eastern Great Lakes	9	435	Oral cavity	IV, unstaged
Greater Delaware Valley	8	199	Oral cavity, larynx	I, II
Illinois	13	519	Oral cavity, larynx	III
Mississippi[b]	2	135	Oral cavity	IV
Northern California	76	907	Oral cavity, larynx	"localized"
Wisconsin	12	254	Oral cavity	I, IV

[a]These data were compiled from the data utilized for the individual case studies.
[b]Represents cases seen in 1974, before network funding, by the University of Mississippi Medical Center and Jackson Veterans Administration Center.

patient pool, and the types of head and neck cancers most frequently treated in each network.

The data on patient characteristics are taken from the first project year and for the prefunding year for Mississippi. They indicate that the number of hospitals contributing patient data and the number of patients reported varied considerably among the networks. The Mississippi network reported the fewest patients and obtained data from only two hospitals. Northern California reported the largest number of patients from the largest network.

There is no distinct pattern, however. The Eastern Great Lakes network and the Greater Delaware Valley network had comparable numbers of hospitals but Eastern Great Lakes reported more patients. This is an artifact of the data-collection process. The contracts with these networks required that they register a minimum of 200 patients per year. Eastern Great Lakes reported all head and neck cancer patients registered in all participating hospitals. Greater Delaware Valley followed the contractual prescription and limited registration to 200 patients. The Wisconsin and Illinois networks had similar numbers of participating hospitals (12 and 13, respectively). Yet Illinois reported almost twice as many patients as did Wisconsin. These figures suggest that the supply of head and neck cancer patients was not comparable across the seven regions and that the number of patients reported was not simply a function of the number of data-collecting hospitals in each network.

Within each network there was usually considerable variation in the distribution of patients by hospital. In other words, the number of patients with head and neck cancer was not equal in all participating hospitals in each network service region at the start of the project. In nearly every network, more than half of the reported head and neck cancer patients came from the headquarters institutions. Usually these were two or three major hospitals where the network principal investigator had his practice. Thus, patients as a network resource were concentrated in, or in control of, only a few hospitals in each network.

The data in Table 4.2 indicate that the most common cancer sites for all network patient populations were the larynx and oral cavity. However, the stage at which diagnosis was made in the first year of data collection was variable. Advanced-stage cancers were more likely to have been diagnosed in Eastern Great Lakes, Mississippi, Illinois, and Wisconsin. Early-stage cancers were more likely to have been diagnosed in the Arkansas, Greater Delaware Valley, and Northern California networks.

The high percentage of cancers diagnosed at the late stage in some networks reflects the impact of the tertiary care center as the dominant source of data in those networks. The high percentage of localized tumors in Northern California reflects their strategy of obtaining data from large number of community hospitals in the region. Similar patterns were followed at Arkansas and Greater Delaware Valley. Moreover, all of these hospitals entered the program in the second year, and among the second-year contractors data collection was not as preeminent as it was among the first-year contractors. The high percentage of unstaged cases in the Eastern Great Lakes and Arkansas data sets is consistent with the fact that these data came from physicians' offices and private records. Stage of disease may not be as carefully recorded in physician offices as it is in hospital registries, where the registrar dutifully records this information from pathology reports.

To summarize, patient demographics and the dispersion of patients across these networks suggests several patterns. Three of the network territories (Arkansas, Mississippi, and Eastern Great Lakes) are largely rural and geographically expansive areas with a single, moderate-size metropolitan area where the network headquarters is located. The populations tend to have fairly low socioeconomic status and, in Arkansas and Mississippi, to have limited education. Within these network areas, head and neck cancer patients received their care in one or two tertiary care centers.

The Wisconsin network also covered a large geographic area and was fairly rural. The patient population in Wisconsin was somewhat better educated and had higher average income than in the Arkansas, Mississippi, and Eastern Great Lakes network regions. Within the Wisconsin Head and Neck Demonstration project the patients were concentrated in large tertiary centers, or in one or two large community hospitals or clinics located in various regions of the state. Thus, the patient concentration was somewhat more dispersed than in the Arkansas, Mississippi, and Eastern Great Lakes networks.

Finally, Northern California, Illinois, and the Greater Delaware Valley were primarily urban centers with large metropolitan centers. The populations in these areas were relatively well off socioeconomically. Head and neck cancer patients were primarily in the care of several major treatment facilities, but a relatively high percentage of patients were treated at community hospitals compared with other network centers.

Health Personnel Resources

In addition to an adequate supply of patients, health care delivery systems are dependent upon the level of specially trained health professionals in the region. The successful implementation of complex and sophisticated treatment strategies, such as those suggested by the management guidelines for head and neck cancer that were developed by these networks, requires an adequate number of qualified medical staff, related professionals, and technicians in the region. The availability and concentration of health personnel in the counties of the network regions is thus pertinent to the success of the network programs. Four indices to measure the presence of health professionals will be examined: the number of practicing physicians per thousand population, the number of otolaryngologists per thousand population, the number of radiologists per thousand population, and the number of personnel per hospital (a measure of hospital labor intensity).

Table 4.3 presents the regional averages and standard deviations for these four measures before the network projects began. The standard deviation provides a rough estimate of the distribution of these resources across the counties in each network demonstration region. The larger the standard deviation, the wider the disparity among network counties in the average levels of each resource available; thus, the more concentrated the resource in one or more counties. Small standard deviations would indicate that the network counties have generally comparable resource levels.

Data in Table 4.3 indicate that Northern California, Greater Delaware Valley, and Wisconsin had high physician/population ratios and radiologist/population ratios. Eastern Great Lakes, Mississippi, Arkansas, and Illinois (Chicago SMSA) had lower ratios, although in Chicago the ratio may be influenced by the very large

Table 4.3. Prenetwork Levels of Health Personnel:
Means and Standard Deviations[a]

Network demonstration project	N of physicians per 1000 population[b]		N of otolaryngologists per 1000 population		N of radiologists per 1000 population		N of personnel per hospital	
	$\bar{X}$	SD	$\bar{X}$	SD	$\bar{X}$	SD	$\bar{X}$	SD
Arkansas	1.3	0.51	0.02	0.02	0.06	0.03	430.5	231.5
Eastern Great Lakes	1.0	0.45	0.02	0.02	0.03	0.03	359.6	189.6
Greater Delaware Valley	2.1	0.90	0.03	0.02	0.06	0.04	533.5	152.08
Illinois	1.2	0.46	0.02	0.01	0.04	0.01	609.9	194.03
Mississippi	1.4	0.84	0.03	0.02	0.04	0.02	369.0	189.6
Northern California	2.5	1.25	0.03	0.02	0.08	0.05	533.8	209.0
Wisconsin	1.8	0.98	0.03	0.01	0.08	0.03	548.5	228.8

[a]*Sources:* These data were compiled from the following materials: American Board of Medical Specialists (1972); American Medical Association (1974, 1975); U.S. Bureau of the Census (1976, 1977, 1978).
[b]The rate of physicians to population was calculated using the number of nonfederal physicians.

population in the SMSA when compared with the other network service areas. There were no marked differences among the seven areas in the ratio of otolaryngologists to the population. The absence of differences probably reflects the general scarcity of these specialists nationwide. Average numbers of hospital personnel per hospital were highest in Illinois, the Greater Delaware Valley, Northern California, and Wisconsin, and relatively low in Eastern Great Lakes, Arkansas, and Mississippi.

The standard deviations in Table 4.3 provide a rough indication of the relative levels of concentration or dispersion of health personnel in the counties of each network area. As with the mean values, the standard deviations of the ratios of otolaryngologists and radiologists varied only slightly. On the other hand, the numbers of practicing physicians appears to be most concentrated in some counties of Northern California and Wisconsin (where the ratios are high) and most equally dispersed in the Eastern Great Lakes region, Arkansas, and Illinois (where the ratios are low). The ratio of personnel per hospital varied slightly among the counties of Mississippi and the Eastern Great Lakes (where the supply is scarce) and in the Greater Delaware Valley (where personnel are abundant). This measure varied markedly across the Arkansas and Wisconsin counties. The distribution of hospital personnel in the Illinois region was moderately dispersed, and Northern California's personnel were moderately concentrated.

The availability and concentration of health personnel in the network service regions are difficult environmental factors to summarize because the regions are not comparable on many dimensions that would affect the summary. Data in Table 4.3 and other information gathered for this study show that Northern California, Wisconsin, and the Greater Delaware Valley were all well endowed with health professionals relevant to managing head and neck cancer, while the other areas had poorer ratios of relevant professionals to their populations. These professionals tended to be fairly highly concentrated in the counties where the network head-quarters were situated. This was especially true in the areas served by the California and Wisconsin networks.

Health Facilities as Resources

The final aspect of environmental resources to be considered here is the supply and concentration of hospital treatment facilities in the network regions. The number of hospitals, the hospital beds per thousand population, and the range of hospital facilities all describe the general capabilities of an area to support complex and sophisticated medical treatment strategies. The average levels of these resources for the counties within the network regions before the network projects are presented in Table 4.4. This table also displays the average levels of facility duplication for the network regions. This variable measures the extent to which hospital facilities (as defined by the American Hospital Association) are available in more than one hospital in each network county. The higher the measure, the greater the saturation of individual counties with duplicate hospital facilities.

The most hospitals per county were found in Illinois and in the Greater Delaware Valley and Northern California areas. The fewest hospitals per county were found in Eastern Great Lakes, Arkansas, and Mississippi. Wisconsin was somewhere between these clusters, although the relatively high standard deviation suggests an uneven distribution of hospitals per county. The Arkansas, Eastern Great

Table 4.4. Prenetwork Levels of Health Facilities: Means and Standard Deviations[a]

Network demonstration project	Average N of hospitals per county		Range of facilities[b]		Duplication of facilities[c]		N of beds per 1000 population	
	$\bar{X}$	SD	$\bar{X}$	SD	$\bar{X}$	SD	$\bar{X}$	SD
Arkansas	3.7	3.16	24.4	6.82	0.35	0.23	7.2	2.76
Eastern Great Lakes	5.8	6.03	26.1	10.67	0.49	0.24	5.8	1.62
Greater Delaware Valley	22.7	20.19	40.3	6.53	0.81	0.09	8.2	3.38
Illinois	22.3	37.92	31.7	9.62	0.66	0.18	6.4	4.24
Mississippi	4.5	2.22	21.8	9.17	0.42	0.22	9.1	6.50
Northern California	13.0	8.31	38.2	7.36	0.70	0.18	5.9	2.89
Wisconsin	9.0	9.29	36.0	5.26	0.54	0.24	8.8	2.95

[a]*Sources:* These data were compiled from the follwing materials: American Hospital Association (1973, 1974); U.S. Bureau of the Census (1976, 1977).
[b]The range of facilities is measured in terms of the number of unique facilities offered by the hospitals of the service area. Every hospital reports those facilities it provides, such as postoperative recovery room, intensive care unit, etc. The 1973 and 1974 *American Hospital Association Guide to the Health Care Field* listed a total of 46 facilities. The range of facilities was thus computed by noting each type of facility provided by at least one hospital in the network service area and counting it only once.
[c]The duplication of facilities is measured using the inverse of the ratio of the range of facilities to the total number of facilities (counting all duplications) in the network service area. The closer this measure $\left(1 - \dfrac{\text{range of facilities}}{\text{total \# of facilities}}\right)$ is to 1, the greater the duplication of facilities in the area.

Lakes, and Mississippi areas had relatively low facility ranges when compared with the other networks. These networks also had the lowest values on the index of duplication of facilities, although Wisconsin had a moderate duplication rate. Greater Delaware Valley, Illinois, and Northern California had highest rates of duplication, indicating that most hospitals in the counties served by these networks offered many of the same facilities.

The average number of beds per thousand population did not follow the same pattern as facilities. The most beds per thousand population were in networks with the smallest populations: Mississippi, Wisconsin, Greater Delaware Valley, and Arkansas. In addition to the relatively smaller populations of these areas, many of the hospitals in these areas (of which there were usually only a few) tended to be large state or regional facilities. As such, this indicator probably does not adequately represent overall levels of health facilities.

An examination of the standard deviations displayed in Table 4.4 reveals that the number of hospitals varied most widely by county in Illinois and Greater Delaware Valely. In these regions, then, it is likely that many hospitals were concentrated in one or two counties. Facilities were also concentrated, although less so, in the Eastern Great Lakes, Mississippi, and Arkansas network areas. Facilities were fairly evenly dispersed among counties in the other networks. Beds per thousand also varied across counties in Mississippi and Illinois, and somewhat less so in the Greater Delaware Valley. Duplication of facilities was fairly even in most networks, although the Greater Delaware Valley network showed greatest homogeneity on that index.

To briefly summarize the distribution of health facility resources, Northern California (where resources were fairly evenly dispersed), Illinois, and the Greater Delaware Valley (where resources were more concentrated) enjoyed rich resources. Arkansas, Mississippi, and the Eastern Great Lakes had concentrated, if sparse, facilities, and Wisconsin's sparse resources were dispersed throughout several counties.

Summary

Figure 4.1 provides an overall summary of the discussion of resource distribution in the various network regions. Obviously, no clear pattern can be established given all three types of resources; no one region falls into the same cell on every dimension. But the definition of several types of patterns that seem to differentiate the various network contexts is yet possible.

Northern California is characterized by an abundance of patients, professionals, and facilities. Both its patients and its hospital facilities were dispersed throughout many counties within the region. The region's medical personnel, however, tended to be concentrated in rather specific locations, such as San Francisco, Oakland, San Jose, and Sacramento, generally considered to be highly desirable locations. This situation is indicative of a fairly mobile medical population capable of practicing at several diverse locations and usually requiring a diverse and high-quality range of facilities at each location.

The Wisconsin network had access to limited resources for treatment of head and neck cancer patients. The distinguishing feature of the Wisconsin network was the fact that the network participants were located in six widely dispersed metro-

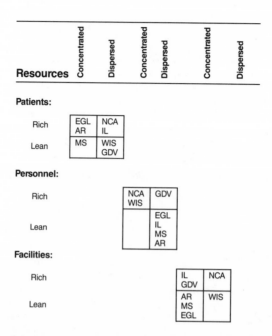

Figure 4.1. Summary of regional resource supply and distribution.

politan areas across the state and thus did not have to compete with each other for resources. The participating institutions had at least adequate facilities to treat head and neck cancer patients following the procedures contained in the guidelines. The region as a whole had an adequate supply of qualified personnel, but more were located in the Madison area (where the University of Wisconsin was located).

Illinois and the Greater Delaware Valley both had dispersed supplies of patients and health professionals (although Illinois had more patients and Greater Delaware Valley had more personnel per capita). Both of these regions also had rich supplies of health facilities distributed among many hospitals in the metropolitan areas they served (Chicago and Philadelphia).

Mississippi, Arkansas, and the Eastern Great Lakes regions represent the final major resource pattern. This pattern is characterized by sparse levels of health personnel and facilities and a relatively large number of head and neck patients (although Mississippi had fewer patients). These three networks served regions that contained predominantly rural populations of low socioeconomic status. Each of these networks covered a large geographic area: all of Arkansas and Mississippi and seven counties in western New York and northwestern Pennsylvania. Each region contained a moderate-size metropolitan area.

In general, we found support for our underlying hypothesis: Network form is dependent upon the regional resource base. Although there is wide variability across networks in their supply and distribution of patients, health personnel, and facilities, two of the three regions that should be characterized as resource-poor developed interpersonal networks: Arkansas and Eastern Great Lakes. The Mississippi network never developed beyond the planning phase. Note, however, that these two interpersonal networks were not lacking in patients; they were lacking in personnel and facilities in local nonheadquarters hospitals to treat patients. This implies that the nonnetwork hospitals were not interested in acquiring a greater number of head and neck cancer patients if expanding the patient base required adding resources to the hospital. This does not mean that our hypothesis concerning the importance of patients is unsupported. To the contrary, the need for patients remains, but, as predicted, it is located in the headquarters institutions and is not an issue for the community hospitals. Apparently, interorganizational networks can take hold without a superabundance of patients, as shown by the Wisconsin network. However, there is a need for an adequate distribution of facilities to support the treatment of patients in these community hospitals, and a wide dispersion of treatment facilities allows each to have an extensive catchment area.

Diversity of Organizational Form

A second major aspect of the networks' environments thought to influence the form of the diffusion channel is the extent and diversity of size and shape of the organizations targeted to participate as network members. Specifically, we hypothesize that interorganizational diffusion channels will develop in those networks composed of organizations that are homophilous on dimensions relevant to the adoption of the innovation. In other words, if target institutions are similar in form, size, goals, or functional specialization to the headquarters institution that is introducing the change into the environment, then direct adoption via interorganizational linkages is most likely to occur. If there is considerable diversity in organizational form (i.e., target hospitals lack needed facilities, certifications, or programs required to implement the innovation), then direct adoption is unlikely to occur, and indirect adoption, via referral to headquarters, is likely to be the pattern. In this case, the diffusion channels will be interpersonal rather than interorganizational.

Table 4.5. Hospital Diversity across Networks (Gibbs-Martin Index/Rank Order)

Network	N of beds	Range of facilities	Percentage with approved cancer program
Arkansas (22 hospitals)	0.69 / 7	0.74 / 7	18 / 7
Eastern Great Lakes (9 hospitals)	0.83 / 3	0.89 / 3	67 / 2
Mississippi (8 hospitals)	0.73 / 6	0.82 / 6	25 / 6
Wisconsin (13 hospitals)	0.86 / 1	0.93 / 1	46 / 5
Northern California (14 hospitals)	0.77 / 5	0.87 / 5	64 / 3
Greater Delaware Valley (9 hospitals)	0.84 / 2	0.92 / 2	78 / 1
Illinois (21 hospitals)	0.81 / 4	0.88 / 4	57 / 4

Diversity in the types of institutions involved in the networks is one way of examining organizational form. Table 4.5 presents the Gibbs-Martin Index of Differentiation (Gibbs and Poston, 1975), along with rank orders for each network on two indicators of diversity of form: hospital size, measured by number of beds, and range of facilities. A third dimension is the degree to which cancer is a program priority for the network hospitals. This is measured by the percentage of network hospitals with approved cancer programs. The Gibbs-Martin index approaches the value of 1 when there is an even distribution of resources across all institutions and 0 when resources are concentrated in a few institutions. Thus, a high value on the index indicates a high degree of similarity among network hospitals, and a low value indicates a high degree of diversity or dissimilarity among the network hospitals.

Network rankings for hospital size and facility mix are, not surprisingly, highly correlated. The most diverse groupings of network hospitals are found in the Mississippi and Arkansas networks, as indicated by their low scores on the index. The two most homogeneous networks are Wisconsin and the Greater Delaware Valley. To some extent, then, our hypothesis concerning the relationship between homophily and form of network is supported since the very diverse networks did not develop organizational diffusion channels and the most homogeneous networks did.

Fairly similar results are found in the proportion of network hospitals with approved cancer programs, our measure of hospital commitment to cancer care in general. We would expect interorganizational linkages to develop in networks where cancer treatment is an active, officially recognized goal of most network members. The smallest percentages of approved cancer programs were found in the Arkansas and Mississippi networks. The network with the largest number of approved cancer programs is Greater Delaware Valley. Northern California and Illinois ranked third and fourth.

An anomaly in these data is the Eastern Great Lakes network, which ranked third on the Gibbs-Martin index for number of beds and range of facilities and second in percentage of hospitals with approved cancer programs. These results indicate a high level of homogeneity among the hospitals in the Eastern Great Lakes network on these important dimensions. Despite this homogeneity, the Eastern Great Lakes network developed along interpersonal lines. The answer to this anomaly lies in the form of the network that developed in the Eastern Great Lakes region. All the hospitals in the network region that were capable of being in the network by virtue of their homophily in structure were components of the headquarters institution because, as described below, the network principal investigator at the SUNYAB component of the Eastern Great Lakes network was chief of otolaryngology at several of the participating hospitals. Thus, it was impossible to differentiate the headquarters from these hospitals for purposes of identifying innovation diffusion channels.

The data in Table 4.5 provide an initial opportunity to examine the diversity across the networks. However, a more complete picture of network diversity can come only from comparisons between headquarters hospitals and the network and nonnetwork hospitals. Our argument is that homophily is a principal factor in the emergence of interorganizational diffusion networks. If this is the case then the issues are these: (1) How similar or dissimilar are the network hospitals to the headquarters? (2) Could the headquarters find a sufficient number of homophilous

Table 4.6. Comparing Headquarters, Network, and Nonnetwork Hospitals

Network	N of personnel ($\bar{X}$)	N of beds ($\bar{X}$)	N of facilities ($\bar{X}$)	Percentage with approved cancer program
Arkansas				
Headquarters (4)	1447	758	25	50
Network affiliates (0)	—	—	—	—
Nonnetwork (26)	325	156	13	8
Eastern Great Lakes				
Headquarters (6)	1490	546	27	86
Network affiliates (0)	—	—	—	—
Nonnetwork (41)	406	250	14	9
Mississippi				
Headquarters (1)	1646	469	35	Yes
Network affiliates (7)	535	247	15	28
Nonnetwork (19)	277	134	10	0
Wisconsin				
Headquarters (1)	1487	626	33	Yes
Network affiliates (10)^a	1106	469	30	40
Nonnetwork (40)	473	253	15	10
Northern California				
Headquarters (4)	1953	570	34	100
Network affiliates (10)	822	317	22	50
Nonnetwork (90)	502	236	17	15
Greater Delaware Valley				
Headquarters (1)	2253	480	35	Yes
Network affiliates (8)	980	403	27	75
Nonnetwork (77)	579	283	17	20
Illinois				
Headquarters (4)	2712	764	35	100
Network affiliates (17)	1280	474	25	41
Nonnetwork (110)	609	305	15	19

^{a}Two hospitals were nonreporting in 1974.

hospitals in the network area to permit direct diffusion? To address these questions we will compare hospital size, facility mix, and percentage of approved cancer programs in the headquarters, in other network hospitals (where relevant), and in other community hospitals in the network region.*

Table 4.6 presents the average number of personnel, beds, and facilities, and the percentage of approved cancer programs for the network headquarters, affiliates, and other nonnetwork hospitals in the region.* A simple "eyeball" com-

---

*The number of hospitals listed here as headquarters and affiliates may differ from previous tables for the Arkansas and Eastern Great Lakes networks. As previously mentioned in the thumbnail sketches in Chapter 2, the Arkansas network was defined as a consortium of four headquarters institutions with a target region of the entire state. Thus, no hospital affiliates were named in the proposal. Similarly, the Eastern Great Lakes network emphasized six headquarters institutions, no organizational members, and a regional target area.

parison of headquarters, affiliates, and other nonnetwork hospitals shows a very consistent pattern. The headquarters institutions are always the largest and most facility-rich institutions in the region. They most frequently have approved cancer programs. Network affiliates tend to be similar to the headquarters, although they are somewhat smaller, with fewer facilities, and less likely to have approved cancer programs. They tend to average about 400 beds, over 750 employees, and about 25 facilities. At least one-third have approved cancer programs. Nonnetwork hospitals tend to average considerably fewer beds and facilities and have fewer approved cancer programs.

Of particular interest in Table 4.6 are the differences in size, range of facilities, and number of approved cancer programs between headquarters and network affiliates found in Wisconsin, Northern California, the Greater Delaware Valley, and Illinois. These differences are much smaller than the differences between the headquarters and the regional hospitals in Eastern Great Lakes, Arkansas, and Mississippi.

The availability of facilities specifically relevant to the treatment of head and neck patients is of particular concern. Eleven relevant facilities were identified and incorporated into each network's thumbnail sketch (see Chapter 2): X-ray, cobalt, and radium therapy facilities; diagnostic and therapeutic radioisotopes; histopathology laboratory facilities; rehabilitation inpatient unit; rehabilitation outpatient unit; social work department; dental services; and speech therapy services. The presence or absence of each facility was ascertained for each hospital in the region, and then each network was ranked according to the percentage of network hospitals with each facility and with an approved cancer program. The result of this ranking confirmed the general pattern described in Table 4.5. As seen in Table 4.7, the higher the percentage in the table cell labeled "network hospitals," the more homogeneous the network hospitals were with the headquarters. The networks that developed interorganizational channels (Greater Delaware Valley, Illinois, Northern California, and Wisconsin) tended to have the highest percentages of these resources available in the network hospitals. Arkansas and Mississippi ranked considerably lower. Eastern Great Lakes had a facility profile similar to that found in the interorganizational networks. As we have noted, however, although the hospitals had the facilities, they had no distinguishable diffusion channels separate from the headquarters; hence, there were no boundary spanners to whom the innovation could be defined and diffused. The hospitals outside the network were incapable of adopting the innovation.

From Tables 4.5, 4.6, and 4.7 a very general sense of the levels of organizational homophily in the interorganizational and interpersonal networks can be ascertained. Clearly, the community hospitals that participated in the interorganizational networks were similar to the headquarters in size, range of facilities, commitment to cancer programs, and access to the resources most central to managing head and neck cancers. The major deviation from that pattern was the Eastern Great Lakes network, but that deviation can be explained by the distribution of personnel within the network and the manner in which the headquarters was defined.

Figure 4.2 shows two patterns of organizational form that roughly correspond to the patterns of distribution of resources observed in the data in the three preceding tables. Outside of the headquarters institutions, the hospitals in the regions

Table 4.7. Comparison of Network and Nonnetwork Hospitals on Availability of Cancer-Care-Related Hospital Facilities

Facilities	Eastern Great Lakes (%)		Arkansas (%)		Greater Delaware Valley (%)		Wisconsin (%)		Northern California (%)		Illinois (%)		Mississippi (%)	
	Network	Other	Network	Other	Network	Other	Network	Other	Network	Other	Network	Other	Network	Other
X-ray therapy	75	23	55	20	89	51	69	38	93	24	86	49	50	27
Cobalt therapy	62	5	50	0	67	18	46	23	57	13	67	16	38	7
Radium therapy	75	18	60	0	89	40	62	33	86	23	86	37	50	13
Diagnostic radio-isotope	88	49	70	20	100	58	92	49	93	67	95	65	75	47
Therapeutic radioisotope	62	15	45	0	89	38	62	33	93	34	90	35	50	13
Histopathology laboratory	100	64	65	40	100	61	100	59	93	78	100	72	63	27
Rehabilitation inpatient unit	38	13	0	0	11	12	38	5	28	11	52	15	0	0
Rehabilitation outpatient unit	25	7	5	0	44	21	38	5	28	17	33	11	0	0
Social work department	88	72	60	20	100	83	85	69	78	67	86	74	75	53
Dental services	75	56	60	50	78	57	62	41	50	50	76	7	25	47
Speech thera-pist services	62	15	15	0	44	38	77	31	43	33	86	7	25	0
Approved cancer program[a]	67	7	18	0	78	20	46	7	64	14	57	19	38	0
N reporting hospitals	8	39	20	10	9	77	13	39	14	90	21	110	8	15
N hospitals[a]	9	43	22	12	9	82	13	42	14	103	21	113	8	19

[a]Percentage of hospitals with approved cancer programs was calculated on the total number of hospitals.

Environmental Characteristics	Network Demonstration Project						
	Interpersonal			Interorganizational			
	Arkansas	Eastern Great Lakes	Mississippi	Wisconsin	Northern California	Greater Delaware Valley	Illinois
Organizational form							
Similar		•		•	•	•	•
Diverse	•		•				
Preexisting linkages							
Density: dense					•	•	•
not dense	•	•	•	•			
Stability: stable			•			•	•
new	•	•		•	•		
Domain consensus: present			•	•		•	•
absent	•	•					•

Figure 4.2. Patterns of organizational form and preexisting linkages.

served by the Arkansas, Eastern Great Lakes, and Mississippi networks tended to be small emergency and acute care facilities with around 300 beds, with limited facilities, and staffed by professionals drawn from a relatively limited range of specialties. These networks were headquartered by one or several large tertiary facilities located in the major metropolitan center of the region. At the headquarters institutions a wide range of treatment and specialized cancer management was available. Thus, the disparity between the headquarters and the other hospitals in the region was great. But, in part, this disparity (at least in Arkansas and the Eastern Great Lakes) was a function of the form of headquarters that was instituted. Because the headquarters were multi-institutional and there was a shortage of hospitals with appropriate facilities and staff in the region, there were no other institutions to which direct diffusion could be directed.

The multi-institutional headquarters format itself resulted from the roles played by the principal investigators in each of these regions. These principal investigators controlled the patients at all the headquarters institutions either directly or through an associate who was directly linked to the headquarters program. Thus, there were no boundary-spanning relationships between headquarters and other eligible institutions that could serve as communication links through which appropriate diffusion channels could be established.

In contrast, the interorganizational channels had service areas that contained a number of large institutions (over 400 beds), which provided a broad range of care and recruited staff from a wide range of specialties relevant to complex cancer management. The headquarters institutions in these areas were uniformly academic medical centers. In Illinois and Northern California they were multi-institutional, reflecting the prevailing cooperative relationship between the medical centers in those regions. Either each of the headquarters had established network relationships with community hospitals based on preexisting programs or they were able to establish these relationships after receiving the network contract. Because these regions contained a broad mixture of teaching centers, community hospitals with teaching affiliations to the medical centers, and small, acute care facilities, it was possible to utilize the ties between the headquarters and the affiliated hospitals for the purpose of implementing a network format for direct diffusion. Since these were institutional relationships that involved interaction between appropriate medical staff at each facility, boundary-spanning roles were in place and could provide the framework for the diffusion channels.

Preexisting Links

The third environmental factor to be considered is the nature and extent of preexisting linkages between the network institutions. The density and stability of those linkages and the extent to which they were perceived as nonthreatening are factors that affect the development of new ties among network institutions. Density refers to how profuse interorganizational linkages were prior to the formation of the network. Extreme density may facilitate the superimposition of new networks upon extant linkages, assuming that the new linkages do not conflict with existing relationships. This is especially likely if these preexisting linkages are highly stable. Stability of linkages refers to how long-lived the linkages are. Successful implementation of a network is likely and stability probable if there is consensus or agreement among the potentially competing organizations that the new linkages do not threaten or encroach upon existing domains of service delivery, expertise, and established referral patterns.

As we noted in Chapter 1, the formation of networks was a signal to all the institutions in the network service area of the intention of one or more of the major educational institutions to expand its influence as a referral center for head and neck cancer. Thus, to institutions that did not participate, the efforts by the headquarters to establish networks could have been perceived as threatening to the stablished referral patterns or preexisting linkages. In Illinois and Northern California this issue was dealt with by inviting all the medical centers to participate as headquarters institutions. Initially in Illinois two of the four medical schools that treated most cancer patients at that time submitted separate applications, although they had communicated with each other prior to the submission. The National Cancer Institute requested that the two organizations merge, which they did under the auspices of the newly established comprehensive cancer center in Illinois. They then invited the other medical schools to participate either as network members or as headquarters units. Two other universities had sufficient interest and participated as headquarters institutions.

In Northern California three medical schools and a college of dentistry had sufficient interest and patients. They also formed their network as part of the consortium that was planning a newly emerging consortial cancer center, similar to that in Illinois. In Wisconsin there was cooperation between the university and the Medical College of Wisconsin, which resulted in participation by hospitals affiliated with the Medical College of Wisconsin as network members. This occurred in lieu of the college's becoming a second headquarters institution. In the Greater Delaware Valley region there was intense competition among the medical schools, and no cooperative relationships were established with other medical schools as part of the head and neck network. Thus, the links that formed the basis for this network were based on preexisting relationships between hospitals that had been affiliated with the headquarters institution for radiation therapy. In the Eastern Great Lakes area the two major cancer treatment programs both submitted proposals and were approved. Like Illinois, they were requested to merge in the second year. They accomplished this merger successfully. In Arkansas the network was formed around a shared radiation therapy facility to which all major treatment centers were contractually bound. There were no competing efforts to establish linkages in the network area. Likewise in Mississippi the formation of a network did not threaten the domain of any competing referral relationships, although, as noted in Chapter 3, Mississippi was the only network to overtly declare an intention to become the tertiary referral center for the region as a network objective.

Thus, in each network area there existed some interorganizational linkages that predated the network program and upon which each network program was established. The nature of these linkages varied considerably. Our analysis of these differences and the patterns of linkage that emerged will focus on three dimensions: density, stability, and consensus. The patterns associated with each dimension are summarized in Figure 4.2. They will be compared to patterns of resource availability, concentration, and organizational diversity to complete our description of the context within which each network program developed.

Preexisting interorganizational linkages outside of the headquarters group were very sparse in the Eastern Great Lakes and Arkansas areas. In both networks the headquarters institutions had linkages with small groups of large hospitals located in the same metropolitan areas. These linkages were based on teaching affiliations, such as residency programs or area health education consortia (AHECS). The network principal investigators usually controlled treatment at these community hospitals through supervision of the procedures or through a direct appointment as chief of the service at the hospital. These institutions were thus functionally part of the headquarters facility and not linked to the headquarters through boundary-spanning relationships. The interorganizational relationships did not provide opportunities for diffusion of new treatment procedures. Outside of these "headquarters extension" institutions, linkages to other hospitals were limited, highly interpersonal, and very unstable. Frequently, the interaction between the headquarters and these community hospitals was limited to continuing education programs offered by the network principal investigator at these hospitals.

This arrangement was most explicit in the Eastern Great Lakes network. The network was constructed around the head and neck programs at two major institutions: The State University of New York at Buffalo (SUNYAB) and Roswell Park Memorial Institute (RPMI). A series of interpersonal ties provided the linkage between the two institutions that permitted the merger. Three individuals were involved in these ties; two held academic and/or staff appointments at both institutions, and the third was a faculty member at SUNYAB and a consultant at RPMI. Aside from these joint appointments, formal relationships between RPMI and local hospitals were virtually nonexistent, although some informal relationships existed and there was some limited referral. When relationships were established they tended to be designed for specific purposes and dependent upon interpersonal ties. Usually these interactions focused on professional and public education, consultation, selective referral for advanced or very rare cancers, or collaborative research with other major cancer treatment centers outside the network area.

In contrast, the clinical programs of SUNYAB were of necessity community-based since the university did not have a teaching hospital, relying instead on long-standing, cooperative relationships with community hospitals. These were contractually established and thus formal. SUNYAB contracted with five public and private community hospitals for its internship and residency programs in head and neck cancer. The chairperson of the department of otolaryngology at SUNYAB was also chief of the head and neck service at each participating hospital.

As we have noted elsewhere in this chapter, the organizational base of the SUNYAB network was sufficient to support an interorganizational network. Within the collaborating institutions, however, individuals crossed institutional boundaries in the routine performance of their tasks, and so there were no boundary-spanning relationships through which diffusion could have taken place. What appeared to be a link between two institutions was actually the activity of a single individual in two organizational settings. Thus, a small core of faculty at SUNYAB provided care for head and neck cancer patients at all the participating institutions.

A similar situation existed in Arkansas, where links between the network headquarters and community hospitals were few and of recent origin. In Arkansas the headquarters consortium had originally been formed to support the development of a community-based radiation therapy facility. The network principal investigator was an otolaryngologist and not a radiation therapist, but either he or his departmental colleagues at the University of Arkansas performed head and neck surgery at most of the hospitals that participated in the radiation therapy consortium. In effect, these institutions also formed a multiunit headquarters.

Outside of this limited consortium of the largest hospitals in Little Rock, the ties between the university and the community hospitals were interpersonal and limited. The principal investigator knew most, if not all, of the otolaryngologists in Arkansas. These acquaintances emerged through his activity in the state otolaryngology association and were strengthened by the fact that he had trained some of them at the university. Others had been with him when he was a resident in another major cancer training program in the region. These acquaintanceships provided a network of interpersonal ties that had been used for referral to the UAMS prior to the implementation of the network demonstration program. These links, however, were not formally established between the UAMS and the other hospitals, as were the SUNYAB links. These were entrepreneurial relationships cultivated for the purpose of stimulating referral, and they had very little to do with institutional affiliations. Functionally, however, they served a similar purpose.

The situation in Mississippi was somewhat different from that in Arkansas and the Eastern Great Lakes. Few preexisting links were present, although network staff at the headquarters in Jackson were involved in patient care at other major facilities in the region in a way that was similar to that described for the Eastern Great Lakes and Arkansas. These sparse links were fairly stable, however, and actually represented interchanges between individuals in boundary-spanning roles. There were links, unrelated to head and neck cancer, that joined the University of Mississippi Medical Center (UMMC) with other institutions in and outside of Jackson. For example, the Department of Pediatrics at UMMC had established neonatal care centers at several network hospitals. A telephone information service based at UMMC provided a link between participants and the university, and staff at UMMC had worked with a variety of community services groups concerned with cancer, usually in conjunction with the Mississippi Division of the American Cancer Society. In general, then, Mississippi represented a program where there was a potential for collaboration through boundary-spanning role relationships.

Yet a third pattern was evident in Wisconsin. As in the Arkansas, Eastern Great Lakes, and Mississippi networks, no preexisting linkages in Wisconsin had been organized specifically for promoting the management of head and neck cancer patients. However, at the time that the NCI was organizing these network demonstration projects, it was also promoting the development of comprehensive cancer centers. The University of Wisconsin was one of the first to be designated a comprehensive cancer center. The Wisconsin Clinical Cancer Center (WCCC) was seeking opportunities to establish ties with community hospitals and the Medical College of Wisconsin as part of their effort to develop a cancer control program, which was required of all comprehensive cancer centers. Thus, initial linkages were formed with the assistance of the cancer control staff at the cancer center. These efforts included approaches to the Medical College of Wisconsin, which had established affiliations with most of the large hospitals in Milwaukee. All the participating institutions had ongoing programs in otolaryngology, and the principal investigator at the University of Wisconsin was well known to most of the otolaryngologists through his activity in the state society. Moreover, he had trained the chiefs of some of these community programs. Thus, there existed boundary-spanning relationships that had their basis in organizations that were homophilous with the university for purposes of diffusion of head and neck treatment.

The University of Wisconsin had strong medical programs and was considered the primary tertiary referral center for Wisconsin. Its designation as a comprehensive cancer center enhanced its legitimacy and further facilitated cooperative relationships. While preexisting organizational linkages specific to head and neck cancer were not present prior to the network effort, the presence of established cancer treatment programs in network hospitals throughout the Wisconsin region indicate that there was a basis for implementing linkages. On the basis of informal interpersonal links, it was possible to identify a group of community-based otolaryngologists who had well-equipped facilities available for managing head and neck patients, and who would be willing to collaborate in a network demonstration program through a regional network.

In northern California a virtual web of relationships between the participating hospitals and the medical centers relevant to the management of head and neck cancer existed prior to the formation of the network demonstration project. These links took many forms. Some were clinical, in which one institution provided services for patients of a neighboring one. Community physicians held clinical appointments at universities, and community hospitals participated in university residency programs. Several hospitals and university centers had been part of a regional cooperative clinical research program, the Western Cancer Study Group, which had just been reorganized as the Northern California Oncology Group (NCOG).

Many of these links were established through foundations that were formed outside of the academic medical centers for the purposes of establishing cooperative research and clinical services. Such cooperation was difficult to achieve organizationally through any single academic center. Other links were newly formed but involved collaboration between several large homophilous academic centers, each of which was a recognized national leader in areas related to oncology. Thus, the possibility for competition was great. Stanford, the University of California at San Francisco, the University of California at Davis, and the University of the Pacific all had affiliations with community hospitals or other forms of outreach. They could easily have competed for more affiliates and used the demonstration project as a way to accomplish this end while at the same time protecting their own domains.

A number of activities in the region forestalled the emergence of a competitive environment. One was the formation of the NCOG. A second related event was the establishment of a corsortium aimed at establishing a comprehensive cancer program for northern California, the Northern California Cancer Program (NCCP). This was headquartered in Palo Alto but was established on neutral territory outside of the Stanford campus. The Northern California Head and Neck Network Demonstration Project followed a strategy similar to that followed in Illinois, and in fact it became the first project of the NCCP. Since the head and neck demonstration project was to be a model of cooperative effort in the region, a neutral, objective third party, the San Francisco Regional Cancer Foundation, was contracted to recruit network participants and organize the program.

A similar pattern was evident in Illinois, although there were some differences. As with the environment in northern California, there were several major medical schools in Chicago and Illinois and each was seeking to establish a major cancer program. In fact, four of these—the University of Illinois, the University of Chicago, Northwestern University, and Rush University—had begun plans to become cancer centers. Eventually, Northwestern and the University of Chicago were funded as specialized cancer centers. In the process it was recognized that none of these centers could meet all the criteria for comprehensiveness without costly duplication of resources. Second, there was a history of cooperation of several sorts. There were well-established referral networks for radiation therapy, surgery, and oncology. There were contractually established community residency programs. Community physicians had clinical appointments at various medical schools. Although the residency programs involved institutional commitments, referral relationships and clinical appointments frequently followed interpersonal ties often based on where the community physician had trained. Of most importance is the fact that all these relationships were well known and accepted by most of the medical community. Through these various ties collaborative research was frequent, and members of various disciplines met regularly in informal clubs to discuss research and new treatment strategies.

Within this context the formation of the Illinois Head and Neck Demonstration Project proceeded in a fashion similar to that of the northern California network. Initially, as we have noted, two contracts were awarded, but because of the preexisting collaborative relationships between the two initial contractors, merger was easily accomplished and the program was opened to other universities. The strategy of forming the network on "neutral" ground facilitated the formation of a comprehensive cancer center, the Illinois Cancer Council (ICC), in the same year that the two contractors merged. The principal investigators requested that the ICC provide the headquarters for the program and assume managerial responsibility. Thus, in Illinois as in Northern California, dense, stable linkages that preexisted formation of the network provided the basis for its formation, and a neutral facility shared by all the participants made collaboration possible.

Dense, stable linkages also characterized the environment in Philadelphia and the surrounding region, which was the site of the Greater Delaware Valley Head and Neck Demonstration Network. However, unlike the preceding programs, the environment in Philadelphia was characterized by competition between the major medical centers there. Thus, each group worked separately to form research and programmatic networks and there was little overlap. For example in Philadelphia the comprehensive cancer center was formed around a cooperative venture between Fox Chase Cancer Center, a free-standing cancer treatment center, and the University of Pennsylvania. Although the grant was awarded jointly, there were in fact two separate programs and little common effort. Hahnemann Medical School, the headquarters for the head and neck program, had no affiliation with the comprehensive cancer center, and none of the participating hospitals were affiliated with that program at that time. Thus, unlike Illinois and northern California, the Greater Delaware Valley did not establish a neutral headquarters in an effort to obtain the cooperation of the other academic medical centers.

Nonetheless, it was formed onto a preexisting research program in radiation oncology. The principal investigator had established this network to standardize radiation therapy dosimetry in the participating hospitals. The boundary-spanning relationships were well established, and it was possible to combine otolaryngologists because of the mutual dependence between radiation therapy and surgery for the management of most head and neck cancer sites at that time. Thus, there were preexisting, dense, and stable linkages within the group that formed the network, but the range was limited to their hospitals. Unlike northern California and Illinois, the Greater Delaware Valley network did not extend to other aspects of oncology or other academic centers in the community.

SUMMARY

The characteristics of the linkages that predated the network program form several distinct patterns that are summarized in Figure 4.2. These patterns vary in linkage density and stability, and in the degree of environmental competition for domain. The patterns of preexisting linkage vary as one moves from left to right across the list of network demonstration projects. The Arkansas and Eastern Great Lakes networks were characterized by an "entrepreneurial" network model: a few unstable, highly interpersonal institutional links based on contracts, but which in effect permitted a small core of actors to deliver services in several institutional settings. Clinical professorships, referral patterns, and other personal–organizational ties common in interorganizational networks were absent in these settings and provided no basis for the type of boundary-spanning role relationships that would facilitate diffusion.

Mississippi and Wisconsin did have substantive interchanges between the headquarters and community hospitals that were based on clinical appointments, referral relationships, and other boundary-spanning relationships. Because there was a single prominent medical center in each network, the issue of domain consensus was not relevant. Mississippi linkages were more stable than those in Wisconsin, although in the latter setting long-standing interpersonal ties among the otolaryngologists facilitated the formation of formal linkages. The linkages were sparse in both locations. Interestingly, in Wisconsin, as in Illinois and Northern

California, the incorporation of the head and neck network as part of a regional effort to establish a comprehensive cancer center was a key feature of the program. Although Roswell Park Memorial Institute was also an early comprehensive cancer center, the head and neck network did not emerge as a central program, nor did the cancer center seek to involve SUNYAB.

In contrast to these four networks, the remaining three networks formed in environments characterized by very dense preexisting linkages and the presence of several major academic medical centers seeking to establish themselves as centers of cancer treatment and patient referral. In each environment efforts to establish a comprehensive cancer center were ongoing as part of the organizational environment. In northern California the linkages between the major competing academic institutions were not long-standing, and in fact there was a history of competition in the region. However, cooperative clinical oncology research had been ongoing in the region and a new cooperative research effort had just been established. Moreover, the major medical schools had agreed to seek a consortial cancer center and had established a headquarters for that activity on neutral ground. So, there was an established pattern of using such neutral bases for collaboration, and this pattern was applied to the implementation of the head and neck network.

Illinois and Greater Delaware Valley established networks on stable, preexisting relationships that existed in environments that can be characterized as densely knit. In the Greater Delaware Valley environment these links were quite narrow and did not extend across the major academic medical institutions. The Greater Delaware Valley network was the only network established in a location where there was a comprehensive cancer center that did not become part of that broader effort. In contrast, Illinois, like northern California, employed the comprehensive cancer center as a neutral headquarters for the network program and was able to attract four of the university medical centers in the region to participate, and with them four networks of community hospitals with boundary-spanning linkages to the headquarters.

Finally, the overall pattern of preexisting linkage in these network environments is not unrelated to the other environmental properties we have examined. Where medical personnel and facilities were scarce and community hospitals were incapable of supporting interorganizational diffusion linkages, the preexisting linkages were very few and unstable. This was the situation in Arkansas and the Eastern Great Lakes region. Further, domain consensus was lacking in these areas. In those regions where resources were more plentiful and fairly well dispersed, and where hospitals were fairly homophilous in form, preexisting linkages were much more prevalent and domain was nonproblematic. Such was the case in Wisconsin, the Greater Delaware Valley, and Illinois, where interorganizational networks developed. Although domain over cancer research and treatment was historically a point of contention in northern California, special efforts were taken to establish cooperative arrangements for the treatment of head and neck cancer, headquartered on neutral ground. As will be seen in the next chapter, the structure of this interorganizational network mirrored those efforts to share domain in the treatment of head and neck cancer patients. Thus, linkage history combined with resource capacity and organizational compatibility to influence the network forms to emerge. In Chapter 5 we will continue our examination of environmental influences on network structures.

5

Network Form, Network Structure, and Boundary Management

INTRODUCTION

In Chapter 4 we addressed our third research question: How did the environment influence the *form* of innovation diffusion network to emerge at each of the seven project sites? Two general network diffusion patterns were evident. The first was an interorganizational pattern in which the diffusion process was initiated directly by dispersing resources to each participating hospital of the network, to enable each to adopt a multidisciplinary treatment strategy. The second pattern was an interpersonal pattern in which diffusion occurred indirectly. Networks whose strategy approximated this model tended to centralize the network resources at the headquarters, and encouraged participating physicians to accept the content of the innovation by referring patients to the headquarters for those aspects of treatment that were not available in their own hospitals. One or the other of these two patterns was more or less approximated by each of the seven network programs.

In this chapter we continue our examination of question 3 by looking at specific structural characteristics of network linkages. We have hypothesized in Chapter 1 that each form of network organization requires a different structural arrangement to accommodate the way in which the network addresses its basic operational problems. For example, within interorganizational networks the structure of linkages between hospitals becomes a crucial boundary management problem. Since network resources are distributed through those links, some care must be taken in deciding what those linkages will look like: What type(s) of interaction forms the content of the linkage, how formalized are those contacts, and how standardized are those contacts throughout the network? Within interpersonal networks, however, other characteristics of network linkages may become more important, such as intensity of contact between network members, and the nature of collegial relationships predating the network projects. In sum, each network interacts with its environment to obtain and manage the resources needed to carry out its central mission, the diffusion of treatment innovation in head and neck cancer. The environment influences network form directly, as seen in Chapter 4, and it also influences network structure, through the linkage patterns adopted by each network in response to environmental constraints.

Our analysis of the relationship between network form and network structure will begin with a discussion of the problem of boundary management. Following an open systems perspective, we argue that all organizations depend on exchanges with the environment for their survival. Those exchanges, however, are often made across institutional boundaries and may require organizations to establish relationships with other organizations. Assuming, then, that resource dependence underlies the establishment of linkages to other organizations, how can such relationships be structured so as to allow for the exchange of resources needed for survival as well as for the maintenance of organizational integrity? On the one hand, there is the need for interdependence among organizations, but on the other hand, there is the need for organizations to maintain separate identities and autonomy, and to be able to respond to disturbances in those relationships that would otherwise threaten the organization's ability to perform.

NETWORK FORM AND BOUNDARY MANAGEMENT

As Scott notes (1987), boundary management by the organization involves both the definition of organizational boundaries and decisions concerning boundary-spanning strategy. Boundary definition involves decisions regarding what (or who) is considered part of the organization, and what is defined as external. It is helpful to think of organizational boundaries as the skin or membrane that surrounds the organization. This skin is of course permeable, since resources must be taken in, and products or services are absorbed back into the environment. Organizations differ, however, in the degree of permeability exhibited by their skins; like people, some organizations are thick-skinned and some are thin-skinned. The degree of permeability is in fact the result of decisions made (either actively by organizational members or passively through historical accident or inertia) about setting oganizational boundaries. Will it be easy or difficult to become a member of this organization? Which is more desirable: tight control over who and what passes through the organization's boundary (i.e., enacting a constrictive or containing boundary) or casting a large net and acquiring many participants (i.e., expanding the organization's boundaries)?

In addition to defining the nature of the organization's boundaries as expansive or constricting, organizations must also decide on strategies for obtaining those needed resources from the environment. These are decisions about boundary spanning. Sometimes, of course, definitional and spanning strategies overlap, are difficult to distinguish, or are made contemporaneously. But for our purposes, we think it is necessary to consider each separately. Although these two types of decisions were not always made deliberately by the network principal investigators or other important actors, they were always made, and they are differentially influenced by environmental constraints. In addition, different combinations of boundary definition and boundary-spanning strategies lead to variations in network structure, as we shall see later in this chapter.

Boundary-spanning strategies include both buffering the organization from disturbing environmental influences and bridging or linking the organization to other organizations. Buffering strategies basically focus on augmenting or adding to internal administrative structures or positions as a means of protecting the organization's core technology or crucial resources from disruptive external events or threats (Pfeffer & Salancik, 1978; Thompson, 1967). For example, when faced with new regulatory requirements, hospitals may respond by adding data-processing personnel in order to extract and manage the data needed to file required reports. Or, legal departments within hospitals may be added or enlarged as a means of coping with more complex regulatory environments.

An alternative buffering strategy would be to augment those more peripheral structures that deal directly with boundary management and interfacing with the environment. In some industries, this might take the form of creating special industry-wide buffer organizations, such as the Tobacco Institute for the cigarette industry, or state "Dairy Boards" in farm states (Dunbar & Wasilewski, 1985; Miles & Cameron, 1982). These types of buffer organizations handle a good deal of public relations activity for their industries and absorb some or most of the "heat" for their industries when public opinion becomes negative, as well as sponsoring and disseminating research in their fields. Within hospitals, governing boards have been recognized as important environmental buffers. Increasing either the size or the community representation of the board has been cited as an effective boundary-spanning strategy (Pfeffer, 1973; Pfeffer & Salancik, 1978). Within the field of cancer research, the American Cancer Society sometimes acts as a "buffer" through its fund-raising and public-interest-building activities. Using these types of buffer organization is, however, potentially more "risky" than augmenting internal administrative structures. Peripheral boundary-spanning units are less amenable to tight control by the organization, and the buffer unit may gain more power than the organization would prefer, becoming quite independent in its actions. The American Cancer Society, for example, is sometimes in competition with the National Cancer Institute for both research funds and control over the direction of cancer research.

Finally, "bridging" strategies represent a completely different approach to boundary spanning since they involve the creation of linkages or dependencies to other organizations, rather than the development of internal structural buffers. External linkages usually imply the loss of some organizational autonomy. For hospitals, bridging strateiges might involve the establishment of external links in at least two different areas. Hospitals could contract with external organizations (whether other hospitals or service agencies) to provide certain clinical services, rather than establishing those services in-house. Radiation therapy services or computerized axial tomographic scanners are two types of clinical services frequently offered on a joint basis by one or more hospitals. Hospitals can also contract for the provision of nonclinical services, such as data-processing, laundry, or other administrative services. Clearly, however, the sharing of clinical services requires a much more active process of organizational linkage than contracting out for laundry services. As part of hospital core technology, clinical services are typically buffered from external influences. Therefore, sharing clinical services constitutes a much greater risk to hospital autonomy. The sharing of administrative services, however, only requires cooperation at the managerial or administrative level (Fennell & Alexander, 1987).

The development of two general diffusion patterns among the head and neck cancer networks essentially represents a choice between buffering and bridging strategies. The interpersonal networks were developed as a means to diffuse management innovations in head and neck cancer, which allowed the headquarters institutions to centralize and maintain control over network resources. Interpersonal innovation diffusion was aimed at encouraging primary health care providers to make a commitment to the innovation by persuading them of the benefits of multidisciplinary care and pretreatment management by a multidisciplinary team. The interpersonal networks were established in environments characterized by lean and/or unevenly distributed resources. Cancer specialists in these areas often treated patients at several hospitals in the headquarters units, and nonheadquarters hospitals saw few if any head and neck cancer patients. These hospitals were unlikely to invest in the resources and staff necessary to manage these kinds of patients. Thus, the rational choice of the headquarters was to buffer; boundary spanning focused on promoting referral of patients into their own facilities, and concentrating use of NCI resources on developing referral networks and augmenting headquarters' facilities and staff.

Interorganizational networks emerged in environments characterized by rich and/or more evenly distributed resources in which several institutions in the network service area had the capability to deliver the innovation. These networks adopted a bridging strategy, through the development of linkages between the headquarters and area hospitals. Network resources were shared with member hospitals in exchange for their commitment to provide state-of-the-art treatment to head and neck patients.

Although the distinction between type of network and type of boundary-spanning strategy may appear to blur considerably, each type of network varied in the definition of its boundaries as either highly permeable or highly constrained. In the case of these networks, the boundary-spanning decisions may have preceded the development of boundary definitions. At the least, spanning strategies were more likely to be clear at the outset, whereas boundary definition strategies were more likely to develop in the process of network planning/development during the first project year.

Once a network was established, boundary definitions differed depending upon the network's approach to solving problems defined as part of its core functions. As we stated above, organizations use boundary definition strategies to manipulate their relationships with the environment, including other organizations and actors. This manipulation is aimed at attaining control over factors likely to influence the organization's performance. Through boundary expansion, the organization tries to improve access to needed resources by absorbing the source of those resources. It may try to secure its markets by establishing captive markets that depend upon it for products or services. For example, manufacturing firms will seek to maintain control over raw materials by purchasing the sources of raw materials. Steel manufacturers buy coal and iron mines, and candy manufacturers seek to control sugar plantations. In the health care industry, hospitals attempt to control patient markets by developing HMOs and other plans that require their clientele to use their services.

Boundary expansion may also be used to combat external resistance to organizational goals through cooptation. Through cooptation an organization's boundaries may be purposively expanded to include groups that are expected to be antagonistic to the organization's objectives. Then the potential opposition is brought into the planning and execution process. It's better to have your enemies inside the tent throwing rocks out, than outside the tent throwing rocks in. Selznick's classic study of the Tennessee Valley Authority (1949) provides an example of cooptation to subdue local resistance to the TVA program among local residents whose land would be flooded by the project. Boundary expansion through cooptation secures environmental support through enlistment of opponents and their indoctrination into the policies and objectives of the organization.

Within the context of this study, interpersonal innovation diffusion was aimed at encouraging local physicians to make a commitment to the innovation by persuading them of the benefits of multidisciplinary care for their head and neck cancer patients. An examination of boundary definition and boundary-spanning strategies in these networks requires a dual-level analysis of both headquarters' strategies (at the organizational level) and network strategy (at the network level). The interpersonal networks were developed essentially as buffering strategies by the *headquarters institutions* to concentrate network resources within their *own* organizational boundaries, and to promote referral by community physicians to headquarters. An appropriate *network-level* boundary definition strategy was to attempt to coopt or bridge to community physicians by offering them membership in the network. In this way the headquarters organization would protect its organizational control over network resources (through buffering), while actually expanding the interpersonal network's boundaries in terms of individual physician members (coopting their support). Moreover, since appropriate patients are usually scarce in such environments, widespread recruitment of many physicians was equally appropriate. Thus, we see a combination of strategies: organizational buffering by the headquarters institutions combined with network bridging to area physicians.

In this type of relationship the nonheadquarters facilities in the environment are weak, and community physicians probably need referral centers if they have not kept abreast of treatment for relatively rare cancers like those of the head and neck. The headquarters then has the problem of motivating physicians and other appropriate health care providers (such as dentists) through educational programs. They must be encouraged to participate in relevant programs to identify patients with suspicious lesions, and to then refer them for treatment. One means of doing this is to make them members of the network and then to reward them for appropriate behavior, often in the form of indirectly granting some of the headquarters' prestige and status through association with it in the network. Since the headquarters seeks resources from these physicians in the form of referrals, the demands made of them as members would be minimal. Hence, network boundaries would be loosely defined with minimal requisites for membership.

Interorganizational networks emerged in richer environments with more evenly distributed resources, where several institutions in the area were capable of delivering the innovation. The headquarters was in a strong position because it had access to resources that would enhance the competitive position of other hospitals in the environment, in return for their participation in the network. When an organization is in a strong position to bargain and controls resources that can be dispersed to enhance the technical core of other organizations in the environment, then network boundaries could be more clearly delineated, and membership criteria more stringent and demanding. The problem of diffusion is to encourage adoption by providing slack resources directly to other organizations in the environment to use to enhance their capability to provide a service—in this case, to treat head and neck cancer patients using state-of-the-art procedures.

Opportunities to participate in the interorganizational networks were in fact limited, owing to the limited resources available in the network programs that could be distributed to participating members. Hospitals that participate therefore may have a competitive advantage over other presumably equally qualified institutions in securing head and neck patients. In creating such a network, boundary definition is oriented toward constraining the size and regulating the form that the network can take. This constraint and regulation ensures that the network does not extend beyond the resources needed to support it, and that only those organizations capable of implementing the innovation are admitted as members. This type of boundary definition is restrictive and designed to control access. Such boundaries restrict entry into the network by raising standards of performance for members, and they impede exit by enhancing rewards for good performance and by appealing to loyalty (Hirschman, 1970). Besides appealing to a sense of loyalty, exclusivity of membership also enhances the value of membership to those who are recruited and invited to participate. If recruiting is selective, entry requirements strict, and membership status highly visible in the community, institutions are more likely to seek membership and are less likely to jeopardize their membership status by failing to perform adequately.

To summarize, all of the networks worked out boundary management strategies both in defining the degree of permeability of their boundaries and in choosing either to buffer the headquarters institutions from external uncertainty or to build bridges to other organizations in their environments. Taken together, these two boundary management decisions give us four alternative strategies, as shown in Figure 5.1. The interpersonal networks chose to develop as buffers for the headquarters institutions, and membership definition could be either very broadly based (the cooptation strategy) or quite restrictive (maintaining a stance of "defensive autonomy"). Interorganizational networks used bridging strategies, with ei-

Boundary Spanning:

	Buffer	Bridge
Expand	Cooptation by Headquarters	Loosely Structured Networks
Constrict	Defensive Autonomy	Formally Structured Networks

Boundary Definition:

Figure 5.1. Boundary management strategies.

ther loosely defined boundaries (a strategy of "loose coupling" among organizations) or more rigid boundaries (the formally structured interorganizational network). As we have discussed, the most likely strategies were those of cooptation within interpersonal networks, and formally structured interorganizational networks. Nonetheless, as we shall see in the remainder of this chapter, each cell is represented by at least one network.

Each of these four boundary management profiles holds implications for the specific structural arrangements developed within the networks. We turn now to an analysis of the various structural forms that emerged in the networks. In describing the structure of these networks we will borrow five different dimensions from several organizational theorists (Aldrich, 1979; Marrett, 1971; Warren, 1967), which have been used previously to characterize the structure of relationships among organizations. These dimensions are used here to characterize the kinds of relationships and the problems faced by each form of network in managing its boundaries and performing its core tasks. They also provide a convenient scheme for elaborating how the constraints imposed by the environment can affect the various patterns of network interaction. Four of these dimensions characterize the individual linkages themselves. These include the degree of formalization of network relations, the intensity of network interaction, the location of decision making within network structures (i.e., centralization or decentralization), and the degree of standardization of network procedures. The fifth dimension characterizes the overall structural patterns of the diffusion networks to emerge (their density, complexity, multiplexity). Finally, we will also examine the shape of the networks after the demonstration projects reached the end of their funding periods, by looking at the structure of more general-purpose linkages, such as the use of shared-service programs, shared-staff programs, and patient transferrals.

BOUNDARY MANAGEMENT AND NETWORK STRUCTURE

Formalization

Formalization of network links refers to the extent to which network relationships are clearly defined and delineated. In practice, formalization can take two forms: It can define the boundary and content of network interactions, and it can define the rights of the participants to network resources and govern the distribution of resources procured by the network. Clearly, formalizing network linkages is one way of restricting network boundaries.

To initially establish a network involving organizational participants, a formal document or contract may be developed to describe the rights, obligations, and rules governing participation in the network. Operating bylaws or a memorandum of understanding usually incorporate these initial agreements into the organizational framework of the network. These documents typically define the planning mechanism, the structure through which plans are implemented, and under what conditions the operating rules can be changed.

The National Cancer Institute required the seven head and neck demonstration projects to develop constitutions and sets of bylaws during their initial planning year. The networks varied, however, in their approaches to network governance.

They differed primarily in three areas: (1) how they defined membership, (2) how comprehensive they made the bylaws, and whether they actually applied to the day-to-day operation of the network, and (3) whether they utilized other contracts to further define rights and responsibilities of various members. Each of these areas represents an opportunity to either expand or constrict network boundaries.

Membership

How membership categories were defined, and how formalized the procedures were for membership application and review differed across the seven networks. Although each network included some mention of membership criteria in its constitution and bylaws, several distinct patterns of membership definition and formalized procedures for application were evident. Table 5.1 summarizes these patterns.

In general, the network's bylaws specified that membership was open to individuals, institutions, or both. The bylaws for the Arkansas and Eastern Great Lakes networks designed both types of membership but actually emphasized only individual membership. These two networks developed primarily along the lines of preexisting interpersonal linkages and, at least initially, were networks of physicians and dentists. The Illinois, Wisconsin, and Greater Delaware Valley networks all emphasized institutional membership and developed as interorganizational networks, using a bridging strategy. The Mississippi and Northern California programs specified both individual and institutional memberships in their bylaws. However, the Northern California network developed primarily as an interorganizational network, whereas Mississippi seemed to be leaning toward a buffering strategy as an interpersonal network.

Table 5.1. Membership Categories and Formalization of Membership Procedures[a]

	Type of membership			
	Individual		Institutional	
Network	Formal	Informal	Formal	Informal
Arkansas		X		
Eastern Great Lakes		X		
Mississippi		X	X (but nonexistent)	
Greater Delaware Valley				X
Illinois			X (among HQ units)	X (within sub-systems)
Northern California	X		X	
Wisconsin			X	

[a]These data were compiled from the data utilized for the individual case studies.

The networks also differed in how formal their procedures were for obtaining membership. The Eastern Great Lakes and Arkansas bylaws on individual membership prescribed that physicians and dentists seeking membership must demonstrate their interest and willingness to participate in network activities. This translated into either a verbal or a simple written expression of interest. Neither network created formal review procedures for the acceptance of new members or the termination of unsatisfactory members. During the implementation years, both of these networks added bylaws allowing membership to be open to nurses, dental hygienists, and other health professionals interested in head and neck cancer. Thus, these two networks clearly adopted a boundary expansion strategy.

The institutional membership criteria established by the Greater Delaware Valley Network were also informal in nature. This network never really developed an actual constitution or set of bylaws: Only an "administrative mechanism" was to govern network activities. Membership was restricted to participants of the preexisting radiation therapy network, and a letter of intent was sufficient to apply for membership. No formal processes were designed to review member contributions, and the principal investigator remarked that the only control mechanism used was "moral persuasion" (personal interview, March 1980).

The Illinois and Wisconsin networks also emphasized institutional membership, but they had formalized procedures for membership application and review. Illinois pursued a methodic plan for enlisting institutional members; the four university centers recruited their own affiliated teaching hospitals or other organizations with which they had less formal ties. Early in this network's history, subcontracts with member hospitals provided for an exchange of network funds for data collection or hiring needed personnel; thus, network membership and responsibilities were clearly formalized for the four university centers. The nets cast by each university center, however, tended to be more broadly based and less formalized.

The Wisconsin network also developed a detailed set of procedures for applicants. Although the founding institutions did not have to apply for membership, all other institutions followed a regular procedure to demonstrate their ability and willingness to comply with the membership criteria. An applicant institution had to submit a formal letter of commitment along with an assessment of its resources and staff available to support network activities, and to provide multidisciplinary care to head and neck cancer patients. An extensive amount of data was required for this application, and review was taken seriously. Full membership amounted to a subcontract with the Wisconsin Clinical Cancer Center (WCCC) and was extended only with a favorable vote by three-quarters of the full membership. Clearly, in this network membership was used as an important boundary-defining mechanism. The granting of membership was intended to be seen as a serious, desirable set of responsibilities that bestowed status on the applicant institution, and the review and voting procedures helped maintain the sense of "group" for all voting members.

Northern California and Mississippi offered individual and institutional membership. Both networks designed fairly formalized application and review processes for institutional members. The principal investigator of the Mississippi network formally invited institutions to apply for membership. Each hospital was to submit a letter of application and designate a specific individual as representative to direct network activities in that organization. Since nothing happened outside of the University of Mississippi Medical Center, however, such a formal invitational process remained moot. In contrast, Northern California institutions actually subcontracted with the network headquarters to obtain network resources.

Mississippi's individual application procedure was quite informal, but this did not result in an expansion of network boundaries. The only participating physicians were clinical staff at the UMMC, and they lost interest in the multidisciplinary clinic during the project's first year. There were no real efforts to recruit members outside of the UMMC staff.

Individual participants in the Northern California network were subject to a fairly formal review process. This network developed two additional membership categories: Participants were categorized as either active or supportive. Active members had to meet fairly rigorous criteria for membership, and a formal review by the steering committee was part of their application process. Supportive members were required only to submit an "expression of intent" to participate in network activities. In a sense, then, the Northern California network used membership definition to cast a broad net (minimal requirements for supportive membership) as well as to define a special, more rigidly specified, inner group of members (active membership).

Network Constitutions and Daily Operation

Another important aspect of formalization of network structure is the degree to which the network's constitution and bylaws were extensive blueprints for the operation and administration of network activities. Moreover, the extent to which the blueprint was actually followed in network operations is equally important. In the discussion to follow we will see that patterns of constitutional specificity and relevance to some extent repeat those concerning the formalization of membership.

Something like a "basic model" of network structure emerges from an examination of all seven networks' constitutions, bylaws, and internal governance mechanisms. This basic model was common to nearly all seven networks, but important deviations can be found in terms of how much detail or complexity was added to the model. The components of this skeletal model included the specification of network directorship or chairperson, an executive or steering committee (with membership and duties defined), an operations and/or data center to administer network activities and coordinate data collection, and several standing committees, such as epidemiology and statistics, rehabilitation, education, and fiscal affairs committes.

The planned structures of the Arkansas and Illinois networks best represent this basic governance model. The Mississippi and Greater Delaware Valley networks exemplify more loosely structured plans, and the Wisconsin, Eastern Great Lakes, and Northern California programs planned more extensively detailed and complex versions of this model. Whether these planned renditions of the basic model were actually followed allows us to estimate the relevance of network blueprints to day-to-day activities.

The constitution and bylaws of the Arkansas network reflected the basic model very closely. A network council was named as the primary governing body, and its membership and duties were fairly clearly defined. Meetings of this council were to be called, as necessary, by the principal investigator. The constitution also specified the organization of an operations and statistical center to oversee network administration, files, and data-collection activities. Standing committees were named in the areas of network cooperation, education, epidemiology and statistics, rehabilitation, and fiscal affairs.

In actuality, however, these governing bodies were infrequently active. The day-to-day operation of the network centered on weekly meetings (during the planning year) of the principal investigator and the project staff. Records indicate that the network council met only twice during the network's entire history, and the committees rarely met, if ever. Decision making and governance were centralized at the project headquarters. Network members constituted the standing committees, but little actual effort was required of them in exchange for network affiliation.

The Illinois network planned a governance structure similar to that of Arkansas, with perhaps slightly more detail. Membership on the executive committee, the network's governing body, was explicitly defined so as to specify the roles of the Illinois Cancer Council (ICC) and the university medical centers in the network's development. A data center and an operations office were called for, and six committees were to be formed in the areas of epidemiology and statistics, education, future planning, cancer detection and control, rehabilitation, and publication. The actual governance of the Illinois network aligned fairly closely with this planned model. The executive committee met frequently and took a strong and influential role in the planning and coordination of the network. Although not all six committees became viable forces in the network, the education, rehabilitation, and data committees were very active, and the overall committee structure was strong.

The Mississippi network planned its internal governance through a memorandum of understanding, which also followed the basic model. Beyond senior offices and a committee structure, however, the organization of this network was not clearly described. The network council was to include the network chairperson and vice-chairperson and representatives of all institutions that had seen a minimum number of head and neck patients in the previous year (actual number never specified). The activities of this body were not described beyond "formulating policy" for the network. Implementation of this rather loose governance structure was even more problematic, owing to the loss of senior officers and the inability of the network to attract and maintain adequate staff to manage the operations and statistical center. Both of these factors were influential in the voluntary termination of this network's contract with the NCI.

The Greater Delaware Valley network deviated the most from the basic governance model in terms of lack of specificity or "blueprint definition." This network did not develop a constitution or sets of bylaws but relied instead upon an administrative mechanism controlled by the principal investigator and the executive director (administrator) of the network. The principal investigator, the coinvestigator, and various hospital representatives were to constitute the board of directors, which was to have some role in policy formulation. The network also planned six committees: an executive committee (function unclear), an audiovisual committee, an education committee, a psychosocial committee, a data committee, and a publication committee.

Actual governance of this network followed procedures that had been previously established (although never documented) for the area's radiation therapy network, led by the same principal investigator and based at the same institutional headquarters as the head and neck cancer network. The board of directors met infrequently, and the principal investigators and the network's data coordinator really made most of the decisions and formulated most network policies. The committees only met informally and did not have much impact on network activities. A small group of individuals who were personally involved in various network programs managed most of the network's day-to-day activities. In general, the Greater Delaware Valley network was rather informally structured and relied a great deal upon preexisting cooperative arrangements among institutions and area professionals involved in the radiation therapy network. The head and neck cancer network's structure remained diffuse and vague since major program activities could be managed within the framework of well-understood, previously accepted cooperative mechanisms. In effect, a diffusion network never developed within this network program; rather, one was borrowed from an older program.

Wisconsin's constitution had all the features of the basic model, plus several additional "options." This network's blueprint was somewhat more extensive and explicit than the four networks we have already discussed. It described the WCCC as the primary contractor with the NCI, and all member institutions were subcontractors with the WCCC. Each member institution was to be represented by its own investigator, who would be responsible for that institution's contractual obligations and activities. The network constitution named the principal investigator as the network chairperson, and the steering committee, composed of the institutional investigators, was to advise the chairperson on policy and planning. Three other standing committees were defined: data evaluation, education, and rehabilitation. The network administrator directed the operations office and was responsible for the organization and coordination of various network activities. The network biostatistician headed the data center and managed all data-related activities.

The actual operation of the Wisconsin network followed its blueprint rather closely. The steering committee met monthly, and meetings were well attended. The other committees met on a less scheduled basis, but still met fairly often. The clarity of membership procedures and obligations allowed this formal structure to function well in the implementation years. Again, this network's structure and functioning represents the ideal typical bridging network, with constrained boundaries. Members were expected to perform and help run the network in exchange for network resources.

The planned structure of the Eastern Great Lakes network also involved a fair degree of elaboration beyond the basic model. Since this network was built upon two separate networks of Roswell Park Memorial Institute (RPMI) and the State University of New York at Buffalo (SUNYAB), the resulting Eastern Great Lakes network contained both preexisting structures and a rather complex governance structure.

The RPMI network was interpersonally based on referral agreements among physicians. There was no formal committee structure or administrative apparatus. The principal investigator of this network maintained total responsibility and control, and RPMI administrative staff handled network administration. The SUNYAB network, however, used a much more elaborate governing structure. Three task forces were formally organized and run by paid staff members. These were the clinical, epidemiology and statistics, and education task forces (much like committees). The principal investigator chaired the clinical task force, which functioned as the policy-making, executive committee of the SUNYAB network. The epidemiology/statistics task force was headed by the network statistician, and a health educator was to be hired to direct the education task force. This elaborate structure was eventually replaced by a simplified plan for the combined networks.

The Eastern Great Lakes memorandum of understanding functioned as the combined network constitution. This memorandum superimposed a unifying structural apparatus on the two separate networks. The two principal investigators alternated in the positions of network chairperson and vice-chairperson. The chairperson was to direct a council that was to function as a policy-developing body. This council was to include representatives of any institution or network that treated at least 20 cases of head and neck cancer in the preceding year, and specific numbers of practitioners in particular fields were to be elected to the council each year by the full membership. The memorandum described four standing committees to cover the areas of network cooperation, education, epidemiology and statistics, and fiscal matters. The administrative office of the network was the operations and statistical center, headed by a director appointed by the network chair.

Although the planned structure of the Eastern Great Lakes network was fairly elaborate and carefully formulated, the actual operation of the network was considerably simpler and much more informal. Neither the steering committee nor the standing committees were very active or effective in shaping network policy or activities. The two principal investigators made most policy decisions, and the staff of the operations/statistical center had responsibility for program implementation. Formal network government played a significant role only in the development of programs in nursing and rehabilitation, for which specialized *ad hoc* committees were established. As in Arkansas, the Eastern Great Lakes network asked little of its members in an attempt to attract as many physicians as possible.

The Northern California network was probably the most complex program, with the most deviations from the "basic model." In fact, the California network structure almost constituted a completely different vehicle. It was built upon a detailed organizational plan, which specified two distinct apparatuses: one for network planning and another for program implementation. This network's blueprint was based primarily on subcontractual arrangements with various organizations to carry out particular tasks. Each undertaking was planned by a network committee together with the contracting organization. Committees were formed for the areas of overall network coordination, epidemiology and evaluation, program planning (with subcommittees on detection, pretreatment, treatment, and rehabiltation), and education (professional and public). Committee membership was planned to reflect the network goals of multidisciplinary, multi-institutional involvement in the network, program decentralization, and geographic representation of the entire region.

The California network was the first project initiated by the Northern California Cancer Program (NCCP). The NCCP guided the network's development and served as the primary contractor with the NCI and with the various subcontracted organizations. Even administration of the network's day-to-day activities was subcontracted out, to the San Francisco Regional Cancer Foundation (SFRCF), which helped in the early planning of the network. During these early days, the committee structure was the major force in policy formation and program preparation. Once planning was completed, the subcontractors took over, implemented network programs, and so became the major foci of activity. The steering committee met periodically during the implementation phase to address network problems, but network documents contained no record of other meetings or any new committee memberships. Since the Northern California network's governance structure took the form of a "flow chart" rather than a blueprint, it is not surprising that it was indeed implemented and adhered to in the various stages of the network's life cycle.

Subcontracts for Resource Exchange

In addition to the specification of membership rules and structural "blueprints," another important indicator of network formalization is the use of contracts to regulate the exchange of network resources, specifically, funds from the NCI. In our discussion of membership and network structure, we have already seen how the use of subcontractual arrangements was important in the organization of several networks. Not surprisingly, only those networks that emphasized institutional membership and a bridging strategy used subcontracts to formalize relations and thus restrict network boundaries. This was evident in the Illinois, Wisconsin, and Northern California networks. The two interpersonal networks, Arkansas and the Eastern Great Lakes, did not use contractual arrangements. The Greater Delaware Valley network also did not use contracts but relied upon the structures of preexisting relationships from the radiation therapy network in that area. These borrowed structures may have served in place of new formal contracts to manage transferring funds for data collection and to ensure the availability of various professionals at each hospital.

In general, both of the interpersonal networks represented fairly centralized structures in which network resources were used primarily to develop and implement programs at the headquarters institutions. Affiliated members were then encouraged to refer head and neck cancer patients to the headquarters for treatment or diagnosis, and to participate in educational programs available at the headquarters institution only. The Eastern Great Lakes network emphasized a modeling approach in which members were invited to learn about management innovations through observing their implementation at the headquarters institutions. The newest procedures developed at RPMI and SUNYAB were in this way transmitted out to the community. Funds were not dispersed throughout the network to help develop similar programs at other locations, so subcontracts were unnecessary. The Arkansas network also chose to centralize available funds in the network headquarters and focused on informing members of the extensive facilities and innovative management techniques available in Little Rock. Network headquarters staff organized educational programs and offered them throughout the state to various professional groups. These programs clearly urged health professionals to refer patients to Little Rock for sophisticated management techniques. This network's attempt to develop multidisciplinary team management outside of Little Rock was fairly limited and not very successful.

The interorganizational networks used two primary types of contractual arrangements to disperse network funds and resources, and thus to constrain network boundaries to specified organizations. The Illinois and Wisconsin networks subcontracted with member institutions to ensure standardized data collection. Funds were provided to member institutions through these contracts to hire necessary data collectors. In the case of Wisconsin, the contract actually delineated all aspects of the relationship between the headquarters and members, including the responsibilities of each institutional representative to attend steering committee meetings, the data-collection activities, and the continued demonstration of the institution's ability to provide multidisciplinary team management of head and neck cancer. Although the Mississippi network indicated plans to establsh contractual arrangements with member institutions for purposes of data collection, the network dissolved before those contracts were finalized.

The Northern California network used the other type of contractual arrangement. Here, subcontracts were awarded to institutions to implement particular network programs. For example, the SFRCF was given a subcontract to provide administrative support for the network. The California Tumor Registry of the State Department of Health received a subcontract to implement program evaluation and manage the network's data system, and the WCCF subcontracted to develop and implement the management guidelines.

Both of these strategies decentralized the use of network funds. Subcontracting with member institutions for data-collection activities, however, did not result in any decentralization of program planning or implementation since the network headquarters still controlled goal setting and program design. Nonetheless, the Northern California strategy of subcontracts awarded on the basis of task specialization did foster a truly decentralized network structure.

The use of subcontracts to regularize and delimit relationships between member institutions and network headquarters generally echoes the patterns of formalization evident in membership application procedures and internal governance mechanisms (Table 5.1). The Illinois, Wisconsin, and Northern California networks tend to rank high in levels of formalization in all three areas of network governance, whereas Arkansas and the Eastern Great Lakes networks were generally less formalized, relying on interpersonal contacts and informal arrangements. The Greater Delaware Valley network seemed to operate very informally, with a rather loosely structured network administration, but it had the advantage of a previously developed, stable, and well-accepted interorganizational network. The Mississippi network exhibited some indications that a formalized structure might have evolved if the program had survived, but boundary management strategies were so unclear at the time of network dissolution that it is very difficult to know.

Intensity of Relations

The intensity or importance of contact between actors or organizations in a network affects a network's stability, and ultimately its success. Intensity theoretically involves both the frequency of interaction between actors and the level of commitment to the relationship (Aldrich, 1979).* Intensity also represents another

---

*In the organizational literature on linkage intensity, the frequency of interaction between organizations and the level of commitment to the relationship are usually assumed to covary, although there have been few direct tests of this assumption (see Galaskiewicz, 1979; Lincoln and McBride, 1985). Social network analyses of interpersonal and interindustry ties, however, have found that these correlations are sometimes negative or nonexistent. Mizruchi and

factor in boundary definition: Networks adopting a boundary expansion strategy are unlikely to develop intense relationships. Boundary constriction through formalized linkages, however, is more likely to result in a network composed of a smaller number of intense relationships. For ties between organizations, commitment would perhaps be measured by the magnitude of resources expended in establishing and maintaining the link; resource commitment is a good indicator of how important the link is and how stable it is likely to be. Similarly, frequently used links are more difficult to break and are thus likely to last longer.

The intensity of relations within the networks, across the networks (network to network), and between the networks and the NCI will all influence the effectiveness of the entire network program. In our examination of intensity of contact within each network, we will consider two important questions: (1) Were important resources of member institutions (such as key personnel) committed to the network for use in implementing network programs? (2) How frequently did intranetwork interaction take place, through either full network meetings or committee meetings?

Interpersonal Networks

Since both the Arkansas and Eastern Great Lakes networks developed as interpersonal networks and did not use contractual arrangements to formalize links within their networks, it is not surprising that the level of resource commitment by network members in these two programs was very low. In Arkansas, individual network members were not required to commit any resources to network programs other than to "demonstrate an interest" in the network's goals and to provide access to patient files. Participating physicians were asked to complete data forms on their patients, but these were so difficult to obtain that the network hired a medical records technician to personally visit physicians' offices and obtain missing forms and follow-up information on all cases.

Network physicians were also encouraged to participate in programs through various committee memberships, but the committees rarely, if ever, met. It was clearly difficult to get members to participate in any way beyond allowing access to data on their patients. But given a boundary expansion strategy where all the network resources remain with the headquarters institution, it would have been inappropriate (and probably ineffective) to pressure physicians into more active, responsible membership roles. The network council convened only twice during the first year, and those attending were the physician members from the Little Rock area. There is no indication that the council met in later years. Full network meetings occurred twice a year, one of which was held each year at the state convention of ear, nose, and throat specialists and was fairly well attended. The nonconvention meetings were not very well attended.

Similarly, membership in the Eastern Great Lakes network was not tied to any type of formal commitment beyond the expression of interest in the problems

---

Koenig (1986), for example, found that increases in the volume of transaction between industries may lead to conflict, rather than consensus. Further, Palmer, Friedland, and Singh (1986) found that tie intensity (the number of redundant board interlocks between two firms) had no effect on the likelihood of tie reconstitution following a disruption or severance in a board interlock.

related to managing patients with cancers of the head and neck. Data entry was not required, although interested professionals were invited to employ the forms and enter cases into the data base. Funding for assistance in data collection was not available, however, and after some initial slight interest, most members did not enter data. Direct involvement in, or support of, other network programs was neither a requirement nor a privilege of membership.

Although the Eastern Great Lakes memorandum of understanding established a fairly elaborate committee structure to provide direction for the network, there was no evidence that the steering committee or any of the standing committees were active or that they met with any regularity. As nearly as can be determined, full network meetings were held following major presentations by outside guest speakers during the fall, winter, and spring. About five of these meetings evidently convened during the implementation years, but no documents report any detail about their accomplishments.

While very low-intensity relationships are characteristic of these interpersonal networks, both networks enjoyed a fairly high level of resource commitment from various *nonmember* community organizations interested in network goals. In Arkansas, for example, the Little Rock Junior League committed both money and volunteers to the establishment and operation of the network dental operatory and screening program. Both Arkansas and the Eastern Great Lakes had the support of local chapters of the American Cancer Society, which provided personnel for educational programs. Another example is the local dentists' and dental hygienists' support of the Eastern Great Lakes network. Dentists affiliated with the network initiated an active program aimed at early detection of oral cancer and at teaching the public the techniques of oral self-examination. Dental hygienists were not members of this network, but they provided crucial support for the program, including endorsement from their professional association. The local dental society also supported the screening program and eventually took it over.

Within the Mississippi network there was a very low level of intensity in relations, which may have contributed to the early failure of this program. Network physicians were clearly unwilling to support or implement the cooperative multidisciplinary team approach. Senior members of this network were unconvinced of the utility of committing resources to outreach and educational programs, which were already supported by other community groups, such as the ACS. Although contracts were to be issued to member hospitals to support data collection, it is not clear whether data were ever really going to be collected in an institution other than the UMC and the Vetedans Administration Center. Some physicians acted as faculty for educational programs and some dentists volunteered to conduct screening programs, but there is no further evidence of any other resource commitment by any other individual or institution. There is no information on frequency of network interaction. According to the principal investigator, this network died from lack of interest.

Interorganizational Networks

The level of resources committed to network projects in the Greater Delaware Valley network seems to have been greater than in the interpersonal networks. However, the real extent of the intensity of member relations is difficult to judge, given the lack of documentation of many of this network's activities and procedures. Clearly, member institutions were committed to multidisciplinary management of head and neck cancer since each member institution adopted weekly head and neck pretreatment planning conferences. Whether these conferences represented an instance of actual resource commitment by the institutions is not clear since data coordinators hired by the network managed these conferences. The network also employed psychosocial professionals to provide services at each member institution. By the end of the funding period, the salaries of many of these professionals had been permanently added to the budgets of the network institutions. The network staff and a small group of highly motivated physicians guided the majority of the network programs. In some instances the motivation of these physicians was personally based, such as the physician whose spouse had cancer of the larynx. Although most of these physicians were on staff at Hahnemann, two key programs were directed by non-Hahnemann physicians, and they represented a fairly significant resource commitment from their institutions.

Since the Greater Delaware Valley network's formal structure was not very relevant to the actual operation of network activities, most interaction was rather informal, and it is also difficult to determine how frequently it took place. The network board of directors met four times during the first year and only infrequently during the implementation years. The special committees met only on an informal basis but probably fairly often. Records of committee membership and meetings indicate that project management was handled primarily by the small group of physicians mentioned earlier. This somewhat moderate level of relational intensity fits a description of this network's boundary management as "bridging in a loosely coupled fashion."

The Illinois Head and Neck Cancer Network developed as a "network of networks." The ICC coordinated cancer-related activities of four of the major university medical centers in Chicago. Linkages between community hospitals across different subnetworks were usually nonexistent, and network linkages between a university and its satellite hospitals were specified by contractual agreement that allocated network funds to individual hospitals for data collection. Commitment of community hospital resources to network activities was negligible, but relations among the ICC and the four university centers were very intense, involving considerable resource commitment and frequent interaction.

The network executive committee, composed primarily of representatives of the ICC and the four universities, was very active in program planning and implementation. The physician coinvestigators, or network coordinators, from each university were members of the executive committee and helped coordinate the institutions within the university's network. Network funds partially paid for the salaries of these physicians, but to a great extent their activities and involvement in network programs represented a substantial resource commitment on the part of their universities.

Members of the executive committee were also frequently members of special activity committees, several of which were very active throughout the network's history. They constitute another important indicator of the intensity of relations between the universities in this network. The development of active rehabilitation teams at three of the four universities further committed hospital resources to network goals, because not all members of these teams were funded through the network. These university teams attempted to organize similar teams in the satellite community hospitals, and members of these satellite teams received no network funds.

In the Northern California network many diverse organizations were involved in the planning and implementation stages; however, of these organizations the NCCP and the SFRCF were the most intensely committed. The most important resource the NCCP contributed to the development of this network was the continued consultation and moral support of its multi-institutional, multidisciplinary board of trustees. To a great extent, the NCCP board made it possible for this network to effectively coordinate such a large geographic area. The major resource the SFRCF committed was the expertise of its staff and their experience in coordinating large regional programs of cancer care. The SFRCF also contributed its neutral identity to coordination of this network, which allowed for cooperative relationships to exist among a large group of potentially competitive organizations.

Resource commitment as an aspect of relation intensity was most characteristic of the planning stage of this network. It was during this stage that the committee structure was most important. Committees were composed of representatives from 35 different organizations. This membership reflected the multidisciplinary, multi-institutional, decentralized, wide geographic focus of the NCCP. The network committees met a total of 26 times during the planning year and devoted more than 1000 hours outside of fomally scheduled meetings. This represents a fairly high level of resource commitment to network relations.

During the implementation stage of this network, the committee structure dissolved and the programs were implemented by specific subcontractors. In some instances, as with the Greater Sacramento Cancer Council and the Bay Area Tumor Institute, the commitment to the network, over and above what was specified in their subcontracts, was substantial. In general, the Northern California network maintained intense relationships with a smaller number of specified members in order to assure performance of its major programs. Again, boundary constriction was used extensively, even though this network was quite large and covered a huge geographic area.

The Wisconsin network was characterized by a generally high level of linkage intensity. Participants subcontracted with the WCCC, and each institution had its own coinvestigator. A committee of the coinvestigators governed the network, and, according to the constitution, each coinvestigator was responsible for group studies, representing his or her institution at meetings of the network, and developing protocol studies at their respective institutions. During the first year of network operation, the coinvestigators met monthly for the purpose of planning the activities of the network. The minutes of these meetings indicate that they were well attended, and if an investigator could not attend, a delegate was usually sent.

As implementation proceeded, it was necessary only for the governing committee to meet quarterly. This central committee continued to govern the overall progress of the network, including data evaluation, professional education, and community outreach. The investigators still interacted with each other regularly because they all participated in specific network programs. Participation in various programs was very active, and meetings were well attended.

A further indication of commitment to the network developed during the second year of data collection. Subcontracts in the Wisconsin network allocated funds to member institutions on the basis of the number of head and neck patients registered. These funds were then used to defray the cost of hiring necessary personnel to collect data. The major problem with joining the network after the initial year of data collection apparently was abstracting data for those past network years. The network budget was not sufficient to fully support this activity, so members joining in later project years had to bear some of this cost. This qualification was a good test of how committed these later joiners were, and it was an effective way to keep network boundaries reasonably rigid.

Another group that provided considerable assistance to the network program was the cancer control staff of the WCCC. A physician with extensive experience in community organization was the chief of the Division of Cancer Control at the WCCC and was able to assist the network in promoting its various outreach programs. Once public and professional education programs had been initiated, they were integrated into the continuing medical education programs at the University of Wisconsin, or into the cancer control programs of the WCCC.

The first column of Table 5.2 summarizes our discussions of linkage intensity for each network. There appears to be a relationship between intensity and network boundary spanning (buffering/interpersonal network versus bridging/interorganizational network) and, looking back at Table 5.1, formalization. Both interpersonal networks, Arkansas and the Easter Great Lakes, were fairly informal in structure and low in linkage intensity. Mississippi was also a low-intensity network. Although the Greater Delaware Valley network was fairly informal in structure, its member relations were fairly intense. Finally, in the organizational networks where structure was formally specified (Illinois, Northern California, Wisconsin), network relationships were all very intense.

If intensity is related to stability and network effectiveness over time, then we might expect the formally structured, interorganizational networks to have an edge over the informal, interpersonal networks. However, the effectiveness of a net-

Table 5.2. Intensity, Decentralization of Decision Making,
and Standardization of Relations

	Intensity (high-medium-low)	Decentralization (high-medium-low)	Standardization (high-medium-low)
Interpersonal networks			
Arkansas	Low	Low	Medium
Eastern Great Lakes	Low	Low	Low
Mississippi	Low	Low	Low
Interorganizational networks			
Greater Delaware Valley	Medium	Medium	Medium high
Illinois	High	High	Medium
Northern California	High	High	Medium high
Wisconsin	High	High	High

work's boundary management strategy depends upon both resources available to start with and how the network defines its mission. Broad diffusion in the interpersonal networks could be achieved only if members were not required to do much in exchange for affiliation with the network. Besides, diffusion for these networks was defined as promoting referral of patients into the network headquarters for treatment, rather than fostering direct adoption of multidisciplinary management by network members. For the former strategy, nonintense linkages made sense; establishing a referral pattern does not require nearly as much investment or commitment, either initially or over time, as would getting community physicians and community hospitals to change their own treatment and management procedures.

Relations with Other Networks and with the NCI

In general, nearly all the network projects reported some degree of interaction with each other. Except for the Mississippi investigator, all network principal investigators attended the national meetings every year, and most reported back to their networks with enthusiasm and some new suggestions for program improvements. The California PI reported that these meetings were only "minimally helpful," but then the Northern California network was the most independent and individualistic of the network projects. They developed their own data-collection forms, management guidelines, and evaluation criteria. The Eastern Great Lakes, Illinois, and Wisconsin networks worked together a great deal on the set of data-collection forms and management guidelines that were at least considered by the other three networks. Further interaction revolved around special symposia held in Little Rock, Wisconsin, and Chicago.

Interaction with the NCI was unanimously considered unsatisfactory. All projects reported that leadership from the NCI was insufficient and unhelpful. As a result, the various network projects developed independently, making comparisons of strategies and outcomes very problematic. Data collection, guideline dissemination, and evaluation criteria were not standard across networks, a situation that might have been avoided if the NCI had provided more direction.

Location of Decision Making

The structure of the decision-making apparatus within each network concerning network objectives and activities constitutes another very important variable of network structure. Typical "bureaucratic" organizations tend to have pyramidal authority structures in which most decisions and authority rights are held by positions at the top of the hierarchy. However, in networks composed of either professionals or professional organizations, such as our head and neck cancer networks, traditional pyramidal structures with centralized decision making would ruffle many feathers and alienate nearly all network members. Relationships within a network that allow for decentralized or at least joint decision making should be more "acceptable," more stable, and presumably more effective.

This traditional view of professionals and decentralized decision making, however, assumes a high level of interest among all network members, and fairly intense linkages. As we have seen so far, that assumption does not hold water for those networks that developed as buffers around the organizational boundaries of the headquarters institutions. These networks cast a broad net for individual members in their areas. These members were not imposed upon unduly in exchange for acceptance of the network's goals. So, one would expect to find decision making on network goals and programs to be fairly well centralized within the headquarters institutions in such networks. Further, we might also expect centralization of decision making to occur wherever resources tend to be centralized, since that sort of structure would then be isomorphic with environmental constraints. In the following section we will examine the extent to which network members were involved in decisions concerning both the definition of network objectives and the implementation of activities.

As with levels of formalization and relationship intensity, decentralization was rather low in both the Arkansas and Eastern Great Lakes networks. In both networks, determining goals was in the hands of the network PIs. A planning committee composed primarily of network staff assisted the Arkansas PI in defining goals, but this committee was mostly involved in program implementation. Network members were not particularly active in determining goals or executing programs.

The same picture of decision making is presented in the Eastern Great Lakes network. Here, the two PIs defined network priorities. Network members did not take an active role in program implementation; they were to observe the practice of the innovation and to be the target of educational programs. Network staff implemented the programs and often involved nonmember institutions, such as the ACS, the Lakes Area Regional Medical Program, and area dental hygienists.

Even though the Mississippi network lasted only one implementation year, there is evidence that network decision making was fairly centralized. The constitution designated a network council to assist the PI in establishing priorities and developing policy, but there is no evidence that the council ever met. Thus, the PI seems to have been the sole policy maker. Program implementation was also very centralized because it was handled completely by the PI's staff.

Goal definition and program implementation seem to have been somewhat less centralized in the Greater Delaware Valley, and member institutions participated to some extent in both tasks. During the planning year, the PI and the coinvestigator met regularly with the network board of directors, which was composed of affiliated institutional representatives. They developed policy and set priorities together. Although less active during the implementation years, the board members represented eight network institutions, and this committee continued to meet frequently during the later years. Network staff and special committees composed of institutional representatives managed the programs. Although the number of those truly actively involved in program management was somewhat small, there was at least some attempt to decentralize decision making and program implementation in the Greater Delaware Valley network.

Decentralization was also evident in the Illinois network, but it did not characterize all network relations. The four universities and the ICC shared decision making and program implementation. Affiliated community hospitals were sometimes represented by at-large members of the executive committee, but the university PIs and coordinators were permanent members of this decision-making body, and the chair rotated between the two network PIs. Similarly, the special committees managed all network programs, and committee membership primarily included staff from the universities. Thus, although shared decision making was institutionalized in this network, not all members were involved in either goal setting or program implementation.

In contrast, both the Northern California and Wisconsin networks were highly decentralized. Each represents a different pattern of decentralization. In California, decision making and program implementation involved many different member institutions and individuals through the vast committee system and the subcontracts. Each of the various committees developed policy for its specific area, and each contracted organization was responsible for following the policy for its particular program.

The Wisconsin network was organized according to a more traditional model than the Northern California network, but it was also highly decentralized. Decision making was shared along general rather than specialized lines. All of the affiliated hospital coinvestigators looked to the network PI for guidance in planning network activities, but these member investigators were still centrally involved in planning and implementing various aspects of their program. The initiative for most of these programs came originally from the network PI or the project staff, but no program was adopted without considerable discussion among, and input from, the affiliated investigators. These individuals identified locations for various educational and outreach projects, defined research questions, and raised queries about subjects affecting their participation, such as the extensiveness of proposed data collection. Following discussion, if the group agreed, the project would be adopted. Although the investigators would most frequently act as advisors and would exercise veto power or influence the direction of a program, on occasion they developed their own interests in certain areas and proposed ideas for network programs.

The general findings concerning the location of decision making are summarized in the second column of Table 5.2. The pattern nearly duplicates that of linkage intensity and is related to formalization of network structure. In general, these structural patterns of network linkage also conform well with patterns of boundary management discussed earlier in this chapter, as well as with patterns of resources availability and concentration. Networks located in rich environments where resources were somewhat dispersed tended to exhibit formalized network structures in which the intranetwork linkages were fairly intense and decision making decentralized (such as in the Greater Delaware Valley, Illinois, Northern California, and Wisconsin). Lean environments with concentrated resources tended to produce interpersonal, informal network structures where linkages were low in intensity and decision making was centralized at network headquarters (Arkansas, Eastern Great Lakes, and Mississippi).

Standardization of Procedures

A fourth dimension characterizing network relations is the extent to which program procedures were standardized. Standardization of procedures helps ensure predictability in network activity and the pursuit of network goals, and to some extent, standardization encourages stability in network interactions. In terms of boundary management, a minimal level of standardization could actually fit either boundary expansion or boundary constriction strategies. Network members probably prefer to think that they are being treated at least as well as all other members, whether they are in large, informal networks or smaller, more formally structured networks. However, beyond this threshold level of standardization, we would expect more standardized procedures to be evident where exchanges are more frequent and intense.

A common goal of all the networks was to transmit new information and technology concerning the treatment of head and neck cancer. Standardized communication procedures would help ensure that the innovation was successfully diffused, and activities surrounding the dissemination process formed the basis for most network transactions. To determine standardization of network activity, we will examine (1) to what extent the network required its members to use standardized treatment protocols, and (2) to what extent the network required its members to use a uniform data protocol. Data forms are of particular importance since their uniform use would allow for the evaluation of innovative treatment interventions.

Physicians in the Arkansas network were not required to use either standard treatment interventions or uniform data forms. Treatment innovations were practiced at the University of Arkansas for Medical Sciences (UAMS), and all physicians were encouraged to refer their head and neck patients to the UAMS clinic for evaluation and treatment. Network members were required to provide access to records of their cancer patients for data-collection purposes, but the network data coordinator actually completed the data forms. This coordinator found it necessary to visit each physician's office to complete and retrieve data forms. Since a standard form was used throughout the network (if not by the members themselves), the Arkansas network did employ at least one standardized transmission procedure.

In both the Eastern Great Lakes and Mississippi networks, the level of standardization was quite low. Standardized treatment interventions were evident only at the headquarters institutions (SUNYAB and RPMI in the Eastern Great Lakes; UMMC in Mississippi). The Eastern Great Lakes network members were "invited" to submit case materials for data-collection purposes but were not required to use standard data protocols. In Mississippi, the UMMC multidisciplinary clinic was the only example of standardized innovative treatment, and it was to serve as a model for other network institutions. The failure of uniform data protocols was tied to the clinic's failure. Participating physicians in each network affiliate were to complete registration forms for the data base in consultation with multidisciplinary teams that were to be modeled after the UMMC clinic. Since the clinic failed, the teams were never formed; and data collection throughout the network was never achieved.

A much higher level of standardization seems to have developed in the Greater Delaware Valley network. Hard evidence of these procedures was unfortunately not available. During the planning year, this network adopted a fairly specific and complex diagnosis and treatment protocol designed at Pennsylvania Hospital. All member institutions reportedly adopted this protocol. This network also emphasized the development of formal multidisciplinary treatment planning conferences at every network institution, and these conferences ensured compliance with the Pennsylvania protocol. There is no way to assess the actual process of these multidisciplinary conferences or their impact on case management. A standardized data protocol was also used by all network members, and each member institution hired a data coordinator to ensure standardized collection. These efforts were not entirely successful, and neither data collection/management nor impact evaluation was a very high priority of this network. It is clear, however, that the utility of the data base for the evaluation of network impact was problematic, owing to inconsistent staging techniques used by some network members.

Standardization was moderate in both the Illinois and Northern California networks, and the patterns of procedural standardization were similar in the two networks. Each network developed an extensive data system based on a uniform data protocol used by all member institutions. In Illinois, employment of the data protocol constituted the major contractual obligation for member hospitals. In California, 76 hospitals adopted standard data forms during the implementation years. These hospitals represented nearly all of the institutions reported by the AHA in each of five northern California counties and the Sacramento area in 1978. Data-collection procedures and quality control measures were explicit and extensive, but neither of these two networks required members to adopt a specific set of standardized treatment interventions. Rather, each chose fairly informal, collegial processes of innovation transmission to encourage the implementation of optimal management techniques.

The PIs of the Illinois network had been involved in writing the national patient management guidelines. They attempted to standardize adoption of, and compliance to, the guidelines through the use of the data forms. Since the physicians were not involved in completing the forms, though, standard adoption was not successful. Transmission of innovative treatment strategies also occurred through frequent interaction among the PIs and coinvestigators, and through the use of the many informal ties between physicians that were already in place before the establishment of the network.

In Northern California, a contract was awarded to the WCCF to disseminate this network's set of management guidelines. The WCCF designed a series of intensive seminars on head and neck cancer management, which in general were poorly received. Their failure was attributed to the fact that they were not integrated into a larger program or activity in the community. No other method for demonstration of the guidelines was developed.

In addition to resistance to the seminars, the concept of guidelines proved to be anathema to many physicians, including those network members who participated in their development. By specifying the action a physician should take in the treatment process, guidelines and other standardized treatment protocols prevented physicians from exercising their own judgment. Thus, guidelines were perceived as an insult to professional autonomy.

On another front, the Northern California network did manage to foster a fairly uniform consideration of pretreatment planning through the development of multidisciplinary pretreatment planning conferences. These conferences were implemented in four areas of Northern California where no such arrangements previously existed. The patient management guidelines were the basis upon which the conferences were structured. To obtain network support (funding for an administrative assistant or coordinator), these pretreatment planning conferences had to meet fairly extensive requirements to guarantee that the conferences would be multidisciplinary, multi-institutional, regularly scheduled, and carefully documented. Where a community head and neck committee did not already exist, the SFRCF staff would identify and recruit interested individuals and institutions. Each committee was responsible for the organization and implementation of its particular pretreatment conference and would make decisions concerning the specific procedures or protocols to adopt and where the conferences were to be held. The conferences were therefore not completely standardized in content.

Standardization of both treatment intervention and data protocols was high in the Wisconsin network. In fact, each activity helped reinforce the other. The Wisconsin network required potential members to demonstrate their ability and willingness to provide treatment as specified in the patient management guidelines. Furthermore, data collection using a standard form constituted the basis of contracts between network headquarters and member institutions. The use of a standard data-collection form served to institute standard procedures for planning and implementing the management strategies for head and neck cancer patients. As part of data management, the treatment procedures each participant used were monitored by use of the forms filed with the data base. The review committee conducted this surveillance and noted instances where the treatment procedures deviated from the guidelines. These deviations were usually discussed with the treating physician. Reportedly, most deviations resulted from patient refusal to accept the recommended treatment plan or from situations where the patient's overall health status contraindicated the standard treatment.

Our findings on procedural standardization are summarized in the third column of Table 5.2. As we have suggested, standardization is to some extent dependent upon both the resource context and the boundary management strategy underlying each network. Specifically, the availability of resources and the strength of the relationship linking headquarters to member units affect the degree to which network procedures for innovation diffusion can be standardized. For example, the Mississippi, Arkansas, and Eastern Great Lakes networks were all located in fairly lean environments where substantial differences in organizational form existed between headquarters and affiliated institutions. In addition, cooptation of physician members was the predominant boundary management strategy. These networks all exhibited fairly low levels of procedural standardization, since network members did not all possess the organizational structures or resources needed to allow uniform transmission of the innovation. Further, the strategy of attracting as many physician members as possible was incompatible with expectations that these coopted members would be willing to individually adopt treatment protocols and fill out data forms. The strength of the network tie between headquarters and physician member was just not sufficiently important to the physician to warrant the effort needed to use either protocols or data forms.

Standardization was moderately high in the Illinois and Northern California networks. Here, resources were in good supply, but network institutions were not all compatible in structure. Both of these networks were located in areas where various prestigious university centers competed for prominence in cancer treatment. In order to establish harmonious, cooperative linkages, allowances for differences in domain and the existence of previous linkages or spheres of influence had to be made. Thus, standardization could not be overwhelmingly high. It was higher than in the interpersonal networks, though, since the bridges built to member hospitals involved the commitment of resources from the headquarters to the affiliate. The resulting obligation thus decreased the tendency to dismiss standard data forms and protocols as "too much bother."

Standardization was a viable strategy in Wisconsin and the Greater Delaware Valley for different contextual reasons. Both areas enjoyed moderate levels of resources. The Greater Delaware Valley network was built upon an extant network structure where cooperation, exchange, and collaboration were already highly developed. With the groundwork in place, a new set of treatment strategies and data forms could be easily adapted and standardized to fit the preexisting network structure. Wisconsin did not enjoy the advantages of a preexisting network structure, but membership criteria (rigid boundaries) ensured that only institutions with at least the minimum level of needed resources and facilities could participate. Further, the rights and obligations of membership clearly set up network membership as desirable, prestigious, and remunerative. If you wanted to be part of the club, you have to pay the dues, and for the Wisconsin club the dues were standardized protocols and data forms.

Characteristics of New Linkages Specific to Head and Neck Cancer

The last dimension of network relations that we will consider is the overall shape or structure of the linkages forming the head and neck cancer networks. Here we will examine the structure of linkages in place at the end of the project period specific to the delivery of head and neck cancer treatment. In the final section of this chapter we will describe the structure of more general-purpose health delivery linkages to remain after the project funding period. Our analysis of ongoing head and neck cancer treatment linkages is primarily qualitative, whereas survey data on general-purpose linkages among network hospitals allows us to attempt a more technical social network analysis of those linkages. For both types of linkage structures we will investigate the influence of environmental characteristics, and correspondence with boundary management strategies.

By the end of the funding period it was possible to construct network diagrams of the structure of head-and-neck-cancer-related linkages for each of the surviving six networks. Three variables of structure were used to construct these diagrams: linkage density, complexity, and multiplexity. Density has already been discussed with regard to preexisting organizational linkages. Complexity refers to the level of stratification or hierarchy present in the relationships among a set of organizations. A complex or hierarchical system is one in which a small subset of dominant organizations can be identified, and each organization has its own subsystem of affiliates. In complex, hierarchical systems there is typically little interaction between units in different subsystems, and what cross-subsystem interaction there is occurs between the dominant organizations.

Multiplexity refers to the context of network linkages. Multiplex linkages between organizations contain more than one type or level of transaction (Gluckman, 1955) and are likely to be more stable than single-focus links. Figure 5.2 summarizes these three dimensions of each network's head and neck cancer linkages for the six surviving networks. Thus, each diagram represents the shape of the network's structure at the end of the implementation period.*

Arkansas was primarily a network of interpersonal linkages centered around the

---

*These diagrams are only symbolic representations of the six network structures; they do not accurately represent the total number of network members. For example, the total of individual members in the Arkansas network by the end of the project period numbered over 100.

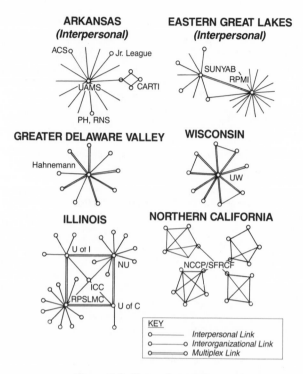

Figure 5.2. Network structures.

principal investigator and other senior staff at the UAMS. A small interorganizational network for radiation therapy, the Central Arkansas Radiation Therapy Institute (CARTI), was associated with the Little Rock nexus of head and neck specialists. During its implementation years, the Arkansas staff focused on establishing relationships with physicians throughout the state who saw head and neck patients. Through patient referrals, these individuals would then have access to all of the specialized facilities and staff in Little Rock that provided multidisciplinary care. Membership grew to 50 members, and links were also established with various community agencies, such as the ACS, the Junior League, and the public health nurses. Linkages were of medium density and were primarily single focus. Individual members provided access to patient data and periodically participated in educational programs. The community agencies typically provided support for one specific network project. The general structure of the Arkansas network was unstratified.

The Eastern Great Lakes network was also primarily interpersonal in nature, although there were ties linking SUNYAB and RPMI, and SUNYAB was linked to a multi-institutional consortium. The primary linkages of this network connected individual physicians to the programs and facilities of these two tertiary institutions. As with the Arkansas network, this network added many individuals as members and established relationships with several community agencies during the implementation years. Typically, the linkages that emerged between the Eastern Great Lakes network and other organizations were highly specific, usually single-stranded, and often formed for a specified duration of time. The aim was for the community organizations to assume responsibility for the program after it had been developed and implemented with network support. This network was similar to the Arkansas network in that it was minimally complex and medium in density, and had uniplex linkages.

Both the Greater Delaware Valley and Wisconsin networks developed simple, nonhierarchical networks of medium density joining organizations to network headquarters with fairly strong, multiplex links. As we have seen, the Greater Delaware Valley network developed along well-established preexisting links. Multiplexity was the result of superimposing head and neck cancer network exchanges on preexisting linkages for radiation therapy. In Wisconsin, however, multiplexity was the result of the careful cultivation of linkages through contractual obligations that operated on several levels: data collection, program involvement, and personal interaction. The Wisconsin network was also somewhat more dense that the Greater Delaware Valley network, owing to the existence of direct ties between some of the affiliated hospitals.

The relationships that developed in Illinois and Northern California were the most complex of any of the network projects, but the nature of their complexity was very different. The Illinois Head and Neck Cancer Network developed as a hierarchical "network of networks." Fairly strong, multiplex links connected the four university centers and the ICC, and each university had ties with satellite hospitals. Linkages within these subsystems were fairly dense and sometimes of multiple focus. Linkages between subsystems were infrequent and usually via the university centers.

The California network was also complex but not in the hierarchical manner as in Illinois. There were strongly dominant organizations involved in management of the network, as with Illinois. Unlike the Illinois universities, though, they were not intermediaries in relationships between community hospitals and the headquarters. Instead, community hospitals related directly to the NCCP. The NCCP and SFRCF provided neutral, decentralized coordination. Stratification of the network took the form of task specialization and geographic differentation. Task areas were delegated to different groups of organizations, usually one task to a geographic locale. Thus, the linkages that developed were not very dense over all the network, but density and multiplexity were fairly common within separate regions. The key organizing concept of this network was the integrated service area. This plan fostered the development of strong, cooperative links between institutions in specific regions and encouraged task specialization so as to minimize domain conflict and squabbling over claims to expertise.

These dimensions of network structure, as represented by the diagrams in Figure 5.2, can be related to characteristics of network context or environment. The fairly simple interpersonal networks based on single-purpose links developed in fairly lean environments with diverse organizational forms. Of particular importance in both areas was the lack of similarity between headquarters and member institutions. These networks developed as centralized structures where network programs were concentrated at the headquarters, and network participants were defined as passive targets to be "coopted" for information diffusion.

The "wheel" structures of multiplex organizational links characteristic of the Wisconsin and Greater Delaware Valley networks developed in environments with medium levels of necessary resources and fairly homogenous organizations. Both of these networks exhibited a minimum level of complexity and a maximum of member involvement. Homogeneity of organizational form in these environments allowed institutional members to directly adopt programs initiated by the headquarters.

Finally, the complex, hierarchical structures developed by the Illinois and California networks were partly a response to the rather rich, complex environments in which both networks were located. Although many organizations in both networks were homogenous in form, there were several factors that seem to have influenced the development of these networks into stratified systems with few linkages between subsystems and many linkages within subsystems. In Illinois, preexisting linkages were fairly dense and stable, and these relationships were characterized by domain consensus. Dominant actors in this setting were easily identifiable. It made sense to structure a network that emphasized strong, cooperative, multiplex linkages between the dominant university centers that controlled subsystems of affiliated hospitals so that each university's domain was unthreatened. In California, however, preexisting linkages were fairly unstable and lacked domain consensus. Thus, the structure of this network allowed specific domains or spheres of influence to develop by emphasizing task specialization and geographic stratification. Rich supplies of resources and many organizations capable of using them could potentially lead to high levels of competition. Northern California's particular form of complexity prevented this occurrence.

At this point we can return to the typology of boundary management strategies presented in Figure 5.1 and attach specific networks to each of the four cells, as presented in Figure 5.3.

Clearly, the interpersonal networks of Arkansas and the Eastern Great Lakes mixed buffering of the headquarters unit with an emphasis on expansion of interpersonal network boundaries. In each network, physicians throughout the region were recruited as members, persuaded to refer their head and neck patients to the headquarters institution for treatment, and rewarded with access to educational programs, association with the university center, and awareness of state-of-the-art management for these patients. The Mississippi network would probably have followed this pattern, but lack of interest and a failure to convince physicians of the benefits of either network association or multidisciplinary management as practiced at UMMC resulted in a buffering strategy with constricted boundaries.

Bridging was used by the remaining four networks, but some opted for expan-

Boundary Spanning:

		Buffer	Bridge
	Expand	*Cooptation* Arkansas E. Great Lakes	*Loose Coupling* Greater Dela. Valley Illinois (among satellite hospitals)
Boundary Definition:	Constrict	*Def. Autonomy* Mississippi	*Formal Networks* N. California Wisconsin Illinois (among university centers)

Figure 5.3. Boundary management in the networks.

sive network boundaries and others for constricted boundaries. Illinois did a little of both; boundary management between the headquarters institutions and the ICC was very tight, formally specified, and intense, whereas within each university's subsystem of affiliated hospitals, the strategy was more open, less rigid, and somewhat less formal. The Greater Delaware Valley adopted a truly "loosely coupled," expansive boundary strategy that relied upon the old network structure for radiation therapy.

Finally, the Wisconsin network typified the strategy of constricted boundaries surrounding a network of formal, interorganizational linkages, centering on the university headquarters institution. Northern California also followed this pattern in general, but with more task specialization and decentralization throughout its broad geographic region.

GENERAL PURPOSE LINKAGES: ANALYSIS OF THE RELATIONSHIP BETWEEN CONTEXT AND LINKAGE STRUCTURE

About one year after the end of the funding period for the second set of network projects, questionnaires were sent to the chief executive officer of each hospital or clinic that had been mentioned in the original proposals to the NCI by the principal investigators of each of the six surviving networks. Information was obtained in these questionnaires on three types of relations among these "network" organizations: involvement in shared service arrangements, the extension of medical staff privileges to medical staff of other hospitals, and patient transfers between hospitals (a copy of the questionnaire can be found in Appendix C). It is important to emphasize that these linkages were in no way directly tied to head and neck cancer network programs, and the CEOs were not questioned about the cancer network programs or activities. Our intent here was to capture information on patterns of general cooperative linkage that may exist among the sets of hospitals originally targeted for involvement in the cancer network programs. Thus, hospital CEOs were surveyed about their hospital's cooperative programs, whether or not the hospital was an actual participant in one of the four interorganizational networks or merely functioned as context for the two interpersonal networks. As described in Chapter 2, the CEOs were given a list of the targeted network hospitals in their region, with which they were to indicate whether the hospital shared services, extended staff privileges, or transferred patients. In addition, additional lines were provided to list names of other hospital exchange partners.

Using these three types of general-purpose linkages among the targeted organizations, we again examined network density and complexity. In addition, we also examined a third aspect of general network structure, one that is perhaps not as easily defined as either density or complexity. We were interested in the extent to which the head and neck cancer programs as action sets (temporary alliances set up around a specific purpose) overlapped with, or developed into, more general-purpose, ongoing network linkages, or whether members of these organizational action sets were more likely to develop long-term linkages with other organizations outside of the action set. The former strategy can be termed *internal viability*, which would be used to describe an action set that is less likely to simply disappear at the end of the federal funding period.

With the use of survey data, density was quantitatively measured as the ratio of the number of linkages observed between organizations to the maximum number possible $(3(N(N-1)))$. Internal viability was measured as the ratio of the number of internal linkages to total linkages indicated, counting linkages to both network and nonnetwork institutions. Thus, this measure indicates the relative frequency of relations outside the action set. It varies from zero to one, equaling zero when no linkages are internal, and one when all linkages are internal.

Our analysis of complexity of general-purpose linkages relies upon block-modeling techniques to uncover underlying network structure. Blockmodeling can be used to identify "structurally equivalent sets" or blocks of actors (Mullins *et al.*, 1977), and to determine the relationships between such blocks. Blocks consist of subgroups of network actors who relate to each other similarly, and who all relate in similar ways to other blocks of actors. Complex networks would be indicated by existence of multiple blocks (or subsystems) that can be ordered or interrelated through different organizing relationships or principles. For example, within networks of hospitals, subsets of hospitals may interact through the transfer of specific, hard-to-treat patients; other subgroups may share administrative functions or laundry services or jointly operate a radiation therapy center; still other groups may share the same group of cancer specialists on staff. Thus, multiple blocks may be identified, and the organizing principles linking blocks to other blocks could follow several different lines: sharing administrative functions, clinical services, production staff, or patient groupings. A structurally simple network would produce only one or two blocks linked to each other along a single dimension.*

We converted our survey data on the three types of hospital linkage into sociomatrices, which are then "stacked" or combined (see Light and Mullins, 1979). Blocks are then identified through a principal components analysis on the stacked data. The advantage of this combined analysis is that the patterns of interaction uncovered more fully represent actual network behavior, since network actors are likely to interact along a number of dimensions within any given time period.

The sociomatrices are partitioned into "image matrices," which allow us to examine interaction patterns among blocks of actors on each of the three types of linkage, shared service arrangements, extension of staff privileges, and patient transfers. The blocking scheme is established by examining all three forms of interaction simultaneously. The disaggregation into image matrices based on the combined linkages, but reflecting each of the three forms of interaction separately, allows more detailed analysis of the actual patterns of network relation.

The image matrices for the six networks are presented in Table 5.3. Matrices composed of all 1's are referred to as "full rank" matrices, indicating that interaction on that dimension occurs throughout the matrix. For example, from Table 5.3, the image matrix on patient transfers within the Eastern Great Lakes network is of full rank. Two blocks of actors were identified in this network, and patient transfers link both blocks. Further, both shared service arrangements and staff privilege

*For more information on blockmodeling techniques, see work by Arabie *et al.* (1978), Bonacich and McConaghy (1979), Boorman and White (1976), Light and Mullins (1979), Mullins *et al.* (1977), and White *et al.* (1976). The more technical aspects of this analysis can be found in Fennell *et al.* (1987). What follows is a fairly nontechnical description of results.

Table 5.3. Image Matrices for Six Surviving Networks

			A Shared service arrangements				B Staff privilege extensions				C Patient transfers		
			I	II	III	IV	I	II	III	IV	I	II	III	IV
Arkansas	Block	I	1	0	0	0	1	0	0	0	1	0	0	0
(n = 22)		II	0	0	0	0	1	0	0	1	1	1	1	1
		III	0	0	0	1	0	0	0	0	1	0	1	1
		IV	0	0	0	0	1	1	1	1	1	0	0	0
			I	II			I	II			I	II		
Eastern Great Lakes	Block	I	0	0			0	1			1	1		
(n = 9)		II	0	1			1	1			1	1		
			I	II			I	II			I	II		
Greater Delaware Valley	Block	I	0	0			0	1			0	1		
(n = 9)		II	0	1			1	1			1	1		
			I	II	III		I	II	III		I	II	III	
Illinois	Block	I	0	0	0		0	0	1		1	1	1	
(n = 21)		II	0	1	0		0	0	0		1	1	1	
		III	0	1	1		1	1	1		1	1	1	
			I	II	III		I	II	III		I	II	III	
Northern California	Block	I	0	0	1		0	0	0		0	0	0	
(n = 14)		II	0	0	0		0	0	0		1	1	1	
		III	1	1	0		1	1	0		1	0	0	
			I	II	III		I	II	III		I	II	III	
Wisconsin	Block	I	0	1	0		1	1	0		0	1	0	
(n = 13)		II	1	0	0		1	1	1		1	1	0	
		III	0	0	1		0	0	1		1	1	1	

extensions are more constrained dimensions of interaction, owing to the absence of linkage between blocks (indicated by zeros). Because each nonzero element of the more constrained matrices is duplicated in the image matrix for patient transfers, the matrices for shared service arrangements and staff privileges can be thought of as contained within the least constrained matrix for patient transfers.

Comparing image matrices across networks gives us information on both the number of blocks identified and which type of linkage was either most or least pervasive. Only two blocks of hospitals were identified in both the Eastern Great Lakes and Greater Delaware Valley networks. Three blocks emerged in Illinois, Northern California, and Wisconsin, and four blocks were identified in Arkansas. Although Arkansas developed as an interpersonal network, 22 hospitals were originally mentioned as potential network members and the network region covered the entire state, so the larger number of blocks is understandable. Again, the least constrained matrix for Arkansas was patient transfers; however, this matrix is itself somewhat constrained, owing to the absence of linkage among seven dyads of blocks.

Three blocks of actors were identified in three of the four interorganizational networks (Illinois, Northern California, and Wisconsin). Once again, interaction along the patient transfer dimension is most pervasive for all three of these networks, and nearly full rank is achieved by the Illinois matrix on this dimension. The remaining interorganizational network, Greater Delaware Valley, presents image matrices quite similar to those of the Eastern Great Lakes network.

The image matrices for each network can then be multiplied (using Boolean matrix algebra) to produce "inclusion lattices," which represent the ordering of the compound relations within each network from the least constrained (image matrix is mostly 1's) downward to the most constrained. The inclusion lattices are shown in Figure 5.4. The letter combinations that form the "nodes" in these lattices represent the various relational components produced from the matrix multiplication. In these lattices, A stands for shared service linkages, B represents linkage through the extension of staff privileges, and C represents patient transfer arrangements. Thus, the product AC represents the pattern of linkage between blocks of actors involving both shared service and patient transfer arrangements. The multiplication process also serves to reduce restrictions on the connections of blocks in the image matrices. Linkages indicated in AC suggest that, in addition to single-step linkages between blocks, there are also multiple-step linkages. Hospitals in Block I may be tied to hospitals in Block III if the Block I hospitals share services with Block II, and the Block II hospitals transfer patients to Block III.

The ranks shown to the left of each lattice refer to the number of ties linking blocks of actors for each relational component. The higher the rank, the more inclusive or pervasive that linkage pattern. In an inclusion lattice, each relational component is fully contained in the one directly above it; thus, all of the interactions represented in the bottom, most constrained, lowest rank elements are included in the next level of the lattice, indicated by a line linking the two components.

Before comparing the six lattice structures, a *caveat* is needed concerning the relationship between network size (number of hospitals surveyed) and lattice complexity. To a certain extent, visual complexity increases with network size. Further, the set of hospitals linked through shared service programs, extension of staff privileges, and patient transfer arrangements as reported in this survey does not always correspond with the set of hospitals and actors identified in our earlier chapters as primary diffusion network actors. We are not looking for a replication of Figure 5.2; rather, we are examining other dimensions of organizational linkage at about the end of the diffusion network programs.

The lattices in Figure 5.4 provide an additional approach for examining linkage or relational complexity in these networks. Complexity in the linkage structure is indicated in the frequency of connections between elements that skip intervening ranks or levels. For example, in the Arkansas network, the chain connecting A to BA skips from rank 6 to rank 13, bypassing elements at ranks 7 through 12, whereas the linkage between C and CA is a direct one, without any jumps. In general, a

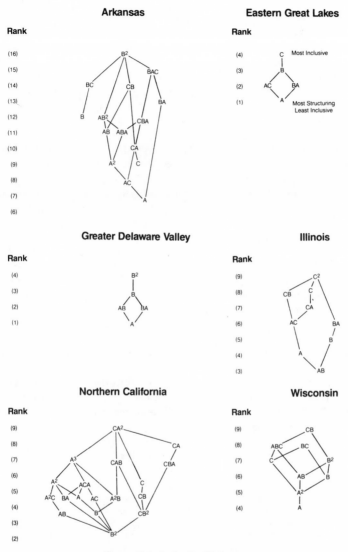

Figure 5.4. Inclusion lattices.

direct linkage in the lattice is interpreted to mean that the pattern of linkage represented by the lower-ranked element is completely included in, or duplicated by, the higher-ranked element. Translevel jumps, however, represent additional linkage complexity since the pattern of linkage of higher-ranked elements does not necessarily reproduce patterns at contiguous lower ranks. In other words, relational patterns in translevel jumps are not predictable by merely increasing the number of connections involved (i.e., increasing rank, or reducing constraints). Translevel jumps indicate that there is probably another variable underlying or organizing the pattern of connections within a network. Thus, the network structure is more complex compared with network lattices composed of all direct linkages.

Building on this notion of underlying complexity, then, we can compute a ratio of the number of lattice linkages between noncontiguous levels to the total number of linkages in the lattice. The higher the proportion of translevel linkages, the more complex the network. We can then compare linkage complexity across networks, as well as comparing which types of relational elements are ranked highest and lowest in the six networks. Table 5.4 summarizes these indices.

First of all, with the exception of Northern California, the highest-ranked elements for all the networks tend to involve either the extension of staff privileges or patient transfers. Share service arrangements rarely occur as a pervasive or inclusive form of linkage among these hospitals sets. Similarly, shared service arrangements are frequently found in the lowest rank of these lattices, meaning that linkages on this dimension are highly constrained, as was evident in the preponderance of zeros in the shared service image matrices. In fact, shared service arrangements are the most difficult types of linkage to effect, of the three examined here. A shared service program involves linking hospitals at the level of facility availability, which in the clinical arena means linking at the technical core (Thompson, 1967). For the non-controlling hospital, this would imply a loss of autonomy and considerable dependence in its relationship with its sharing partner. Of the six networks, only Northern California seems to have used this type of linkage to any great extent, probably because of its reliance upon the integrated service areas concept, which may have fostered the development of shared service programs between institutions in specific locales.

Also from Table 5.4 we see that Arkansas exhibits the highest proportion (0.55) of translevel jumps, followed by the Illinois network (0.40), Northern California and Wisconsin (0.33 and 0.31, respectively), and finally the Greater Delaware Valley and Eastern Great Lakes networks (0). Thus, the Arkansas network actually shows the highest level of complexity in its general-purpose linkages, followed by Illinois and the remaining networks. These complexity rankings (using the propor-

Table 5.4. Inclusion Lattice Characteristics

Network	Highest-ranked element[a]	Lowest-ranked element	Proportion of translevel jumps
Arkansas	B^2	A	0.55
Eastern Great Lakes	C	A	0
Greater Delaware Valley	B^2	A	0
Illinois	C^2	AB	0.40
Northern California	CA^2	B^2	0.33
Wisconsin	CB	A	0.31

[a] A = shared service arrangements, B = extension of staff privileges, C = patient transfers. Exponential notation means that the pattern of linkage involves multiple blocks of actors on that dimension.

tion of lattice linkages between noncontiguous levels) actually correspond fairly well with what we know about the general structure of the head and neck cancer action sets, especially the use of multicentered headquarters in both Arkansas and Illinois.

Although the Arkansas network evolved primarily as an interpersonal network, we know that four of the major hospitals in Little Rock, including the University of Arkansas for Medical Sciences, formed a legally binding joint venture to construct a centralized radiation therapy institute. The principal medical staff of the institute held joint appointments at the university and enjoyed staff privileges at the other three major hospitals. The rest of the hospitals in this network were linked primarily through interpersonal ties among physicians and patient transfer agreements to the four major institutions and to the radiation therapy center for the provision of specialized cancer care. The lattice structure for general-purpose linkages in Arkansas shows a somewhat similar pattern. The most inclusive type of linkage (highest rank) concentrates on the extension of staff privileges across blocks of actors, and shared service arrangements tend to concentrate in the lower right side of the lattice (fewer shared service programs link blocks of hospitals). Similarly, in the Illinois network, the underlying organizational principle, which is reflected in the high proportion of translevel jumps, was a multiple-centered system of four major university medical centers and their satellite hospitals, all linked to the state comprehensive cancer council.

The inclusion lattices for the Wisconsin and Northern California networks show many single-rank jumps and a lower proportion of multiple-rank jumps. In Northern California this might again reflect the use of the integrated service areas, which fostered the development of strong, cooperative links between institutions in specific locales, and encouraged task specialization among different groups of hospitals within the diffusion network. ISAs were likely to influence both general patterns of hospital linkage and the development of the diffusion network. In Wisconsin, the head and neck cancer network took a simpler form, in which nearly all member hospitals were directly linked to the network headquarters. Recall that this structure was the result of a careful management of network boundaries through contractual obligations that operated on several levels: collection of data on cancer patients, program involvement, and personal interaction.

Finally, the simplest inclusion lattices are found in the Greater Delaware Valley and Eastern Great Lakes networks, with no translevel jumps in either lattice. Both of these networks were composed primarily of single-stranded exchanges, linking member hospitals or physicians to the tertiary care center in their area. In the Eastern Great Lakes network, most specialists at the university center held appointments at the member hospitals, and all other institutional linkages were essentially contained within physician linkages and physician arrangements for transferring patients among institutions. The Greater Delaware Valley network actually developed along the pattern of a preexisting network for sharing radiation therapy staff and facilities.

Thus, the structural pictures provided by the inclusion lattices of the general-purpose linkages among network hospitals are fairly comparable with the network diagrams presented in Figure 5.2. Arkansas represents the one potential deviation. Apparently, general-purpose linkages among the hospitals in the network area were more complex than the head and neck cancer network structure. This would suggest that the network could have possibly been built around linkages between hospitals, rather than between physicians. However, two things need to be remembered here. First, the resource situation for the delivery of multidisciplinary treatment for head and neck cancer would still have presented a major obstacle in developing a diffusion network around hospital linkages. Outside of Little Rock (in fact, outside of the four institutions of the Central Arkansas Radiation Therapy Institute), there were neither the hospital facilities nor the staff needed to allow for direct innovation adoption or the building of bridges between the headquarters and potential member hospitals. Second, the complexity found in the Arkansas inclusion lattice primarily represents the linkages among the four institutions composing CARTI; CARTI was considered an extension of the UAMS in its role as headquarters institution for the head and neck network.

The results of our blockmodel analysis and our computations of network density and internal viability were used to produce rank orderings of the six networks. In addition, rankings were computed for several resource variables compiled from secondary data sources, using data for years prior to the beginning of the network projects. These resource variables were computed for each network region, defined as those counties in which a member hospital was located, or considered part of the network service area by the PI. These variables include the number of patients in the network regions over age 65, the ratio of specialists to GPs, the distribution (or level of concentration) of these two resources, the degree of similarity or homogeneity in hospital sizes (based on number of beds) within the network, the ranges of facilities offered by network institutions, and the degree of homogeneity in hospital staff sizes within the networks.

These rank orderings afford us a simple method to quantitatively examine the relationship between network environment (resource availability and dispersion) and the network structures of ongoing general-purpose linkages. All network structure and resource rankings were arrayed from least to most: the more dense/complex/internally linked, the higher the ranking; the larger the resource supply, the higher the ranking; the more evenly dispersed the resource, the higher the ranking; and the more homogeneous the hospitals, the higher the ranking. Because our variables consist of ordinal level rankings on a series of individual units, Spearman's rho can be used to evaluate the magnitudes of the various relationships. Although there are a number of measures of association appropriate for this type of analysis, rho was chosen because it is sensitive to the magnitude of the differences between the ranks, rather than simply being an enumeration of concordant and discordant pairs of ranks.

Table 5.5 summarizes the correlations between environmental and network structure variables. Again, structure here is defined in terms of the general-purpose linkages reported by hospital CEOs for patient transfers, shared service arrangements, and the extension of staff privileges. Although very few of these correlations reached levels of statistical significance (as might be expected with a sample of six networks), they can be used to tentatively examine how network context and ongoing network structure are interrelated.

From the first column of Table 5.5 we see that density has a weak positive correlation with the supply of elderly patients and a moderate negative correlation with the supply of specialists. Conversely, density is moderately linked to both the

Table 5.5. Correlations among Network Structure
and Environmental Variables[a]

| | Network structure | | |
Environmental dimensions	Density	Complexity	Internal viability
Resource availability			
N over 65	0.200	−0.147	0.486
Specialists/GPs	−0.429	−0.294	−0.086
Resource dispersion			
N over 65	−0.657	0.147	−0.086
Specialists/GPs	0.600	−0.265	0.486
Homogeneity within network on			
N of beds	0.429	−0.647	−0.714[b]
Range of facilities	0.429	−0.647	−0.714[b]
N of staff	0.543	−0.971[c]	−0.657

[a] Source: Fennell, Ross, and Warnecke (1987).
[b] $p < .10$.
[c] $p < .05$.

dispersion of elderly patients and the dispersion of specialists, but the former is negative and the latter is positive. In practical terms, this means that hospitals are more likely to cooperate in areas where specialists are evenly distributed, and where the patient supply is concentrated in specific locations, rather than distributed throughout the area. Density is also moderately correlated with the three measures of hospital homogeneity; thus, interhospital linkages are somewhat more dense where hospitals are similar in size and range of facilities.

Our different signed correlations between density and the distribution of patients and physicians suggest that these two types of environmental pressures may lead to different strategies of hospital cooperation. Clearly, patients and specialists represent different constituencies for interorganizational transactions, and perhaps different foundations for the development of linkages among hospitals. An area's elderly population functions as an important justification or "need" for many hospital services, especially cancer treatment facilities, since this is the segment of the population that is most frequently hospitalized and requires the most labor- and technology-intensive treatment for a variety of illnesses. If this "supply" of patients is not evenly distributed throughout an area, it is likely that hospitals will find it necessary to cooperate or align with other hospitals in order to share this resource, either through patient transfers or shared service programs.

Specialists, however, are a different constituency for hospitals in that they often act as organizational members of many different hospitals or boundary-spanners among several hospitals. As such, their distribution throughout a region may provide a basis or blueprint for interorganizational linkages, rather than functioning as a type of resource to be exchanged. As a professional community, specialists refer patients to other specialists and to various hospitals in a region; thus, the more evenly dispersed the region's supply of specialists, the denser the resulting set of institutional linkages based upon interpersonal ties. Organizational networks, then, to some extent may be structured along patterns defined by professional networks (see Hall, 1986).

Earlier we demonstrated the considerable variation observed in complexity across these six networks, and we rank-ordered them on the basis of the relative number of translevel jumps found in their inclusion lattices. The second column of Table 5.5 shows almost all negative correlations between network complexity and the environmental variables. Again, the size of the correlations linking the specialist population to complexity is about twice the size of the correlations with the elderly population. Although none of these correlations are of great magnitude, these results do suggest that as the population of medical specialists becomes more concentrated, hospital linkages may become more complex. Using inclusion lattices to measure complexity, we find that sets of hospitals may become more fragmented and indirectly linked to other groups of hospitals in regions where specialists concentrate in certain areas.

Of some interest, however, is the fact that the correlations between complexity and the hospital homogeneity indicators are of substantial magnitude and are consistently negative. Thus, it would seem that the dispersion of different types of hospitals is a better predictor of complexity than is resource availability or dispersion. The more heterogeneous the hospital set, the more complex their linkages.

The third column of Table 5.5 displays the correlations between the environmental characteristics and the internal viability of the networks. Internal viability was defined as the ratio of within-network linkages to total linkages. A moderate positive correlation is found between the supply of elderly patients and internal viability, and there is no relationship with patient dispersion. Again, an even distribution of specialists tends to be found in network areas with relatively high proportions of within-network linkages, repeating the type of association found between specialist dispersion and network density. If the normative pressures of specialists function through the development and structure of professional networks, then this result makes sense. An even distribution of the professional labor force may result in not only more interorganizational linkages in the area (density) but also a larger proportion of within-set linkages to total organizational linkages (viability).

Further, we also find large negative correlations between hospital homogeneity variables and internal viability, as was true for network complexity. In other words, within-set linkages (for patient transfers, shared service programs, and staff privileges) are the more pervasive type of organizational linkage reported by the hospitals in those sets where hospitals are very dissimilar in size or facility mix. Highly differentiated sets of hospitals (in terms of either goals, size, or function) may be more locally interlinked in general owing to the development of interorganizational divisions of labor. In some respects, these results fit well with our examination of homophily in the development of diffusion linkages. Linkages to share hospital services by definition mean that one hospital actually possesses a particular service, while the sharing partner does not. Recall that direct innovation transfer is possible only where hospitals are suitably equipped to directly use the innovation. Shared service linkages imply the exact opposite. Thus, homogenous sets of hospitals are less likely to be interlinked to share services, transfer patients, or extend staff privileges, but they are more likely to diffuse innovation to each other directly.

SUMMARY

In Chapter 4 we examined the influence of network environment on the network form to develop, as either interpersonal or interorganizational. In this chapter we have seen how network environment continues to influence the actual structure of network linkages, whether interpersonal or interorganizational, in an important way.

In the first part of this chapter we examined the case histories of each network in order to qualitatively depict the emergence of various boundary management strategies and their implementation as network structures. Choice of boundary definition (as expansive or constrained) and choice of spanning strategy (buffer or bridge) together influence the emergence of network structures in terms of the level of network formalization, the intensity of relations, the location of decision making, and the level of standardization. By and large, what we found was that resource availability and concentration are clearly linked to choice of boundary management strategy, and together they influence nearly all of these dimensions of emergent network structure. Networks located in rich environments where resources are somewhat dispersed are appropriate for bridging strategies among organizations in which linkages are formalized and fairly intense, decision making is decentralized, and programs are moderately standardized. Lean environments with concentrated resources tend to facilitate buffering strategies by headquarters institutions and interpersonal networks that are broadly cast and informal in structure, with low-intensity linkages. In such networks, decision making and network resources are controlled by the network headquarters.

We also examined the structure of both the linkages that were in place at the end of the project period specific to the delivery of head and neck cancer treatment, as well as more general-purpose linkages to remain after the project period. Our qualitative diagrams based on the case histories and our more technical block-models of general-purpose linkages paint fairly similar pictures. In general, environmental complexity in how resources are distributed and what the target hospitals look like encourages the development of similarly complex network structures.

In Chapter 1 we introduced the assumptions of resource dependence as a useful framework for understanding how and why linkages among organizations develop. Resource dependence starts with the assumption that organizations are not completely self-sufficient: in order to acquire the resources they need for survival they may have to engage in interaction and/or exchange with other organizations (i.e., "bridging" strategies may be necessary). Further, what those linkages look like, how dense, complex, formal, internally focused, and intensely used, may depend upon the resource picture facing organizations.

Our analyses in this chapter on network structure confirm the utility of a resource dependence approach. In addition, they suggest one respect in which the approach could be further refined. Not all resources or environmental constraints appear to be equally important in shaping the structure of interorganizational networks or defining the boundary management strategy to emerge. For health organizations, organizational homogeneity seems to be particularly important in the development of diffusion linkages. Formally defined connections between hospitals to diffuse innovations seem to occur only where hospitals are sufficiently well equipped to begin with to easily permit the direct transfer of new treatment techniques in exchange for specific services. Thus, although organizations are not completely self-sufficient, they can't engage in exchanges with other organizations without something of value to offer (such as patients for research). If the "payoff" is innovative technology, they must possess the facilities needed to adopt innovative techniques.

6

Variation across Hospitals in Network Program Participation

Penny L. Havlicek

INTRODUCTION

Throughout this book we have emphasized the influence of the environment on the development of the individual head and neck network demonstration projects. We demonstrated in Chapter 3 how hospitals in these networks established agendas and how their participation was influenced by these agendas. Two types of participating hospitals were identified. Academic medical centers sought new sources of patients for research and training and to estbablish themselves as regional cancer centers. Community medical centers sought to establish oncology programs that would attract young oncologists and their patients.

We have used the resource dependence perspective to demonstrate how these networks formed and attempted to diffuse components of the innovation in their service regions. In the preceding chapters we have argued that a major issue in network development is the ability of participating organizations to access needed resources while preserving their autonomy. In Chapters 4 and 5 we discussed how the activities of member hospitals shaped the way these networks developed, but from a network viewpoint. In this chapter we will consider factors that influenced participation by individual hospital members in these network programs, to determine whether their reasons for participating were consistent with the agendas described in Chapter 3. We will, in effect, examine how the community hospitals balanced network participation against organizational autonomy, answering our research question 4: What explains variation in participation by individual hospitals?

We posit two primary explanations for network participation: organizational power and organizational interest. From a resource dependence perspective both

PENNY L. HAVLICEK • Division of Survey and Data Resources, American Medical Association, Chicago, Illinois 60610.

explanations address the issue of access to resources. The power perspective addresses access to resources from the standpoint of exchange and centrality. From the interest perspective, access to resources is a function of commitment to the shared organizational objective of treating patients with head and neck cancer.

ORGANIZATIONAL POWER

Power is an elusive concept. It has been defined and studied in a multitude of different approaches. In this chapter we will conceptualize power in three ways: as a property of social relationships, as a function of the organization's position in a network through which resources flow, and as a function of access to resources external to the system.

Power and Exchange

As a property of social relationships power is situation-specific (Emerson, 1962): An organization or an individual powerful in one situation may not be powerful in another. From this standpoint, power results from an imbalance or a dependence in exchange relationships. Dependence results from control by one actor of resources needed or highly valued by another. Dependence is enhanced when these resources are available nowhere else in the environment (Cook, 1977; Emerson, 1962).

The availability of scarce or highly valued resources has been a key factor in investigations of how environments can control organizations (Jacobs, 1974). Control, like power, is exercised through exchange relationships. The powerful or controlling organization is strategically located in the sector of the environment where other organizations are most dependent. In exchanges between organizations two factors become crucial: (1) the essentiality of the item being exchanged, and (2) its availability from other sources.

Power and Centrality

An alternative approach to defining organizational power emphasizes the organization's centrality or its position in a network of multiple social relations. Power results from the organization's strategic location in the network (somewhat like Jacob's notion described above) and the position of the organization with respect to others in the organizational milieu. Centrality also emphasizes control. Centrality is the ability of the organization to control resource acquisition by other organizations through control of "strategic contingencies" (Benson, 1975, p. 233) that might otherwise be available to other organizations in the environment. Such control may result from a monopoly on vital goods and services, access to vital markets for products, or the ability to legitimize activities performed by other organizations or to certify their value.

In contrast to exchange theory, centrality focuses on the use by the powerful organization of its position in the environment to control the resource flow within a network, rather than on the exchange relationship (Benson, 1975). Centrality in a network is positively related to referral flow, communication flows, attribution of influence by others in the environment (Boje and Whetten, 1981), and the perceived potential for mobilizing resources controlled by others (Galaskiewicz, 1979).

Power and External Linkages

A third dimension of power emphasizes the options that an organization may have for acquiring resources. External linkages may provide avenues for further resource acquisition, making the organization less dependent on any single exchange relationship. Thus, as we noted in Chapters 4 and 5, organizations with multiple linkages, such as community hospitals with links to more than one medical school or tertiary hospital, may be less dependent on any one tertiary center, and the centrality of network headquarters may be less dominant than in environments where the linkages are all single-stranded and the headquarters represents "the only game in town."

Exchange and centrality conceptions of power differ primarily in the emphasis they place on relationships. They also differ on the relative emphasis placed on how control is exercised. The exchange theorist views power as a function of the direction and flow of resources in a relationship. The centrality approach places more emphasis on the position of the organization in the environment relative to resource flows. Both perspectives concur that power within a relationship or network is influenced by linkages outside the relationship, because these other links represent alternative access to vital resources that could potentially alter the internal balance of control.

We have already discussed in Chapter 1 how the resource dependence perspective relates power to participation in network activities. According to this perspective, organizations must compete for scarce strategic resources. To obtain these resources they must enter into relationships with other organizations. In these relationships some organizations inevitably become dependent upon others, although the goal is to minimize dependence and maximize autonomy (Aldrich, 1979). The possession of resources that are the basis of exchange and dependency relationships is the basis of power. Although no assumptions can be made about the relative importance of each, the distribution of resources and the kinds of exchange relationships through which they are exchanged both within and outside the network can be used to specify the organization's power.

Assuming organizations are so motivated, it is likely that a powerful organization will participate in network activities in order to consolidate or enhance its position in the network service region. Its position may be enhanced in a number of ways. Through joint participation in new programs, the organization may learn of innovations in the industry (Aiken and Hage, 1968). By establishing relationships or alliances with other organizations that can provide services or resources, the powerful organization can maintain control by dictating or managing the flow of resources of information within the region. Also, participating with others in a joint program may enhance the organization's prestige and hence its power in the dependency relationship (Perrow, 1961; Pfeffer, 1972).

INTEREST STRUCTURE

Another way of looking at why hospitals would participate in network programs is from the standpoint of common interest, or what is sometimes called the "collective good" (Olson, 1975). This conception follows from the resource dependence perspective. It assumes that the organization acts consistently with its interests and decides to participate when it determines that these interests can be enhanced by participation in the program. As discussed in Chapter 3, these interests are reflected in the organization's agenda. If the network can provide resouces that are of common benefit to all members, then these resources are a collective good for the network members, and once achieved or maintained, they cannot be denied to any member in good standing. In contrast to power theory, then, it is commitment to the common good, rather than power, that generates compliance with network objectives.

It may be assumed that provision of state-of-the-art treatment to head and neck cancer patients was a common interest of the participating hospitals in the networks, although, as we have already indicated in Chapter 3, there were other latent agendas. The networks received slack resources from the National Cancer Institute to pursue this common interest. The headquarters was empowered by NCI to require its members to perform certain functions, specified by the network bylaws, and aimed at enhancing the introduction of state-of-the-art treatment in the network service region. In return, the participants were given access to a portion of the common good, which took the form of funds provided through the contracts, as described in Chapter 5. Thus, there was a common interest (delivering high-quality care) and a common good (network financial support received from the NCI). Compliance with the network program can therefore be hypothesized as a function of commitment to the common interest and a desire for a share of the common good.

If this hypothesis holds, participation would be assured because of the nature of the contractual relationship. Since network activities were periodically reviewed and evaluated, it was possible for the network, and the individual participants, to lose the common good if they did not comply with the contract. Thus, the benefit was either for all or for none. Moreover, although all members of the group or network may have a common interest in obtaining the collective good, they have no common interest in paying for it. Rather, they may prefer to permit others in the group to pay while minimizing their own costs. Consequently, provision of the good is a function of factors related to the value of the good to the group, its cost, and the likelihood that the individual members will receive a reasonable share in return for their participation.

There were varying demands made upon network members for their participation. As discussed in Chapter 5, these demands depended upon the nature of the network and the amount of interaction required for diffusion to occur. However, a direct share in the good in the form of funding given directly to the participating member did not usually occur. In fact, only Wisconsin, Northern California, and Illinois actually funded staff at the participating hospitals, and even in these networks the amount of funding varied. In the others, the funds were used either to develop regional resources that could be shared by all members or to initiate programs that would communicate the state of the art to participants in the network.

Commensurately, as shown in Chapter 5, the degree of commitment required of participating hospitals was related to the demands made of them for the common good. Generally, the fewer demands, the less their share of the good. However, it can be argued that hospitals that participated benefited in other ways besides receiving a direct share in the good. This could occur in several ways: (1) A hospital may benefit in reputation owing to its public affiliation with the network project; (2) a hospital may benefit as its staff acquires special knowledge not available to other hospitals' staff who do not participate; (3) by participating in the present program with the headquarters institution the community hospital may be invited to participate in other programs where the good may be more extensive; and (4) the existence of the network may serve to attract other programs to the region, which may benefit the participants disproportionately because of their current participation.

Certain characteristics of the group and its membership may influence how the good is distributed and the benefit perceived by each member. One factor is the size of the network or group. Size determines how much of the good is needed. Small groups may be better able to provide the collective good than large ones because there is more to go around when the total gain needs to be divided among a few members (Olson, 1975). For this reason there is a high probability that in a small group the return to each member will exceed the cost of participating. By contrast, in large groups the collective good cannot be provided without reliance on coercion or other inducements since the individual member's return rarely exceeds the cost of participation.

Size of the member also affects whether the good is provided. A member's size may reflect level of interest in the good. A small member may have less interest in the good and, therefore, less incentive to pay the costs of providing the good than a large member. Similarly, a large member would pay a disproportionate share of the costs of obtaining the good and expect to benefit disproportionately.

Where the members of the group have a disproportionate interest in the good, the probability of achieving it is high. In such groups the members with the most interest will benefit so greatly that they will have much to gain from seeing it is provided, and they will ensure that it is provided even if they have to pay all the marginal costs of so doing (Olson, 1975).

In this analysis, the hospitals in each network with the most interest in instituting the network and disseminating state-of-the-art care were the headquarters institutions. These hospitals participated disproportionately in the network programs and provided the major share of the network resources. Contractually, this was their obligation, and if they were not motivated to participate, the network would not exist. Thus, the participation of the headquarters hospitals is taken as a given, and our interest in this chapter is in explaining variations in participation of the community hospitals and how they defined the "common good."

MEASURING POWER, INTEREST STRUCTURE, AND PARTICIPATION

Power as Resource Centrality

Two indicators of a particular hospital's access to strategic resources are used in this analysis: the range of hospital facilities (varying from one to forty-six facilities) and the number of hospital staff. Both measures were described in Chapter 2. Control over high levels of each of these resources would enable a hospital to better control resource flows within its network, thus affording it a more central position.

Power and Exchange

The exchange rate between hospitals is defined in terms of both the mutual extension of staff privileges and the exchange of head and neck cancer patients. To develop this measure a questionnaire was sent to the chief executive officers (CEOs) of all network hospitals, and each CEO was asked to describe the procedures by which staff privileges were extended between it and other hospitals in the network. A hospital could report that no privileges were extended or that privileges were extended through various mechanisms. Each hospital was also asked to indicate the hospitals in the network to which it transferred patients for the treatment of head and neck cancer and the hospitals from which it received patients. An exchange was defined as favorable when (1) staff at a participating hospital received staff privileges at other hospitals more frequently than it gave staff privileges to staff at other hopsitals, and (2) more patients were received in transfer from other hospitals than were transferred by the hospital to others. A surplus in these exchanges implies that the hospital with the surplus has a special facility or resource not available uniformly in the network since their staff is in relatively greater demand and other hospitals are more likely to transfer patients to it.

Power and External Linkages

The linkages an organization has to organizations external to the network are defined in terms of shared services. Shared services are those functions, clinical or administrative, used jointly by two or more hospitals for their mutual benefit and at their mutual cost (Astolfi and Matti, 1972; DeVries, 1978). Hospitals participate in shared service programs as a way of improving services and gaining access to scarce resources that could never have been acquired on an individual basis and to realize economies of scale (Alford, 1976; DeVries, 1978). Shared services take a variety of forms. Hospitals share services when they agree to offer different services, when one hospital is contracted to provide a service to other hospitals, when hospitals jointly purchase services or products, or when they pool manpower or capital resources (Astolfi and Matti, 1972).

These data were also obtained from the survey of CEOs. As part of that survey they were asked whether their hospital shared services with other organizations. If they indeed shared services, they were asked to select from a list of 39 services those they shared and to indicate the name of the organization with whom they shared the service. Other kinds of organizations besides hospitals, such as blood banks, and hospital associations were included on the list. Since the linkages to organizations outside the network are of primary interest in an analysis of power, a hospital's shared service linkages were grouped into the following categories for analysis: (1) the number of hospitals outside the network with which it shared services, (2) the number of network hospitals with which it shared services, (3) the number of other shared service organizations with which it shared services. The percentage of all organizations with which a hospital shares services that are outside the network was used as the indicator of linkages to organizations outside the network.

Measuring Interest Structure

Three factors relate to the group's ability to provide itself with the collective good: (1) the size of the group, (2) the variance in the group's interest in the good, and

(3) the individual member's level of interest in the good (Olson, 1975). The size of the group and the variance in the group's interest in the good are contextual properties of the hospitals (Lazarsfeld and Menzel, 1961). The operationalizations of size of the group and the level of interest of the individual members are relatively straightforward. The size of the group is simply the number of hospitals in the network. The level of individual member interest in network activities is measured by the number of head and neck patients treated at the hospital. The more head and neck patients treated, the more relevant the network program is for the hospital.

The coefficient of relative variation (CRV) of the head and neck cancer admissions to member hospitals is used to operationalize the network's variance in interest. This measure is calculated as

$$CRV = [AD(Md)/Md] \times 100$$

where AD is the average absolute deviation from the median or mean. The median (Md) is used as the origin because it is the point around which the sum of deviations is smallest.

This statistic has several advantages. Since it expresses variation as a percentage of its origin, the interpretation of the resulting coefficient is straightforward. The larger the coefficient, the greater the variation in interest among the hospitals in the network in head and neck cancer. Also, expressing the variation as a percentage of its origin eliminates the effect of scale location (Mueller et al., 1970).

Participation

The dependent variable examined in this chapter is the degree of participation by community hospitals in network activities. Hospitals could participate in two types of network activity: program planning and program implementation. Programs were planned in network committees and implemented by member organizations or their representatives. The way we have operationalized these measures of hospital participation distinguishes between these two types of activity. Both measures are drawn from network documents and attempt to reflect hospital participation over time.

Committees were charged with developing operative and regulative rules and procedures. Operative rules and procedures refer to regulations pertaining to an organization's tasks or its production process. Regulative rules and procedures refer to governance or the internal functioning of the organization (Zey-Ferrell, 1979). The committees made decisions regarding operative rules and procedures when they planned network projects and decided how these projects were to be carried out. The committees made decisions regarding regulative rules and procedures when they developed criteria for membership and policies regarding member reimbursement. As we described in Chapter 5, the regulative rules were generally established early in the network history and were very dependent upon the type of network and manner in which members participated in the overall program of the network.

The documentation produced by the networks that described the committee structures and composition varied greatly in completeness and in how recently it was compiled. Some networks never described their committee structure in a single document, making it necessary to glean information about committee structure and activity from various reports and other documents. Others described their committees once and not again. Still others periodically provided lists of committees and their members, but only by comparing reports could one tell that there had been changes in size and composition. Still, even allowing for the uneven quality of the data, it was possible to arrive at two measures of committee participation that capture both the depth and the breadth of a single hospital's participation.

Depth of participation is measured by the percentage of members of the network's executive committee or other governing body that represented affiliated community hospitals. Although the networks had committee structures of varying composition, all networks had a governing committee of some sort. If this committee was described only once, that description was used. When it was described more than once, the description of the committee during the time of peak committee activity in the network's history was used. If a member represented more than one hospital, then each hospital was counted as represented.

Breadth of participation by a hospital was measured by the percentage of network committees ever formed on which the hospital had a representative. This measure attempts to circumvent the unevenness of the data available by accepting whatever information on representation is available. If the hospital is mentioned as being a member of a committee, it is counted as being represented on that committee.

Programs implemented by the networks were rich in variety because the contractors were given great latitude in determining their programmatic emphases. Moreover, even programs with similar emphases implemented their programs differently. There were common patterns that emerged and appeared to be patterned by important factors related to how and why each network was organized. These are described in the next chapter.

In spite of this variation, there was sufficient commonality in program objective that, allowing for the variation in expression, it was possible to develop two measures of variation in participation. Two program areas were sufficiently common among the networks that such measures could be devised. These were (1) the provision of high-quality, multidisciplinary care, and (2) the conduct of regional educational programs aimed at medical and lay community members and designed to promote the provision of the multidisciplinary care.

Allowing for diversity of specific program content, high-quality, multidisciplinary care for head and neck cancer patients was generally promoted by the networks in two forms: (1) by establishing multidisciplinary, pretreatment planning conferences at which treatment plans and rehabilitation concerns were presented, and (2) by organization of multidisciplinary treatment teams that attempted to follow the written guidelines. The multidisciplinary planning conferences were frequently held in the community, and community physicians were invited to attend and present their cases. The patients presented were reviewed by a multidisciplinary panel, which then made treatment recommendations. Treatment teams, on the other hand, were generally limited to a participating hospital. They developed treatment plans and delivered the treatment themselves. They were frequently set up in the university hospitals as models for community hospitals to follow. Both vehicles emphasized multidisciplinary evaluation prior to treatment.

A single measure of participation in multidisciplinary care was devised that accepted participation in any form. A hospital was defined as participating in such care if (1) it had representation at the pretreatment planning conference or (2) it had established a multidisciplinary treatment team.

The education programs developed by the networks had various purposes, depending upon the type of network and the network's objectives. However, all networks offered educational programs as part of their activities aimed at diffusing state-of-the-art multidisciplinary care into community settings. These activities took several forms: (1) talks to community and professional groups given by individuals affiliated with the network; (2) community education events, such as lectures to students or senior citizens regarding oral self-examination, or special health fairs held at shopping malls or state fairs; and (3) formal professional education presentations or seminars.

Five measures of participation in educational activities were developed. The first refers to community education and is defined as the number of community educational events given or attended by a representative of a participating hospital. Participation in informal professional educational activities was defined in two ways: (1) the number of presentations given by a representative from a participating hospital, and (2) the number of presentations hosted by a participating hospital. Two additional measures were developed to assess the extent of participation in the third category of events, formal lectures or seminars. These are (1) the number of such lectures given by a representative of a participating hospital, and (2) whether the participating hospital hosted any formal lectures or seminars.

POWER AND PARTICIPATION

In the analyses presented here we examined the relationship involving the three sets of power variables (associated with exchange, centrality, and external linkage) and participation in network activities by the community hospitals. The results are summarized in Table 6.1. As can be seen in this table, the exchange variables (exchange of staff and exchange of patients) are not consistently related to participation. Exchange of staff privileges is unrelated to any of the participation variables. Community hospitals that experienced favorable exchanges of head and neck patients are more likely than those without a favorable exchange of patients to be represented on committees of the network. However, a favorable exchange of head and neck patients is not related to participation in any of the other types of network programs or activities.

When the centrality variables (number of facilities and size of staff) are examined, resources are related to participation. The number of facilities is positively related to membership on network committees, participation in multidisciplinary activities, and hosting formal and informal professional education programs. Size of staff is unrelated to committee participation but is related to the likelihood that the hospital will participate in hosting informal professional programs.

Finally, the percentage of ties or linkages to organizations outside the network is inversely related to one aspect of program participation; as the percentage of external ties increases, staff participation in formal educational activities decreases. External linkage is unrelated to the other participation variables. This suggests that

Table 6.1. Zero-Order Correlation Coefficients of Power and Participation, Community Hospitals

	Committee			Participation variables program				
Power variables	Percentage on steering committee	Percentage of committee	Multidisciplinary activities	Percentage of community education	Percentage of informal professional education	Host informal professional education	Percentage of formal professional education	Host formal professional education
No. of hospital facilities	-0.04	0.32[a]	0.35[a]	-0.06	0.17	0.34[a]	0.14	0.44[a]
N	64	62	64	64	64	64	56	64
No. of staff	-0.10	0.26	0.24	-0.03	0.06	0.38[a]	0.04	0.14
N	64	62	64	64	64	64	56	64
Exchange of staff	0.03	0.22	0.06	0.13	0.09	0.17	0.18	0.07
N	51	49	51	51	51	51	45	51
Exchange of patients	0.07	0.35[a]	0.07	0.05	0.18	0.10	0.12	-0.06
N	66	64	66	66	66	66	58	66
Percentage of extranetwork ties	-0.24	-0.15	0.25	0.04	0.03	-0	-0.37[a]	0.10
N	46	44	46	46	46	46	38	46

[a] $p < .05$.

the more independence the hospital has, the less likely it will be to participate in network programs. However, this association is not strong. It would appear that the best predictor of participation among the power variables is the control of resources in the form of facilities and staff. Thus, centrality seems to be the best predictor of participation. Community hospitals that are involved in patient exchanges are likely to serve on network committees that set policy for the networks. This undoubtedly reflects their importance to the network and particularly the ability of the network to register the number of patients required by the NCI. Finally, the percentage of shared service ties to organizations outside of the network was negatively associated with participation, although the association was weak. It suggests, however, that access to alternative resources may lessen the need for participation in the network and give those hospitals with access to external resources greater autonomy in compliance with the network program.

Overall, the power analysis suggests the following pattern: Community hospitals with large resources of patients, facilities, and staff are likely to be important for the network because of what they contribute to the network's activities, and hence, they will participate in decision making. However, they are likely to participate in network activities only to the extent that they are linked to the network for their resources and patient access. Control of resources (the centrality variables) were most predictive of all forms of participation.

INTEREST STRUCTURE AND PARTICIPATION

The relationship between interest structure and participation by community hospitals is examined in Table 6.2. In this table size of the network is inversely related to participation. In smaller networks, community hospitals are more likely to be represented on committees. Moreover, in these smaller networks, community hospitals are more likely to participate in multidisciplinary activities, community educational programs, and informal professional education programs, and to host formal educational programs.

Interest as measured by the number of head and neck cancer patients is also positively associated with committee participation. The positive association means that community hospitals with larger numbers of head and neck admissions are more likely to be listed as being represented on network committees. Also, community hospital interest (number of patients) was associated with participation in network activities, including multidisciplinary treatment activities and hosting informal professional education programs. The fact that the community hospitals most involved in treating head and neck cancer patients were also involved in multidisciplinary treatment and in hosting professional activities indicates that these networks may have been having the desired effect of diffusing state-of-the-art treatment to the community.

An inverse relationship existed between variation of interest in the network and committee participation. This suggests that the network context has an important impact on hospital participation in network governance. It seems consistent with a line of reasoning that community hospitals are likely to be involved in network governance only in those networks where they are equal partners as

Table 6.2. Zero-Order Correlation Coefficients of Interest Structure and Participation, Community Hospitals

Interest structure variables	Committee		Participation variables program					
	Percentage on steering committee	Percentage of committee	Multidisciplinary activities	Percentage of community education	Percentage of informal professional education	Host informal professional education	Percentage of formal professional education	Host formal professional education
Size of network	−0	−0.29[a]	−0.45[a]	−0.31[a]	−0.29[a]	−0.17	−0.25	−0.35[a]
N	67	65	67	67	67	67	59	67
Interest of hospital	0.05	0.42[a]	0.33[a]	0.02	0.14	0.49[a]	0.26	0.08
N	56	54	56	56	56	56	48	56
Variance in interest in network	0.18	−0.53[a]	−0.33[a]	−0.25	−0.18	−0.28[a]	−0.17	−0.25
N	56	54	56	56	56	56	48	56

[a] $p < .05$.

defined by similarity in the number of patients treated. Where there is great varia-tion in interest (i.e., the head and neck cancer patients are unevenly distributed), then perhaps the network hospitals can be presumed to have less interest and are less willing to contribute their resources to the "common good." It would imply further that the headquarters dominate and therefore receive the most benefit and hence contribute the most. As we have seen in Chapter 4, an absence of homophily (indicated here by variation in interest) tends to be most common in the interper-sonal networks where the headquarters institutions chose to centralize decision making and governance, and where resources were less likely to be distributed to the community.

SUMMARY AND CONCLUSIONS

Power and interest structure were both directly associated with participation by the community hospitals in the networks. This would be expected, given that the programs were directed toward them as a primary audience. Not only did power and interest structure correlate with participation, but they influenced vari-ous types of participation in consistent yet different ways.

Interest was more consistently related to participation than was power. The most significant correlations with participation were size of the network, hospital interest, and variance in network interest structure. Among the power variables examined here, the number of facilities was most strongly associated with participation.

Nonetheless, the power variables and interest variables can be combined in a model that treats them as complementary factors. In small networks community hospitals were more likely to participate, and participation was most likely, when the hospitals in the network had the appropriate facilities. Consistent with these observations was the fact that community hospitals with high interest (i.e., greater numbers of head and neck cancer admissions) were more likely to be involved in both governance and program activities. These patterns in the data suggest that community hospitals seemed to use their network participation to enhance their position and access to the "good," defined as access to a greater share of patients. But participation is unlikely unless the networks have access to resources that enable participation. This conclusion is consistent with the finding that where potential network organizations were quite dissimilar, participation by community hospitals was low.

In conclusion, these findings suggest that community hospital participation in networks may depend on the presence of certain combinations of power and in-terest factors. Community hospitals are most likely to be involved in networks when the network is itself small, and when the community hospitals have the capability to participate fully (i.e., facilities and patients are at adequate levels).

7

Definition and Diffusion of the Innovation

INTRODUCTION

Following Rogers's (1983) discussion of organizational innovation diffusion, we argued in Chapter 4 that innovation adoption in organizations follows a series of steps. These are (1) agenda setting, (2) matching identified problems in performance with possible solutions or innovations, (3) defining or restructuring the innovation to fit the organizational setting (reinvention), (4) clarifying the meaning of the innovation for the core activities of the organization, and (5) routinizing the innovation as part of the regular activities of the organization.

The innovation that is described here had three components. Its software included an innovative approach to cancer management emphasizing multidisciplinary input. Diffusing it called for defining the state of the art in multidisciplinary care and then formulating that care definition into a structured format. Finally, transmitting the innovation from research to community settings called for creation of a new organizational form, networks. In Chapter 3 we discussed agenda setting and how the agenda defined by the National Cancer Institute was matched to the agenda established by each participant. Chapters 4 and 5 dealt with reinvention of the network component of the innovation, thus answering research question 3: How did the environment influence the form and structure of the innovation diffusion networks to emerge at each of the seven project sites? In this chapter we will again employ the concept of reinvention, focusing on the way multidisciplinary, state-of-the-art patient care was defined by each program and then reformulated for dissemination. Our analyses here respond to research question 5: How did the environment and network form affect the way in which the innovation was introduced and initially tried?

We will also consider how the networks interpreted the innovation's meaning for their core activities, and so structured their diffusion activities. Then we will examine how the form of the innovation affected the way in which it was defined and structured to fit its organizational setting, and the meaning it had for network activities.

The basic concepts of multidisciplinary care contained in the underlying software of the innovation were consistent across the seven networks. However, local contingencies played an important role in how the innovation was defined and formulated for dissemination. In addition to local contingencies, there were two factors common to all networks that influenced how the content of the innovation was formulated and the form of the innovation diffusion process. These were the form of network and whether the contract was awarded in year 1 or year 2 of the program. Thus, the actual content and mode of dissemination chosen by each network was influenced by the organizational context in which each program was developed and the headquarters' interpretation of the meaning of each aspect of the innovation for its core activities.

DEFINITION OF THE INNOVATION

The establishment of the head and neck demonstration projects was based on several premises. The first was that head and neck cancer patients required multidisciplinary management that included pretreatment planning by a team of specialists, consisting of surgeon, radiation therapist, maxillofacial prosthodontist, speech therapist, and dietician. The second was that there was general consensus about state-of-the-art treatment for most forms of head and neck cancer, and so experienced clinicians could formulate treatment guidelines incorporating this consensus. Third, it was assumed that such written guidelines would be accepted by community physicians.

The contracts that established these networks did not require that the networks develop a common set of guidelines. However, the planning group that had been convened by the NCI to develop guidelines for the entire cancer control program had recommended that common guidelines and data forms be developed if network programs were initiated. The contracts required that each network develop some form of local guidelines containing state-of-the-art management principles for head and neck cancer and a plan for their dissemination. Each network was also required to demonstrate its capability to obtain data on a minimum number of patients.

At an early meeting of the principal investigators awarded contracts in year 1, it was decided to formulate a common set of guidelines and a common data set. Following the practice of the cooperative research groups, they agreed to devise a common set of data forms. During the remainder of that first planning year the first-year contractors, Eastern Great Lakes, Illinois, and Wisconsin, met, drafted a set of guidelines, and agreed upon the common data items that would be used to assess compliance with the guidelines. However, they were unable to agree on a common data form, a point to which we shall return.

The draft guidelines contained an introductory section and nine site-specific sections. Each section was organized around four common themes: the epidemiology, etiology, and natural history of the disease; diagnosis and pretreatment planning; treatment; and rehabilitation. The guideline content reflected the professional orientation of the first-year contractors and the state of knowledge at the time they were written. Surgery was described as the "treatment of choice" when factors such as tumor size and location and the patient's overall condition are considered. Radiation therapy was the second preferred treatment modality. Chemotherapeutic regimens that are now well recognized had not been evaluated for head and neck cancer and so were not mentioned in these early formulations of the state of the art.

In all but one section, the guidelines were intended to be nonprescriptive because it was assumed that a consensus existed about state-of-the-art treatment. That one section, however, clearly intended to communicate appropriate management techniques to community physicians and other health care professionals who might be the first to encounter the head and neck cancer patient. This section was a list of 17 and, after final revision, 19 common errors in the management of head and neck patients observed by the principal investigators. For the most part these errors related to early detection, diagnosis, and preliminary work-up of these patients, but they also included some frequent treatment errors and errors in follow-up care. The list was also intended to convey the importance of prompt and informed response to such cancers for improving the posttreatment morbidity and mortality associated with these cancers. Second-year investigators were asked to comment and suggest revisions. They did this, and ultimately the list of common mistakes in treatment was increased to 19, a section on managing thyroid cancers was added, and a set of recommended data-collection forms was appended.

After the guidelines were written, reactions were sought from professionals treating head and neck patients. Through this period the contractors tried to achieve widespread dissemination of the guidelines. The first-year investigators wrote most of the guidelines. Comments were also requested from other medical staff at the network institutions. Drafts were circulated by the principal investigators to medical staff affiliated with the program at headquarters and in the participating community hospitals. Rehabilitation professionals were specifically asked to review the guidelines and comment since they had not written any of the rehabilitation sections and rehabilitation was an important theme. The principal investigators made some effort to broadly disseminate the guidelines to community physicians in their network service areas. They also agreed to try to obtain feedback from health professionals in their local communities who were not directly affiliated with the network, but who were most likely to first encounter a head and neck cancer patient and make initial treatment decisions. Copies of the draft guidelines were mailed to local physicians. When educational programs were conducted, the guidelines were distributed and discussed. Those who received the guidelines were requested to communicate their reactions directly to the principal investigator.

Obtaining feedback about the guidelines was the primary mode of dissemination utilized by the networks during the demonstration contract period. The final guidelines, published under the title "Management Guidelines for Head and Neck Cancers, 1979" (U.S. DHEW, 1979), were not distributed until February 1980, six months before the end of the contracts. So there was really no time for dissemination of the final draft during the contract period. However, the final 1979 draft did not change appreciably from the earlier draft.

REINVENTION: ALTERNATIVE DEFINITIONS OF THE INNOVATION

Physicians

Only the first-year networks used the guidelines as the primary vehicle to stimulate community interest in the concept of multidisciplinary management of head and neck cancer patients. Through their efforts to obtain community feedback, the first-year network investigators attempted to create knowledge that the guidelines were available and that they contained useful information about how to manage head and neck cancer patients. The diffusion process was initiated through preexisting channels in the network communities and had the explicit sponsorship of the headquarters institutions. Much of the guideline content could be tried without major investment by the practitioner or the practitioner's hospital, assuming the necessary facilities were already available. There was ample opportunity for feedback, and the first-year networks set up support programs to assist those community physicians who attempted to adopt the guidelines.

Among the network principal investigators, differences regarding the relevance and validity of the guideline content became increasingly evident as the second-year network programs were implemented. There was common ground among them regarding the underlying concepts incorporated into the ideas surrounding multidisciplinary management. This agreement, however, did not extend to the formulation of written guidelines as a way of disseminating these concepts. Although all seven networks reviewed the 1977 draft guidelines and provided commentary used in the revisions, they did not share a common enthusiasm for the written guidelines. The first-year contractors were the authors of the guidelines that were hammered out in several meetings during the first contract year. The second-year contractors had not been part of that process, and they had different ideas about both the substance and form of the ideas to be disseminated. They were particularly skeptical about the need for, and acceptability of, a written document among community physicians.

The second-year networks reinvented the notion of multidisciplinary treatment planning according to how they saw the whole innovation (i.e., multidisciplinary care, formulation of state-of-the-art management principles, and networks) influencing their agenda and core activities. The agenda for the second-year contractors, like that of the first-year group, was to implement regional cancer control programs to support their developing cancer centers. However, unlike the first-year contractors, the second-year networks were more likely to be organized around shared community facilities, such as radiation therapy units, clinics, or other satellite organizational units. In some instances, pretreatment planning conferences were already being held; in others, the setting or organizational form was conducive to such a format and they were initiated. Thus, for these second-year units, the pretreatment planning conference was highly preferable to the written guidelines as a diffusion channel because it brought community physicians into direct contact with physicians and facilities at the headquarters.

A further difference between the two groups of contractors was their varying perceptions of the acceptability to local physicians of written guidelines as the final word on state-of-the-art treatment of head and neck cancer. Local antipathy to the idea of written guidelines was reported by most of the second-year networks. The principal investigators felt that local physicians would not accept written guidelines. Hence, alternative formulations of the state of the art had to be devised so as not to jeopardize the basic agenda of building a regional cancer program.

The critical role of local acceptance is exemplified in Mississippi, which had explicitly defined as its agenda becoming the tertiary cancer referral center for the region. They intended to accomplish this by establishing their newly formed multidisciplinary clinic as a model treatment facility and source of information about state-of-the-art patient management procedures for local community hospitals. Using network resources, the clinic staff planned to develop protocols that would reflect local treatment practices and preferences but would also encompass the state of the art. Although Mississippi acknowledged the existence of the guidelines, they were not adopted as treatment guidelines in the clinic. It became increasingly evident that no agreement would be reached within the clinic about what constituted state-of-the-art treatment, and ultimately, the concept of the clinic as a regional resource proved to be unworkable. When this occurred, the entire program was terminated by the university. It was clear that the Mississippi network was unable to stimulate community interest in the innovation in any format.

The Northern California and Greater Delaware Valley networks also reinvented the component of the innovation that required formulation and dissemination of the multidisciplinary, state-of-the-art treatment strategies. As with Mississippi, these networks discovered that local practitioners were reluctant to accept written guidelines purporting to define "state of the art." The Greater Delaware Valley network developed a single patient management protocol as an alternative to site-specific guidelines. This protocol clearly reflected the influence of the radiation therapists who constituted the network leadership. The Northern California network subcontracted the development and dissemination of guidelines to a local foundation, headed by a radiation therapist. After subcontracting, however, they discovered that the local practitioners would not accept any form of written guidelines, and eventually the subcontract was terminated. At this point the 1977 guidelines were disseminated for informational purposes without endorsement.

Neither Northern California nor the Greater Delaware Valley ever intended that written guidelines would be the main vehicle for diffusion of the concepts of multidisciplinary care in their service areas. Both planned to implement some form of pretreatment conference as the primary vehicle for disseminating the concepts. In the Greater Delaware Valley network these conferences were held on a rotating basis at participating hospitals. Northern California contracted their organization to local cancer planning groups. Both these networks viewed these pretreatment planning conferences as a more flexible approach to diffusion than the written guidelines. The pretreatment conference enabled the physician to consult with other physicians and to develop specific patient management strategies tailored to the specific case. This approach was consistent with community norms and fit better with other components of organizational interaction within the region. However, one outcome of this alternative approach was that the treatment concepts employed by these networks were never explicitly formulated in hard copy. Hence, there was no basis for defining what exactly was diffused.

Arkansas participated more extensively than the other second-year contractors in preparing the revised guidelines. The principal investigator was a coauthor of the added section dealing with thyroid tumors. Nevertheless, like the other second-year principal investigators, he distributed the guidelines but did not endorse their content, saying only that the guidelines were available as suggestions for managing head and neck tumors. Like Greater Delaware Valley, Arkansas was organized around a radiation therapy center established in Little Rock. Like those in Northern California and Greater Delaware Valley, the investigators in Arkansas also chose the pretreatment planning conference as the primary channel for disseminating the content of the innovation. Efforts to expand the pretreatment conference outside Little Rock proved unsuccessful. Thus, all content about multidisciplinary care and pretreatment planning was disseminated through the principal investigator's personal contacts with primary care providers. This approach was consistent with the interpersonal network form of diffusion that characterized the Arkansas network.

Rehabilitation Specialists

The principal investigators from the second-year programs dissented from the concept of written guidelines. Other groups of professionals involved in the management of head and neck cancer patients disagreed with the content of the written guidelines. Although rehabilitation was a prominent feature of the guidelines, the rehabilitation professionals in the networks were dissatisfied with the discussion of rehabilitation. In their view, the guidelines did not adequately incorporate state-of-the-art rehabilitation procedures as specifically required by the network contracts.

Following their review of the 1977 draft, the various network rehabilitation specialists convened a two-day rehabilitation conference to discuss the rehabilitation components of the guidelines. The results of the conference were formulated in a series of recommendations for revising the guidelines to emphasize specific rehabilitation procedures appropriate for certain site-treatment combinations which were neglected in the draft guidelines, and which had been evaluated and were ready for diffusion. It was recommended that these techniques be incorporated into an appendix to the guidelines to be written by the rehabilitation specialists. An outline of the proposed appendix was prepared and funds requested from the NCI to support its preparation. When these were not forthcoming, further effort to revise the rehabilitation content of the guidelines was abandoned, and like the second-year principal investigators, the rehabilitation specialists did not employ the written guidelines for diffusing the state of the art in head and neck patient rehabilitation.

Nurses

The oncology nurses were also dissatisfied with the content of the written guidelines. As with the rehabilitation specialists, their dissatisfaction resulted from the failure by the first-year contractors to consult them about nursing management of head and neck patients. Consequently, the guidelines contained nothing about nursing care for these patients. The nurses tried to produce written guidelines for managing head and neck patients. But, as with the rehabilitation specialists, support for the effort could not be obtained. The effort failed, leaving another group of specialists, and another discipline required for multidisciplinary care, dissatisfied with the content of the written guidelines.

In all, the various efforts made to reinvent the basic concepts incorporated in state-of-the-art, multidisciplinary care for head and neck cancer patients arose from differences among the innovators about how such concepts should be formulated and disseminated. There were also differences in how the networks perceived the innovation would fit with their agenda and core activities. Reinvention was successful when the network investigators found ways to meet their contractual requirements and yet remain consistent with the local agenda.

For the most part, efforts to formulate alternative written guidelines failed. There were two reasons for the failures. First, there was no agreement among the principal investigators about the effectiveness and acceptability of written guidelines; so, understandably, strong support for expanding the written guidelines could not be obtained. Second, those who proposed expanding the written guidelines were not physicians and could not force the issue of support among the principal investigators.

Efforts at reinventing the innovation in other formats proved more successful. The alternative formulations illustrate the importance of the environment and the compatibility between the form of the innovation and the overall organizational agenda. The pretreatment conference had several attractive features for the second-year contractors. It was compatible with organizational approaches to diffusion that were already in place. It did not impose a preformulated approach to treatment on the community physicians. Instead, it provided a context within which the patient could be discussed and treatment options considered. Then the referring physicians could feel that they had some input into the final recommendation. It also provided an opportunity to establish links to community physicians and local hospitals where none previously existed. Moreover, the links were tied to core activities of the network, usually radiation therapy, which provided some sense of stability.

IMPLEMENTATION STRATEGIES

Knowledge/Awareness Stage: Organizational Strategies

The strategies chosen by each network to disseminate the innovation varied by how they defined the innovation and by the more fundamental difference of whether they were interorganizational or interpersonal networks. The first stage of the diffusion process requires that the target audience be made aware of the innovation and its relevance to their needs or to the needs of the organization they represent (Rogers, 1983). From the organizational standpoint this includes *matching* problems with the solution represented by the innovation, *reinvention*, or redefining and restructuring the innovation to fit with the organization's needs, and *clarifying* the meaning of the innovation for the core activities of the organization. We have seen how the headquarters reinvented the form and content of the innovation in order to increase its fit with their agenda and core activities. Now we turn to how they initiated the process of diffusing the innovation from the headquarters to the community practitioners.

The knowledge/awareness process began for all networks with the issuance of the program announcement by the National Cancer Institute and the preparation of a response. An acceptable proposal had to demonstrate that the headquarters institution could reach the target audience, defined as a network of community hospitals. In preparing the proposal, each principal investigator had to initiate discussions with community clinicians about the project, its organization, and its objectives, in order to generate interest and obtain their agreement to participate. Through this process the principal investigator or his surrogate initially defined the network, established membership criteria, and defined the concept of multi-disciplinary care.

This initial process proceeded in different ways depending upon the characteristics of the environment. The results indicated the form the network would eventually take. All applicants proposed some form of interorganizational network, and each investigator provided evidence of support from community physicians, usually in the form of letters expressing interest in the project and general support. The content of these letters varied widely in their specificity, however. For example, letters of support from hospitals where interpersonal networks eventually developed were generally from hospitals that eventually became components of the headquarters of the network. Thus, they did not actually express commitment from targeted potential adopters of the innovation. In contrast, letters from community hospitals associated with networks that eventually took the interorganizational form were more often from community physicians who ultimately became participants in the network.

Whichever form the networks took, participating organizations viewed the effort required to write the application and organize the network as a good investment. Each application had to indicate the potential for the program to continue after the contract terminated. Thus, each applicant had to consider from the outset how it would use the network resources to establish and maintain long-term influence over state-of-the-art delivery in their regions, and through this influence establish a regional cancer control program. There were clear differences in the orientation of the interpersonal and interorganizational networks regarding how they expected to continue their programs after funding ended. These differences influenced how each stage of the innovation diffusion process was initiated.

Interpersonal Networks

The primary objective of the interpersonal networks was to promote the visibility of the headquarters unit as the tertiary referral facility for all head and neck patients in the network service region. From the earliest planning stages, this underlying objective affected the implementation of programs in these networks. As a result, two distinctive features were common to both interpersonal networks. These were (1) the manner in which the innovation was introduced to the target population, and (2) the way the networks defined their target audiences and established linkages for diffusion.

As described in Chapter 5, boundary management and resource allocation were ways in which the networks manipulated their environments to achieve diffusion. In the interpersonal networks most network resources were centralized at headquarters, where they were used exclusively for education and demonstration programs. In addition, educational endeavors were a means of introducing the innovation to community physicians, who were then invited to observe demonstrations at the headquarters institutions. However, no resources were exchanged to implement the innovation in the community. It was expected that community practitioners who identified cases would refer them to the headquarters.

Consistent with that expectation, most of the pilot or demonstration activities the interpersonal networks initiated were intended to strengthen some aspect of the headquarters facility to make it a more attractive referral site. Thus, facilities or services that were added to the headquarters unit were in most cases related to pretreatment or rehabilitation. For example, the Arkansas network hired a maxillofacial prosthodontist and a medical illustrator to design facial prostheses. In addition, a nurse, a speech therapist, and a social worker were added to the headquarters staff. The nurse was assigned to coordinate the pretreatment conferences held at the University of Arkansas and at the central radiation therapy facility in Little Rock.

Both headquarters units of the Eastern Great Lakes network established demonstration programs related to nontreatment aspects of management. At SUNYAB, these programs included a dental clinic at which screening for head and neck cancers, pretreatment dental management, and postoperative care were carried out. Student hygienists rotated through the clinic and received practical training in conducting oral examinations. A nurse was employed and assigned responsibility for coordinating pretreatment conferences at the surgical center. Two programs were initiated that employed social workers to coordinate social support for patients and their families.

At the Roswell Park Memorial Institute two demonstration programs in nursing and rehabilitation were initiated. The major effort in nursing was to develop patient care booklets describing various aspects of self-care following surgery. Eleven booklets were produced and circulated locally and nationally. A second rehabilitation demonstration focused on experimental surgical reconstruction of the larynx, and organized swallowing clinics for patients recovering from the surgical removal of all or part of the tongue.

The interpersonal networks also created knowledge and awareness among community health professionals through boundary manipulation to recruit members. Recall that in Chapter 5 we noted that interpersonal networks defined their boundaries very loosely and their audiences very broadly. To understand how they implemented their programs the process of boundary definition requires further consideration. For example, as described in Chapter 5, membership criteria were inclusive rather than exclusive. Few demands were made of recruited members, because the purpose of recruitment was to stimulate them to participate in network programs and to refer patients to the headquarters for treatment. Lists of members were compiled mainly for promoting participation in network educational and demonstration programs such as symposia, clinics, special demonstrations, or community outreach programs. No resources were distributed to members directly for the purpose of implementing programs at their own institutions, so no specific contractual requirements had to be initiated.

The interpersonal networks also used collaborative efforts between the headquarters and other nonmedical community organizations to stimulate knowledge and awareness of the availability of multidisciplinary patient management strategies among community physicians. Programs were initiated with local units of the American Cancer Society; with professional associations like the local dental and medical societies, hygienists association, and nursing and pathological societies; and with service or quasi-service organizations like the Junior League in Little Rock or the Regional Medical Program in Buffalo, New York. These organizations provided both facilities and membership lists. They offered contacts that could be used to promote the network programs to the target audiences. Through these contacts they helped the headquarters create community outreach networks that enhanced their objectives in cancer control.

As an example of collaboration with community organizations, the Eastern

Great Lakes Network and the Erie County Dental Society sponsored local exhibits at the county fair and a special oral health education week during the winter. The theme of these programs was "Meet Your Mouth," and they featured public education activities and screening clinics. Initially, the network implemented and supported these programs, but as the dental society became more involved and committed to the program, it eventually took them over. In Arkansas, the dental society and the public health nurses' association also participated in similar types of programs and eventually assumed some responsibility for their conduct.

To summarize, the knowledge/awareness phase of the innovation diffusion process in interpersonal networks focused on boundary expansion and on the development of demonstrations of specific innovative aspects of patient management at the headquarters. Boundary-expansion activities included recruitment of community professionals and establishing linkages with community organizations to obtain resources that could be used in reaching the targeted community professional.

Interorganizational Networks

The knowledge/awareness phase in the interorganizational networks was already under way when the contracts for planning the networks were awarded. As we have noted, in most networks it began with preparation of the response to the request for proposals. In some others the linkages between headquarters and the community hospitals preceded the program announcement and were the result of prior innovation diffusion activities. Most of the network principal investigators were recognized leaders in the management of head and neck cancer. Where the links were preexisting, the main initiating activity was their adaptation to use for diffusion of state-of-the-art patient management strategies. Where they did not preexist, they had to be established expressly for the head and neck program during the initial planning phase.

As with the interpersonal networks, the strategy of boundary definition and manipulation played a key role in the initiation of the diffusion process. However, unlike membership in the interpersonal networks, membership carried with it specific expectations and an explicit commitment of resources to the program. Thus, as was shown in the preceding chapter, membership criteria were key elements in the network building strategy. They incorporated formal procedures, including subcontracts that specified the terms of exchange between headquarters and the community hospitals.

The range of interactions covered by the contracts or memoranda of understanding varied with the network. The extent to which contracts were used tended to be most clearly associated with the extent of preexisting linkages. In general, the most inclusive contracts were employed by the newest networks, Wisconsin and Northern California, where there was little or no prior history of interorganizational cooperation or linkages.

For these two networks the demonstration project provided the opportunity to establish broadly based linkages. In Wisconsin there was no competition for agreements with community hospitals to become affiliated with teaching institutions (as in Illinois). There were only two major medical centers in the state, and they did not compete for patients or domain. In California, the community hospitals did not participate in the network via links with the major medical centers, but related directly to a consortial headquarters, the Northern California Cancer Program. The subcontractual arrangements defined the institutional domains and so limited competition.

In contrast, the preexisting linkages between medical schools and community hospitals in Illinois and the Greater Delaware Valley were so dense that their domains had to be carefully delineated for each new project. Thus, potential network linkages available for the head and neck networks were limited by the preexisting organizational relationships. Participating institutions frequently had links to different institutions for different program areas that were often based on ties with former medical students, reisdents, or fellows who were now practicing in these community hospitals. In Mississippi, no head and neck links with community hospitals were ever established, although there were some preexisting relationships.

A second common feature of the interorganizational networks was their use of educational activities as a means of stimulating knowledge and awareness of network programs. Earlier in this chapter we described the ways the various networks reinvented the concept of multidisciplinary care. The first-year networks, Illinois and Wisconsin, used their educational programs as a way of disseminating the draft guidelines for comment, thus stimulating awareness of the guidelines among community physicians. The second-year networks did not use their educational programs to disseminate the guidelines or to promote community awareness of the content of the innovation. Instead, they incorporated these activities into the pretreatment planning group meetings that were implemented in place of guidelines.

The Wisconsin educational programs were organized and presented through participating network hospitals. They were specifically directed to encourage practitioners in the service region to refer their patients to physicians in the participating community hospitals who were part of the network. The Illinois network offered programs jointly with the Illinois Institute of Family Practice and reached a very large audience through this collaboration. As part of these programs, network physicians distributed the guidelines and conducted presentations about them throughout the state. The actual referral routes were never discussed, probably because of the strong preexisting domains in the region. These were absent in Wisconsin, so referrals could be explicitly discussed and manipulated.

Because a major focus of the Illinois network was rehabilitation, a large percentage of educational programs in Illinois addressed rehabilitation. In fact, this was the single most frequent topic of their educational presentations. The target audiences for these presentations were community physicians with a wide range of specializations and, of course, rehabilitation specialists.

Among the second-year contractors, the educational focus was different, reflecting the way they had reinvented the innovation. Northern California organized extensive educational programs addressed to patient and dental care, rehabilitation, early detection, and screening. Mississippi also addressed its educational programs to the community professional. But these were often nonphysicians who worked in the community and were most likely to be the first to identify patients with suspicious conditions that might require further diagnosis and treatment at the multidisciplinary clinic. In neither Mississippi nor Northern California were educational programs used as channels for diffusing the guidelines, although both emphasized multidisciplinary management and, through pretreatment conferences or similar programs, attempted to communicate what was considered to be state-of-the-art head and neck cancer management.

The Greater Delaware Valley network offered very few educational programs.

Those offered were clearly directed at professionals *within* the network and not at the community professional. They were usually general symposia, covering the entire spectrum of tumors of the head and neck. They generally featured outside speakers knowledgeable about the latest treatment approaches for these cancers. This network focused most of its resources on later phases of the diffusion process because the participating units were already aware of the innovation.

To summarize, the way the interorganizational networks used their educational programs to create knowledge and awareness of the innovation related to how they had reinvented the innovation and their choice of boundary-spanning strategy. Overall, the knowledge/awareness phase of interorganizational innovation diffusion focused on definition of linkages and formalization of membership responsibilities and privileges.

PERSUASION

The second stage of the innovation diffusion process is persuasion. At the individual level, persuasion involves convincing the target audience that they should try the innovation. At the organizational level, persuasion includes legitimizing the innovation and establishing a rationale for its incorporation into the organization's operating procedures. It also implies a commitment of some level of organizational resources. Whether diffusion occurs at the personal or organizational level, it occurs between individuals. Persuasion, more than any other phase in the innovation diffusion process, depends upon interpersonal contacts. However, it is also heavily dependent upon the use of data to document the efficacy of the innovation. Interpersonal contacts are used to reinforce the relevance of the data for the particular problem.

Data Collection: The Protocol as a Vehicle for Diffusion

Data collection was a special requirement for all of the networks. It was viewed in the early planning stages as the means to evaluate the program. In terms of the diffusion model, data on performance, which we define here as the effects of the innovative treatment strategy, would be used in the persuasion stage of the diffusion process. We have indicated elsewhere in this book that a limitation of the project was the absence of prior clinical trials data or other unambiguous data to support the concepts of multidisciplinary care. Thus, evaluation was considered to be an important component of the network demonstration program. The data-collection activity in the diffusion process also served in some instances as a way of focusing interpersonal contact on the efficacy of multidisciplinary treatment.

The request for proposals issued by the NCI required each network to develop specific plans for data collection, management, and analysis, including an assessment of current community practice in managing head and neck cancer patients. As with the guidelines, there was no contractual requirement that all networks collect the same data. Each contract required an evaluation and data collection plan by the end of the first year and the capability to collect data on 200 new cases each year.

At the time when the first-year contractors met to develop common guidelines, they also agreed on common data items and decided to develop a common set of data-collection forms that would parallel the guidelines and be useful as a protocol for assessing compliance with them. A common staging procedure (TNM, or Tumor, Number of Nodes, Metastasis), developed by the American Joint Committee for Cancer Staging and End Results Reporting to categorize how advanced and widespread tumors were at the time of detection, was also adopted. Pathologists affiliated with the networks worked with this system to ensure common staging of head and neck cancer patients prior to treatment. This staging system was to be incorporated into the data forms that were being developed.

When the proposed data forms were circulated for review the three original contractors could not agree on a common form. Ultimately, four different data-collection forms were adopted by the three first-year groups (the two headquarters units at the Eastern Great Lakes network adopted different forms). The diversity of data-collection forms increased when the second-year contracts were awarded. Arkansas and Greater Delaware Valley adopted forms similar to the one being used in Illinois. Mississippi devised an entirely different form based on the registry at the University of Mississippi, but because of its premature termination, Mississippi never collected data. Northern California decided to link its data-collection activity to the ongoing, established, population-based registry in northern California. By so doing, California not only adopted a different data-collection form and strategy but also employed staging criteria that were totally incompatible with those being used by the other networks.

From the standpoint of the diffusion process, such incompatibility was a logical outcome of the process of reinvention that was ongoing during the early contract years. The priority assigned to data collection as part of each network's agenda was reflected in the willingness of the network to commit resources and integrate data collection into its overall program. Where the guidelines were adopted as the primary vehicle for diffusion of the concepts related to state-of-the-art, multi-disciplinary patient care, data collection was accorded a high priority and efforts were made to collect data consistent with other networks. This was the case in Wisconsin, Illinois, and Eastern Great Lakes.

In Wisconsin the data-collection form was actually used as a protocol to guide implementation of the guidelines. Thus, among the interorganizational networks it represents the clearest model of the use of data as a vehicle for persuasion. Community physicians were contractually required to complete the data forms and return them to headquarters, where they were reviewed by the network principal investigator (an otolaryngologist), a radiation therapist, and a pathologist for completeness and conformity with the guidelines. Monthly meetings were held with these community physicians during which the principal investigator reviewed any variations from the guidelines that were evident. Attendance at these meetings was also contractually required.

In Illinois data collection was also contractually required. Unlike Wisconsin, however, the physician was not required to complete the form, and in fact, substantial network funding was allocated to support data-collection staff. The objective in Illinois was to establish a common data base that could be used for publications. The headquarters unit responsible for data management and quality control also had the objective of establishing a multipurpose data center. Because the data-collection activity was not linked to the diffusion activity, contracts were extended to more hospitals than could be supported with the funds available. Hence, the quality of the data declined as the amount of data obtained increased, although the data ultimately were used for publications.

The rehabilitation professionals in Illinois did use data collection as a protocol for persuading institutions to establish uniform rehabilitation procedures. A short form was locally developed, and the rehabilitation staff voluntarily completed the form on all patients that were treated and/or referred. The data were reviewed by the rehabilitation coordinator for the network, and feedback was provided to the network professionals.

Eastern Great Lakes was an interpersonal network. The data-collection strategies there focused on documenting the use of multidisciplinary patient management, and both headquarters units established elaborate computer programs to content-analyze the data collected. However, because this was an interpersonal network, data collection was carried out only at the headquarters units; hence, the data collection did not advance the diffusion process beyond headquarters.

Among the second-year contractors data collection had a much more variable set of objectives. In Northern California, data collection was linked to an elaborate evaluation plan. However, as we have already noted, the data obtained were incompatible with those obtained by the other networks. Thus, the evaluation was limited in generality. Also, Mississippi never collected data, and the Greater Delaware Valley network complied with the data-collection mandate in their contract, but data collection had no other purpose and therefore was given low priority.

Although Arkansas was an interpersonal network, the principal investigator used the data form as a protocol for communicating to community physicians his assessment of how they were managing their patients. Much like Wisconsin and the rehabilitation specialists in Illinois, data collection was combined with interpersonal communication as a tool for persuading the community physicians of the importance of the application of multidisciplinary treatment strategies. Data were collected from the offices of physician participants by abstractors hired by the network. The principal investigator then reviewed these data and communicated to the physicians either by telephone or through the network newsletter, where he had a column that discussed various problems encountered in the management of head and neck patients. Through this mechanism he was able to expand his referral network and his influence on the management of these patients.

Educational Programs in Interpersonal Networks

While both the interpersonal and interorganizational networks used educational strategies to persuade the targeted professionals in the community to adopt multidisciplinary management procedures for head and neck cancer, their objectives differed because adoption of multidisciplinary treatment meant different things in each network form. For the interorganizational networks it implied diffusion of technology to community hospitals; for the interpersonal networks it implied referral of patients to the headquarters. As we have already indicated, when the diffusion channel was interpersonal, creating awareness of the facilities available at the headquarters was an essential first step in getting the patients into the appropriate treatment setting. Thus, the interpersonal networks had to emphasize programs addressed to these primary care sources who by virtue of their positions in the health care delivery system were the first to see the head and neck patient. Second, these programs had to convince the community physicians that there was a limit to what could be done in the community without referral to the headquarters.

Because of these concerns, educational programs sponsored by the interpersonal networks focused on programs for the community professionals who could most effectively implement early detection and screening procedures. Among those targeted were dentists and hygienists, who were most likely to see an early lesion as part of their routine work activities. Both the Eastern Great Lakes and Arkansas networks organized educational programs for dentists and dental hygienists. These programs had both in-service and student components. For in-service training of community dentists, we have already described how the SUNYAB component of the Eastern Great Lakes network cooperated with the Erie County dental society to help train dentists in detection. This in-service program was introduced as part of a larger cooperative program of public health education aimed at promoting community awareness of head and neck cancer. They also worked with the School of Dentistry at SUNYAB and incorporated a segment in which dental students were rotated through the oral pathology laboratory and given a special course in identifying suspicious and potentially cancerous oral lesions.

Arkansas paid special attention to the public health nurse, who had frequent contacts with the largely rural poor population that might be at risk for head and neck cancer. In cooperation with the state health department, special training programs were initiated. These programs included a required rotation of all public health nurses through the head and neck clinic at the University of Arkansas Medical Center. The program emphasized the need for multidisciplinary planning for the management of head and neck cancer.

We have indicated that the interpersonal networks did not attempt to diffuse the actual multidisciplinary management strategy to the community hospital. However, they did interact with community hospitals as part of the diffusion process. Characteristically, that interaction occurred through in-service educational programs in which staff from the networks traveled to community hospitals to present rounds or other educational programs. These programs had the purpose of persuading the hospital staff of the need to refer these patients to the tertiary center for treatment. In addition these programs frequently resulted in lasting interpersonal relationships between the community hospital staff and staff from the network. In both networks the primary targets of these programs were the nursing staff, although network physicians attended and interacted with the house staff. In Arkansas, in-service programs were also conducted for rehabilitation staff in the community hospitals.

As part of sustaining those interpersonal linkages, both networks established telephone "hot-line" services that enabled community professionals to obtain telephone consults with the staff at the tertiary hospitals. Although incomplete records were kept, it appears that as many as two or three calls per week may have been placed to the headquarters staff at each network.

Another effort to stimulate interpersonal persuasive contacts was through the publication of network newsletters. The newsletters publicized the hotline and also attempted to communicate the elements of the innovation to the community physicians. Of the two, the Eastern Great Lakes network newsletter was more formal. Its content mainly included information about the activities of the network, such as symposia, demonstration activities at headquarters, and, after it was formed, news about the Eastern Great Lakes Head and Neck Oncology Association, which was organized to maintain liaison with physicians in the region who treated head and neck cancer after contract funding ended.

The Arkansas network's newsletter was more in the nature of a personal communication between the network principal investigator and the community physicians. It contained a regular column by the principal investigator that addressed common errors made in managing head and neck patients. These columns paralleled similar sections of the written guidelines. The material for these columns and for other articles in the newsletter frequently came from data that had been abstracted from the records of the community physicians who participated in the network data program. Thus, through the relative anonymity of the newsletter the principal investigator could communicate with the community physicians on the basis of information about their patients.

A major difference between the Arkansas and Eastern Great Lakes networks was use of the data. The Eastern Great Lakes network did not collect data from their members. No network resources were allocated to obtain data from community physicians, although they were welcome to submit data if they were abstracted according to the data-collection format contained in the guidelines. In contrast, the principal investigator at the Arkansas network spent considerable resources and energy collecting case data from community physicians. Members of the Arkansas network were individual physicians and they were expected to contribute data to the network data base. These data were usually abstracted by network staff.

The Arkansas principal investigator regularly reviewed these data and used them in several ways. As noted, they were used for his column in the newsletter. Sometimes the principal investigator communicated directly with a physician about a patient who appeared to have been mismanaged, given the patient's record. This was done very subtly to avoid offending the physician. In whatever way it was used, the data form provided a highly personalized link between the principal investigator and the community physicians who participated in the network.

The persuasive efforts of the two interpersonal networks were similar in their approaches to the nonphysician community professionals. Both networks recognized that their link with the patient would often be through the dentist, hygienist, nurse, or other health care professional who might see a patient with a suspicious lesion before any physician did. The advice these professionals gave the patient was clearly recognized as significant in determining how the patient would be treated and whether he or she would receive state-of-the-art care.

However, the two interpersonal networks differed in the way each related to community physicians. Their approaches reflected basic differences in how the innovation was defined and, more precisely, whether the guidelines were regarded as the primary vehicle for diffusing the innovation. The Eastern Great Lakes network relied heavily on the guidelines and interacted with community physicians through programs that were didactic and required only a passive response by the community physician. Although the Eastern Great Lakes Head and Neck Oncology Society was organized to promote professional interaction, few community physicians joined, and participation was light among those that did. Didactic lectures and offers to provide telephone consultation did not stimulate direct interaction between the network physicians and the community doctors. Even the newsletter reflected the general distance between the network and community physicians.

In contrast, the Arkansas principal investigator more actively involved local physicians in network programs and, through his personal contacts, attempted to influence how they managed their head and neck cancer patients. Consistent with the approach of all the second-year contractors, the concepts of the innovation were defined through the interpersonal contacts between the PI and the local physicians. Discussion of patient management strategies was occasioned by the use of the data form, the newsletter, the telephone conference, and pretreatment conferences at the radiation therapy facility. Regular attendance at the state oncology society meetings afforded additional opportunities for persuasion through interpersonal contact.

Persuasion in Interorganizational Networks

Persuasion in the interorganizational networks occurred through interpersonal linkages between headquarters staff and professionals in the participating hospitals. Although the interorganizational networks attempted to reach the community-based professionals such as dentists, hygienists, nurses, and rehabilitation specialists, the effort was frequently initiated by community hospitals within the network and was directed at promoting diffusion by stimulating referrals from community professionals to the community hospitals that were part of the network rather than directly to headquarters. In Wisconsin, for example, the educational programs aimed at early detection were sponsored by the network hospitals and encouraged dentists and others to refer suspicious lesions to these community hospitals rather than to the headquarters.

However, the links that received most attention were those between the physician, and in some cases between rehabilitation personnel, located in the headquarters and participating network hospitals. These links, developed during the knowledge/awareness phase of the diffusion process, were often in place before the network contracts were awarded. The contracts formalized these preexisting links and usually incorporated some formal expectations regarding what was to be exchanged. These formal ties provided structure to the persuasion process that was not present in the interpersonal networks. In effect, the formal nature of the links legitimized the persuasive activities within the organizational context.

As with the interpersonal networks, there were marked differences between the first- and second-year contractors regarding use of the guidelines as the diffusion channel. In Wisconsin and Illinois the network activity centered about the guidelines, and, as already described, data collection was used as a tool to monitor guideline compliance. Among the second-year networks, direct contact between the network staff and community physicians in network hospitals defined the innovation and persuaded the community physicians of the importance of multidisciplinary treatment planning. Hence, data collection was not a high priority.

As we have shown, because the Wisconsin and Illinois networks were heavily committed to implementation of the 1977 draft guidelines, they committed network resources to presentation of the guidelines to community physicians and discussing their content with them. Second, these networks attempted to implement and monitor compliance with the guidelines through their data collection activities. Data collection was so central to these networks that it became the major boundary-spanning activity. However, because each network approached data collection differently, its usefulness as a means of persuasion was quite different in the two settings.

In Wisconsin, the principal investigator stimulated interest in the guidelines'

content by involving coinvestigators in the design and development of the guidelines, and by integrating data collection into their ongoing interaction. At regular
monthly meetings drafts of the guidelines were discussed. Moreover, by involving
them in the development of the data form, he obtained their commitment to use it
even when the other networks refused to accept it. Thus, from the outset the
members of the Wisconsin network were committed to the guidelines and to the
data forms.

Wisconsin illustrates clearly the interplay between the formal and informal
elements of the network communication process. Persuasion occurred through
both components. First, there was strong commitment by key network staff, including the principal investigator, biostatistician, pathologist, radiation therapist,
and coinvestigators to implement the data-collection activity. Participating physicians from the community hospitals in the network agreed to code the staging
information themselves, using the TNM staging procedures, and to instruct the
data coordinators in the use of TNM staging criteria at their monthly meetings. The
headquarters team regularly reviewed the completed forms. Forms that were incor-
rect or incomplete were returned to the coinvestigator for correction.

The contracts provided the formal support for this interaction. If the forms
were not being completed correctly or in a timely fashion, the principal investigator
could and did confront the recalcitrant participant and, through a combination of
moral suasion and threats to terminate the contract, could obtain their renewed
cooperation. The fact that the principal investigator could do this without damag-
ing the basic network linkages indicated the strength of his personal ties to the
participants and his persuasive power.

Beyond the persuasiveness of the principal investigator and the potential
threat of withdrawing the contract, there was among the Wisconsin participants a
commitment to securing quality data. Several meetings were held to plan analyses
based on the data. Papers based on the data were published by the coinvestigators.
Thus, the interactions across organizational boundaries were intense and reciprocal
in Wisconsin. Through the regular contact and common commitment, strong interpersonal bonds developed. Behind those bonds was the force of the formal contract, which was invoked when the underlying agreements on which the network
was based were not being observed. The relationships were reciprocal, and the
coinvestigators had real input into network policy. These arrangements gave legitimacy to the network activities that facilitated diffusion.

In Illinois, contractual relationships also established that data would be collected systematically in exchange for network resources. However, the participating clinicians in the Illinois network were not directly involved in the formulation of
the network guidelines and data forms. Because of the size of the Illinois network,
meetings such as those held in Wisconsin were impractical. A governing board
composed of representatives from the headquarters and representatives from the
newly formed comprehensive cancer center was responsible for setting policy and
directing the ongoing activities of the network. After the formal contracts were
negotiated, data collection was carried out by network staff. The network physicians did not play a direct role in the process of data collection, and the data were
not directly used in network activities. Thus, while considerable investment was
made in data collection, and it could not have happened without the consent of the
coinvestigators, it was not a boundary-spanning activity in the same sense as we

observed in Wisconsin. Moreover, there was little direct involvement by the physicians in other aspects of the network activity. They were not involved in setting policy or in deciding how the data would be used. As a result, persuasive contacts did not arise through the boundary-spanning activities of the network, as it did in Wisconsin.

Boundary interaction among the rehabilitation specialists in Illinois more closely reflected the process of collective innovation diffusion observed among the physicians in Wisconsin. The interaction associated with the rehabilitation activities of the network provided a high degree of legitimation for implementing state-of-the-art rehabilitation procedures. These interactions took place around the development and implementation of a regional rehabilitation program for head and neck cancer patients. Initiated during the planning year, these interactions evolved when the rehabilitation coordinator at one headquarters unit developed a rehabilitation team and offered to provide consulting services to meet the NCI rehabilitation requirement for the entire network. Minimal data were collected to document the level of service provided. It soon became clear that this single team could not meet the great demand for rehabilitation services within the network. As a result, teams were established at other headquarters institutions and at several of the community hospitals. Overall, the impact of these links was quite dramatic, and consequently, rehabilitation patterns were altered in the region. Eventually these teams were supported from local patient funding and became integral components of head and neck care in the region.

The successful second-year interorganizational networks, Northern California and Greater Delaware Valley, sought to exert persuasion through the pretreatment conferences established in community settings. These conferences were designed to persuade community physicians of the importance and legitimacy of the multidisciplinary approach to patient care. The way these conferences were organized and the role of headquarters staff in their implementation varied largely because of the projected role of network linkages in the long-range plans of the two networks that implemented this strategy.

The agenda of the Northern California network was to implement an interorganizational framework that became a regional comprehensive cancer center and cancer control program. A preliminary concern was to formally define the domain of each major participant and, through this formalization, ensure that no single unit could use the network to achieve dominance over the others. This was accomplished through a series of subcontracts that governed the distribution of network resources in a way that allowed local physicians to retain control over the management of their patients and yet benefit from interaction with the university-based network staff.

The primary contracts supported implementation of pretreatment conferences. In some cases, these were located in teaching hospitals. In others, local groups formed the conferences under contract with the network. In either case, the concept was to develop community-based planning groups that would establish their own format but would follow a common protocol for discussing patients. Eventually, five conferences were formed, two at academic medical centers and three in community hospitals. In addition to following a common protocol, the contracts required documentation of attendance and the procedures followed at each conference. Data were compiled on all conferences, and reports based on the data detailed the frequency with which they were held, attendance, number of patients presented, and recommendations for treatment. Thus, underlying the program was a common format and data were obtained to document performance. Although the content was flexible, the process by which the innovation was introduced basically followed a standardized plan.

Unlike Wisconsin and Arkansas, there was no single individual who played a central role in the Northern California network. The principal investigator was responsible for administrative and general programmatic activities but not for the diffusion of the basic concepts. This was performed by several members who served as conveners of the pretreatment conferences. These were usually well-established local physicians in each region. The conferences were supported by network staff. Three maxillofacial prosthodontists supplied the rehabilitation input to the pretreatment planning conferences, and one of them attended each conference.

Boundary exchange and persuasion occurred when physicians presented their patients at the pretreatment planning conferences for review and discussion. At each conference, various management strategies might be presented and discussed by those attending. The team would then submit their final recommendations to the referring physician in writing, but the referring physician made the final decision about the treatment strategy to be employed. Thus, as with Wisconsin and Arkansas, the community physicians had input into the process by which the innovation was defined and were able to ensure that their input was taken into account in the final treatment recommendations. Because there was no official answer and the physician was not bound to accept the recommendations of the planning conference, professional autonomy was preserved.

Like the Northern California network, the Greater Delaware Valley network departed from common guidelines in favor of a more flexible approach that took into account local treatment preferences. A multidisciplinary protocol was developed and then supplemented with specific protocols for maxillofacial prosthetics, psychosocial counseling, and speech and audiology therapy. These protocols were implemented through network-supported pretreatment planning conferences.

The Greater Delaware Valley pretreatment conferences were located in community hospitals and coordinated by a nurse or social worker hired with network funds. Although the reports do not specifically indicate, given the history and general focus of this network, these head and neck conferences were undoubtedly conducted as part of general radiation therapy planning conferences. Thus, legitimacy for such innovation already existed.

In summary, persuasion occurred through exchanges across organizational boundaries. These boundary exchanges took several forms. Among the first-year contractors, persuasion activities were based on the guidelines that were used as protocols. These formed the basis for various types of educational activities that were introduced into the community as a way of expanding on the information contained in the guidelines. In some instances, data collection was used as a second persuasive tool within the network to communicate to the community physicians the meaning of multidisciplinary management. In other cases, the headquarters institution developed specific protocols for the pretreatment conferences. These addressed issues of general patient management and the specific treatment strategies recommended for each site. In addition, there were often regular meetings of

Table 7.1. Summary of Network Diffusion Strategies

Network	Definition of innovation	Knowledge/awareness building	Persuasion
1st-year contracts			
Eastern Great Lakes	Management guidelines	Passive boundary expansion Demonstrations of techniques	Didactic seminars Data collection at HQ only
Illinois	Management guidelines	Educational programs	Data collection Rehabilitation teams
Wisconsin	Management guidelines	Boundary expansion through contracts Educational programs	Data collection to foster guideline implementation Personal contacts of PI
2nd-year contracts			
Arkansas	Pretreatment planning conferences	Boundary expansion through PI contacts Demonstrations of techniques	Data collection to foster guideline implementation Personal contacts of PI
Greater Delaware Valley	Pretreatment planning conferences	Cloning of previous RT network	Minimal data collection Cloning of RT planning conferences
Mississippi	Multidisciplinary clinic	Non-MD educational programs	No data collection Network failure
Northern California	Pretreatment planning conferences	Subcontracts	Data collection for evaluation
	Non-MD educational programs		Pretreatment conferences with customized format

key network staff both at headquarters and at network hospitals where further treatment planning took place, and which were designed to further persuade key network staff of the importance of this approach.

Finally, the differences between Mississippi and the other networks were both structural and environmental. The environment of the Mississippi network did not allow for the development of linkages that would permit diffusion. They were not in place prior to the network contract and could not be put into place afterwards. Structurally, the network leadership did not appear to have the support of the key staff within the headquarters institution and could not make commitments that would remain in force, even in response to community pressure. The result was failure of the network. It was unable to get beyond the knowledge/awareness phase.

SUMMARY

Table 7.1 provides a summary of the various strategies used by the networks from definition of the innovation through persuasion. Clearly, how each of the networks chose to define the innovation was dependent upon local contingencies and the extent to which the network PIs were involved (and invested) in producing the management guidelines. Then, at the knowledge/persuasion stage, choice of strategy was influenced both by the definition adopted by the network and by the form of the diffusion network as either interpersonal or interorganizational. At this stage, the two interpersonal networks (Eastern Great Lakes and Arkansas) had more in common than did the three first-year contracts. Then again at the persuasion stage, the choice of innovation definition comes into play once more, as the use of data collection as a boundary-management technique and control strategy is quite evident in both Illinois and Wisconsin. It was also used in Arkansas, combined with the personal contacts of the PI, to persuade and teach network physicians appropriate management principles, even though the guidelines were not openly endorsed by the PI.

In general, the first-year networks were located in fairly rich environments (or, for the Eastern Great Lakes region, what resources existed were concentrated among the headquarters institutions), so that much of the guideline content could be tried without major investment by the practitioner or the practitioner's hospital. These PIs worked together to develop the guidelines, and undoubtedly their network strategies were somewhat influenced by pride of authorship. The second-year network programs did not share their enthusiasm for the guidelines, and there was much more variation both within and across these networks in resources needed to implement the guidelines' content. For these second-year units, the pretreatment planning conference was preferable as a diffusion strategy, in that it brought community physicians into direct contact with headquarters staff and facilities. And, given the preference of the second-year networks for customized pretreatment conferences, it is not surprising that data collection played a minimal role at the persuasion stage in most of these networks.

8

Network Outcomes
Transformation, Survival, and Institutionalization

INTRODUCTION

In Chapter 1 we briefly discussed the problems associated with evaluating network performance, and we have now reached the point where performance must be considered in some detail. We have approached this analysis assuming a contingency relationship involving context, structure, and (implicitly) performance outcomes. Following this framework we have explored how the networks reinvented the innovation and defined its content to meet the constraints and opportunities present in their particular organizational settings. We then showed how the networks adopted various diffusion strategies appropriate to their environments and consistent with the agenda of the funding agency that provided the necessary resources.

In Chapter 3 we discussed the perceptions of "performance gap" at varying levels of organization and showed how the environment of each network influenced first these perceptions and then the agenda that followed. In this chapter we will examine outcome/performance data in the context of the agenda and performance deficits identified by the networks.

As the title of this chapter suggests, we see network outcomes as related to three issues: transformation, institutionalization, and survival. In Chapter 6 we considered how the individual participating hospitals related the meaning and content of the innovation to their own core activities, and how that influenced their participation in key aspects of the diffusion process. In Chapter 7 we discussed how the innovation content and diffusion strategies were reinvented to accommodate the network environments and yet be consistent with the different agendas set by the funding agency and the networks. This reinvention process was the beginning of what we refer to here as transformation. Following contingency theory, we will consider transformation both in the organization of the networks and in the environment. In examining transformation, we will ask several questions: (1) Was the environment changed by the presence of the network? (2) How was the network organization transformed after funding terminated? (3) What effects did that transformation have on network survival? And finally, (4) how was organizational transformation affected by the environment?

In this final chapter we will consider how the various networks routinized different components of the demonstration program, and how these routinized elements became institutionalized as part of other regional cancer programs. In those instances where the network became part of a regional cancer program the network structure survived, although in each case the form of the network changed and programmatic emphases were expanded. Where this expansion did not occur, it was usually because other, stronger network links were present that constrained how the network survived after the program ended. Each of these patterns was evident in the six networks that completed the program.

The outcomes of this program were not limited to either the organizational or regional levels of analysis. The networks had discernable implications at the national level that are evident in subsequent programs sponsored by the National Cancer Institute. The discussion of transformation, institutionalization, and survival would be incomplete if we did not consider the impact that this program had on subsequent efforts to transmit state-of-the-art treatment approaches to community physicians. In many ways, these national level outcomes represent the most dramatic effects of the network program.

THE NATURE OF THE ORGANIZATION AND ORGANIZATIONAL EFFECTIVENESS

In a recent review of assessing performance in health care organizations, Scott and Shortell (1983) summarized both conceptual and measurement issues that must be resolved before performance evaluations can be done. All of the issues are relevant to the task at hand. Included among the conceptual questions are these: (1) What is the nature of the organization? (2) Which constituency should be used as the referent for assessments of performance? (3) At what level of analysis should performance assessments be made? (4) How does time enter into the analysis of performance? Finally, the measurement issue concerns choosing among measures of performance process, structure, or outcome.

Other authors have warned, however, that different conceptualizations and measures of performance may not necessarily correlate in any particular performance assessment (Kanter & Brinkerhoff, 1981; Scott, 1977; Steers, 1975). The absence of correlation should not be too surprising, however, given possible variations in the nature of organizations, relevant constituencies involved in performance assessments, various levels of analysis possible, and the absence of a single time frame within which the evaluation occurs. We have argued all along that network form and context affects agenda and outcome. Just looking at the varying constituencies and their agendas, each of which might influence the evaluation of these network projects, also illustrates this point.

As shown in Chapters 3 and 6, the agendas formulated by the network participants resulted from the headquarters' perceptions of performance gaps in acquiring the patients needed for training and research. The community hospitals' agendas resulted from perceived limitations in providing modern treatment facilities for newly trained physicians. Thus, the agenda for the participants focused on either altering referral relationships or establishing the necessary resource base for implementing regional cancer control programs. The agenda set forth by the National Cancer Institute, however, resulted from perceived performance deficits in the delivery of state-of-the-art care to patients treated in community hospitals. The NCI's agenda was then to ensure greater uniformity in treatment and community access to state-of-the-art treatment. A second agenda was to establish a regional cancer control program.

While these agendas are certainly not identical, they are also not incompatible. But they do set different priorities for action, and without some specification of priority, one could easily arrive at different assessments of performance. In short, what might appear to be a high performance outcome according to one set of priorities would represent merely adequate performance against another criterion.

At first glance it may seem sensible to try and assess just what, if anything, the network projects accomplished with five years of federal support. Unfortunately, a direct assessment of accomplishments may not produce a straightforward answer. Achievement of network goals, performance of networks activities, and meeting the objectives set forth by the funding agency are all slightly different definitions of network accomplishment, which, however defined, cannot be directly assessed.

The very availability, and certainly the quality, of measures necessary for conducting an evaluation depends upon the agenda set within or between organizations. To illustrate this point, let us look again at data collection by the networks. The Wisconsin network used data-collection forms for communicating the guideline content to participating community physicians. Other networks also had agendas that required data. Arkansas used data to guide physician behavior and thus collected data necessary for this task. The form and quality of data required in Arkansas and Wisconsin differed, however, because the agenda differed. In Wisconsin a complete data set was important, and priority was given to collecting data on every patient in each participating hospital. In Arkansas the data were used to counsel individual physicians. Although data collection was carefully done in Arkansas, completeness was less important than finding good clinical material. Northern California also had plans for their data, but transmission of the guideline content was not among those plans. Accordingly, the Northern California format for data collection did not have to resemble a clinical protocol. Since this network intended to use a state tumor registry, selected data items were designed to be compatible with that plan.

Even within networks the data obtained reflected differences in agendas among various constituencies. In Illinois the physicians collected data for research and publication. The rehabilitation specialists used data collection as a protocol similar to the way it was used in Wisconsin. Because each group had a different agenda, the form and method of data collection varied between the two groups. Thus, the collection of performance data is itself a political process (Kanter & Brinkerhoff, 1981). Even for a single network project, analyses will not necessarily yield a consistent picture. For this to occur, the goals of the project have to be clearly specified and data collection and quality control managed by nonpolitical, objective actors, such as might be found in an independent data center.

Finally, in assessing organizational performance it is necessary to clarify what is meant by performance. Organizational performance refers in general to the analysis of how the organization is doing. Specifically: Is the job getting done? Is is getting done well? Or poorly? To answer whether the job is getting done usually invokes the issue of effectiveness or the degree to which organizational goals are being met. Whether or not the goals are clear or commonly shared by various organizational members are, of course, equally important questions that usually need to be answered before making this determination. The issue of quality—that is, whether the organization is performing well or poorly—involves assessment of both effectiveness and efficiency but depends more heavily on the latter. Efficiency is the ratio of outputs to inputs or the cost of producing the organization's product or service. Effectiveness and efficiency are not interchangeable but they are frequently interrelated. An effective organization does not have to be efficient or highly productive, and conversely, an efficient organization does not have to be effective.

In the health care sector there have been increasing calls for cost-effective delivery of services, which means we want the job to get done (meet health care goals), and we want it done efficiently (at lowest cost). Unfortunately, both effectiveness and efficiency present their own particular measurement problems for health care organizations. What exactly are the goals (effectiveness problem)? What exactly are the units of output (efficiency problem)? When the two are combined into one composite measure (cost effectiveness), the measurement problems are more than doubled. Efficiency, productivity, and cost effectiveness are usually easier to ascertain in non-human-service sectors, where profitability is clearly the "bottom line." The organizations that have been the subjects in this study are human-service organizations, and as such, profitability has not traditionally been the "bottom line." Moreover, since these networks were formed to test an innovation using slack funds provided by the federal government, efficiency is not as relevant an issue as effectiveness.

In this study of the head and neck cancer demonstration networks, we would at least like to get a good handle on levels of effectiveness. We can think about efficiency later. Nonetheless, even assessing effectiveness requires definition of the organization's goals. In the last paragraph we handily rejected one possible set of goals: to make a profit. Determining organizational goals involves just that sort of analysis. However, that analysis depends upon one's conception of the nature of the organization: profit versus not-for-profit, or human service versus manufacturing.

On an even more fundamental level, the analytic approach for assessing organizational performance depends upon the image or understanding of the nature of organizations as complex social structures. Are organizations rationally designed tools to achieve specific purposes, systems intent upon survival, or resource-acquisition systems (Scott, 1987)? The framework we chose for this book (and that has guided our preceding analyses) has consistently emphasized resource dependence and contingency. Thus, our analysis of network performance should include an examination of how successful network actors have been in acquiring scarce resources or perhaps creating more sources of support in the environment, and how the environment constrained that resource-seeking process. Secondarily, the network goal was to establish continuing cancer control programs in the network service regions. The success of this objective must also be assessed.

To some extent, however, we should recognize the fact that network performance among this set of seven networks will probably not vary enormously. As described in Chapter 1, these networks were established through contracts awarded after a competitive proposal review process. Presumably that review process screened out applicants who were less likely to succeed, at least in terms of the goals emphasized by the NCI. Given that screening mechanism, the existence of performance variation on any dimension should be examined closely.

There are other kinds of analyses that would derive from somewhat more mechanistic conceptualizations of network goals. For example, was the innovation disseminated? Did patient treatment change as a result of the network projects? Did head and neck cancer outcomes change as a result of successful/unsuccessful innovation diffusion? Each of these issues could be examined, as well as assessing resource acquisition accomplishments. In considering these issues, however, it must be clear that they represent only the agenda of the funding agency and are less relevant to the agenda set by the networks. Again, different constituencies relevant to the network projects would be more or less likely to accept any one of these issues as a measure of network performance.

Further, reliable and valid data to assess treatment-related outcomes of the network projects are simply not available; they do not exist. The reasons why these data do not exist will be explored in this chapter. Nonetheless, we should forewarn the reader that our most conclusive analyses of network performance relate more to organizational concerns of resource acquisition and environmental contingency than to actual changes in health outcomes or care quality for head and neck cancer patients.

MEASURES OF EFFECTIVENESS

Whether one uses structure, process, or outcome measures of effectiveness will depend to some extent on the perspective one holds on the organization's goals. Structural measures tend to emphasize the organization's potential for effective work. Assuming that the existence of certain structural features or arrangements increases the probability of better performance (e.g., staff qualifications, certifications, number and types of special equipment), the structures themselves can be used as indirect measures of effectiveness. Since structural features of an organization are more likely to be under the control of administrators within the organization rather than any other constituency, structural measures are more likely to be preferred by administrators and managers.

Process measures highlight the actual activities carried out by the organization in the pursuit of goals. Qualities of those activities, such as accuracy, speed, appropriateness, extensiveness (or intensity) of care received, and skill or technical virtuosity are all types of process measures. Within hospitals, process measures such as autopsy rates and nursing and patient chart audits are commonly used. Since process measures emphasize the qualities of the actual performance, these measures tend to be preferred by performers. Performance outcomes are often affected by factors beyond the control of organizational performers, as is the structure within which work is performed. But qualities of the performance process are presumably more within their control.

Lastly, outcome measures are based on changes in characteristics of the work "object," or actual results achieved. In medical care, outcome measures typically focus on mortality, morbidity, and recovery rates. In some sense, outcome measures are more directly related to goal achievement than either structure or process measures, since they focus on results obtained. Client groups (patients) and external review agencies are probably most concerned with performance outcomes and actual results.

These three types of measures also differ in the degree of difficulty each presents for data collection. Structural measures tend to be the most readily available of the three, but they are also the farthest removed from actual performance. Reliable process measures are more difficult to obtain since they require on-site inspection of ongoing performance, or sophisticated record keeping to enable reconstruction of prior performances. Self-reported measures of process are to some extent readily available once the researcher gains entrance and acceptance by organizational members. However, self-report measures (including report documents such as quarterly reports to funding agencies) are subject to obvious bias. Outcome measures are usually the most difficult to obtain since they usually involve sensitive information that most organizations are not willing to divulge for fear of being held accountable for mistakes and/or poor judgment. Hospitals do not routinely release financial data, patient charts are confidential, and schools do not routinely publish standardized exam results. Given this variation in ease of data recovery and political sensitivity, the existence of either reliable process or outcome measures usually involves some amount of effective lobbying or influence by constituencies other than management or administrators. For the head and neck networks, this would probably mean influence over the design of network evaluation mechanisms by someone other than the network PIs and their projects staff.

NETWORK CONSTITUENCIES

Although a multitude of agencies, organizations, and actors were involved in the head and neck cancer networks at one time or another, there were three groups that we would consider most central in planning and implementing the networks. These three groups can be identified by their roles in the diffusion process. The National Cancer Institute, specifically the Division of Cancer Control and Rehabilitation,* was the change agent in the diffusion process. The local influentials or boundary spanners were the academic medical centers that applied for network funding. The community hospitals and physicians were the intended audience for the innovation. As we have shown throughout this book, these three groups differed in many ways, specifically in the degree to which they constituted cohesive interest groups with shared agendas. Of the three, the NCI was the most formally organized and recognized interest group. As shown in Chapter 6, the community hospitals and physicians were the least cohesive group and had the most within-group interest diversity. However, it was also clear in Chapter 7 that the academic groups had varying interests that depended upon the year in which they received

*Now the Division of Cancer Prevention and Control.

their contracts and whether they were organized as interpersonal or interorganizational networks.

Identifying the goals of the NCI for the network program is the most straightforward task. At a general level, using the agenda discussed in Chapter 3, we can also identify the goals of each academic center. However, identifying the goals of the individual member community hospitals and physicians is most problematic and can be done only at the most general level presented in Chapter 6. Nonetheless, we can establish that at the aggregate level each group's goals were different. Thus, their assessments of program outcomes are likely to differ as well.

The Change Agent: The National Cancer Institute

The change agent plays a very important role in innovation diffusion (Rogers, 1983). The change agent is usually positioned outside the social system into which the innovation is to be introduced and is linked to that system by ties to influentials in the social system whose opinions are valued by others in that social system. The change agent often provides key information about the innovation and also special resources that facilitate its diffusion. In this case, those resources took the form of funding from the cancer control program. The Division of Cancer Control and Rehabilitation initiated the network programs to accomplish two goals: (1) to facilitate dissemination of multidisciplinary treatment of head and neck cancer patients in community hospitals, and (2) to establish a cancer control infrastructure on which to build other cancer control initiatives.

Early cancer control outreach programs were loosely patterned after national cooperative research groups, which had been established earlier in the history of the National Cancer Institute, to bring together clinical investigators and to provide access to large numbers of patients for the investigation of new treatments. Although several disciplines were represented in these cooperative groups, the major actors in these national cooperative groups were medical oncologists, and the primary research focus was chemotherapy.

At that time, medical oncology was a relatively new specialization, and few medical oncologists were board-certified. Medical oncologists were regarded with some suspicion by surgeons, who were the major group treating cancer patients since surgery was at that time still the treatment of choice for most solid tumors in adult cancer patients. Also, many surgeons did their own chemotherapy. Medical oncologists typically received patients on referral from surgeons or radiation therapists; hence, the concept of multidisciplinary treatment was well recognized by the oncologists. Other specialists, such as surgeons or radiation therapists, typically either handled the entire therapy themselves or called in other specialists as needed, and usually only after the primary treatment had been delivered. Thus, there were differences in perspective based upon specialization as to the meaning of multidisciplinary care, and these differences affected the outcome of the program. Because the network demonstration projects were based on a model derived from medical oncology, it was expected that there would be multidisciplinary input into treatment planning in the networks. Implementing this was part of the agenda established by the National Cancer Institute.

As we described in Chapter 1, achieving a place for cancer control in the formal, mandated program of the National Cancer Institute was the result of a battle that had been waged over many years (Breslow, 1977). With the passage of the National Cancer Act of 1971, cancer control became a mandated component of the National Cancer Program, and suddenly there were funds allocated and a demand for a program. There was considerable pressure from the public, from Congress, and from the president* to deliver the best available cancer care to the public. Many highly visible public figures supported this initiative. Thus, programs that promised to deliver to the public the results of the research programs of the NCI were in great demand, and the Division of Cancer Control and Rehabilitation was responsible for delivering these programs.

Two network demonstration projects were initiated at this time as part of the congressional mandate for cancer control via the 1971 act. In addition to the head and neck demonstration project, a breast cancer network demonstration program was also established, although the participants were a different group of hospitals. During this same period, the Division of Cancer Control and Rehabilitation also sponsored other cancer control outreach programs that followed a network format, the Cooperative Group Outreach Program (CGOP). The CGOP provided funding to the cooperative clinical research groups to develop linkages between academic hospitals and community hospitals. These linkages made it possible to enter community hospital patients on NCI-approved clinical trials. These programs had the dual purpose of introducing cancer control into established program areas and building links between this newly created division and the centers of academic cancer research.

The second aspect of the NCI goals for the newly established cancer control program was to establish regional cancer control outreach initiatives as part of the comprehensive cancer centers. Thus, the head and neck demonstration networks were part of a broad cancer control initiative. The economic support provided by these programs was directed at the major centers of cancer research in the United States. Clearly, an aspect of the agenda at this time was to legitimize the cancer control program and to defuse the notion that the cancer control dollars would be drawn from funds that supported the main mission of the NCI, which, in the view of academic medicine, was clinical and basic research.

Diffusion of modern treatment out "into the field," i.e., into the community hospital setting where most cancer patients are initially seen, helped advance the second goal of building a cancer control infrastructure. Coincidental with the network demonstration projects, the NCI was also trying to set up regional comprehensive cancer centers across the country. Designation as a comprehensive center could provide both actual and symbolic legitimation to an institution trying to gain dominance as a center for cancer research. Participating in the diffusion of the multidisciplinary treatment concept was an entry point for certification as a comprehensive cancer center. Any institution interested in such certification needed to demonstrate its eligibility through the implementation of such outreach programs. In the development of these comprehensive cancer centers a set of criteria of "comprehensiveness" were devised, and maintaining a cancer control outreach program was one of the criteria specified for review. Without such a program a center could lose its designation and with it access to several sources of funding.

*Recall that the president, Richard Nixon, had made finding a cure for cancer his administration's equivalent to "walking on the moon."

Thus, the NCI had to establish programs that would support cancer control initiatives by the centers. The head and neck cancer and breast cancer networks were early components of the initiatives.

From the NCI's perspective, then, an effective network was one in which multidisciplinary treatment was enacted both within the academic medical center/network headquarters institution and at the community treatment centers in each network region. Data from the case histories of the six networks summarize whether such activity was demonstrated during the networks' project years.

Table 8.1 summarizes five strategies or levels of enactment of the multidisciplinary treatment goals found among the six operative networks (Mississippi excluded). Although these five levels approximate a Guttman scale conceptually, since higher levels presume the incorporation of previous levels, empirically they do not fit that pattern. The "simplest" or least costly strategy was merely to report multidisciplinary treatment as a focus for planning network activities. This was specifically designated as a goal by three of the network programs: Eastern Great Lakes, Wisconsin, and Northern California. All six networks implemented multidisciplinary treatment/planning teams at the headquarters institutions, and all but one network (Northern California) clearly indicated that these headquarters teams were to be used as "models" or examples for other network members to follow. Northern California also proposed a modeling approach, but it was to be done through community-based programs and not at headquarters.

All of the interorganizational networks, Illinois, Wisconsin, Greater Delaware Valley, and Northern California, made some effort to establish and implement multidisciplinary treatment interventions in their network hospitals. How they approached this activity varied and was constrained by the environment. Wisconsin targeted the community hospitals that participated in its network program. Through the network contracts they were required to establish and implement multidisciplinary treatment planning. Data collection in Wisconsin was used to

Table 8.1. Implementation of Multidisciplinary Treatment

Network	1 Primary focus of planning years	2 MD teams operative at HQ	3 HQ teams used as model for network emulation	4 Network funds used to establish teams outside of HQ	5 Network funds used to establish and monitor MD teams throughout network region
Arkansas		X	X		
Eastern Great Lakes	X	X	X		
Wisconsin	X	X	X	X	X
Northern California	X	X		X	
Greater Delaware Valley		X	X		
Illinois		X	X	X (Rehab only)	X (Rehab only)

monitor the implementation of this program, which employed the written guidelines as the protocol. Northern California did it by subcontracting multidisciplinary treatment-planning conferences to community hospitals in the various regions served by its network. Physicians in hospitals in the area drew upon the expertise of the pretreatment planning councils.

The Greater Delaware Valley network was built upon an existing network initially established to ensure uniform standards for radiation therapy in the region. The participating hospitals were encouraged to implement a multidisciplinary treatment strategy, and the headquarters used their contract funding to hire a maxillofacial prosthodontist to provide rehabilitation input to the program. In Illinois the introduction of multidisciplinary treatment was led by the speech pathologist network implemented during the network project. These individuals pushed the physicians to include them in pretreatment planning. Thus, the multidisciplinary strategy was implemented in those hospitals that hired speech pathologists. These tended to be the academic medical centers and larger community hospitals. However, to the extent they received referrals from other hospitals, these speech pathologists were in a position to encourage multidisciplinary treatment planning in other network hospitals.

The interpersonal networks were unable to influence community hospitals that were not part of the headquarters because the appropriate linkages were absent, and the community hospitals were not equipped to adopt the innovation. They tried to implement the innovation by encouraging referral. This was more successful in Arkansas than in Buffalo, in part because Arkansas was more committed to a multidisciplinary approach than was Buffalo, and in part because there were more established linkages between the Arkansas network principal investigator and other local physicians who would be likely to refer. Similar links existed in Buffalo at the SUNYAB component, but they were confined to hospitals that were already part of the headquarters.

From the NCI's perspective, the interorganizational networks came closer to meeting its definition of effectiveness. Wisconsin, Northern California, and Illinois ultimately established comprehensive cancer centers, and the Head and Neck Demonstration Network provided resources for early cancer control initiatives in these regions. The regional approach was most completely developed in Illinois and Northern California, where consortial cancer centers were established following models initiated with the development of the head and neck programs. Wisconsin's center was based at the University of Wisconsin and did not develop as a consortium.

The Greater Delaware Valley Network was constrained by the inability of the various academic centers in Philadelphia to form a consortium such as occurred in Illinois and Northern California. It remained largely a radiation therapy network. Within that constraint, however, it did introduce a protocol for multidisciplinary planning for head and neck cancers, but it did not fulfill the broader aspects of the NCI agenda in that no further cancer control programs were built on the network structure.

The interpersonal networks would probably be judged less successful by the NCI criteria of effectiveness. The Roswell Park Memorial Institute component of the Eastern Great Lakes Network did become a comprehensive cancer center. Educational and epidemiological research were emphasized. These activities built on links established during the demonstration network period, although the direct connection with the head and neck program is difficult to demonstrate from the data available. Little further cancer control programming resulted from the SUN-YAB component, although there is a strong program in preventive medicine with a major emphasis in cancer epidemiology at SUNYAB. However, this program did not link very strongly to the head and neck program.

In Arkansas there are more vestiges of cancer control outreach that may be consistent with the stated goals of the NCI. Through CARTI the headquarters institution continues to influence cancer care in the region. However, no cancer control framework in the form of either a cancer center or other network activities ever emerged.

Boundary Spanners: The Academic Medical Centers

Although official NCI goals were usually given some prominence in official pronouncements, for the academic medical centers and the participating physicians involved there was really only one operative goal. Domain establishment or enhancement as a regional center for cancer research was the primary inducement for nearly all of the participants, except perhaps for the Greater Delaware Valley network and the SUNY Buffalo component of the Eastern Great Lakes network. In the cases of Illinois, Wisconsin, and Northern California, the objective was clearly the implementation of a comprehensive cancer center. For Arkansas, the objective was to build a referral network for the headquarters institution.

The exceptions are of some interest. Recall from Chapter 2 that the Eastern Great Lakes Head and Neck Demonstration Network was the result of a merger of two first-year contracts with the State University of New York at Buffalo (SUNYAB) and Roswell Park Memorial Institute (RPMI). Within the SUNYAB component, community hospitals formed a network that provided residency opportunities for the medical school at SUNYAB. The chief of the otolaryngology service at SUNYAB was the principal investigator and with two associates, also on the faculty at SUN-YAB, did all the head and neck surgery. Thus, they controlled a high percentage of patients treated in the community hospitals, and domain was not an issue. The RPMI component was a free-standing cancer center established and maintained by New York State. It was viewed with suspicion by local physicians and was unable to establish a local network for treatment, although it did (and still does) maintain programs in continuing medical education and public health education aimed at early detection and prevention of cancer in the region. Thus, in effect, there were environmental constraints that limited the potential for domain enhancement and forced this network to focus primarily on public health education and patient referral by dentists.

Environmental constraints also existed in the Greater Delaware Valley network region that limited the extent to which domain enhancement was possible there. Philadelphia, like Chicago and San Francisco, had several major academic medical centers with interests in treating cancers. Two of these centers, the University of Pennsylvania and Fox Chase Cancer Center, decided early in that period to apply for designation and support as comprehensive cancer centers. They were ultimately encouraged to merge and for a while maintained a limited form of consortial arrangement. However, the other medical schools, including Hahnemann Medical School, which was the network headquarters, did not participate in this arrangement. As a result, each medical school maintained separate domains, and these were very well defined and delimited. Because the Greater Delaware Valley Network was built upon an established network of hospitals, little effort was made to expand beyond the radiation therapy field since it was the primary focus of the preexisting network.

Within the context of the network demonstration projects, establishing one's research dominance in the region could take several different paths. As we have seen in previous chapters, a primary path used by nearly all of the networks was to somehow centralize patient referrals in the region, either directly under the control of the headquarters institution, as in Arkansas or the Roswell Park component of the Eastern Great Lakes network, or indirectly through the use of a "neutral" third party, such as the Illinois Cancer Council in Chicago. Another related strategy was to establish a formally accepted definition of each competing institution's "turf," by centrally organizing an institutional division of labor. Network funds were used in a number of regions to set up such divisions of labor, such as in Wisconsin, where contracts between headquarters and member hospitals formalized who was responsible for what activities. In Northern California the contracts differentiated types of programs to be developed by formerly competing centers.

Finally, a somewhat less frequently used strategy for building institutional domain was to establish coalitions in a region between the network institutions and other relevant organizations. In Northern California this was done extensively and produced a truly community-based network that involved both hospitals and other organizational forms, such as foundations. The result was to eliminate competition between the powerful academic medical centers through the establishment of "neutral turf." The Illinois network was also able to do this by creating a "super-headquarters" at the Illinois Cancer Council (ICC). Like the Northern California Cancer Plan, the ICC was located in a neutral location and was governed by a director, hired by a consortium of the medical schools, who was not viewed as competing for either students or clinical resources with the established cancer programs in the region. This pattern of consortial interaction did not occur in Philadelphia, and this more than anything else distinguished the Greater Delaware Valley network from the others that were located in areas where there was potential competition among major academic centers for these resources.

In Wisconsin and Arkansas, the question of domain took a different form. In these two networks the problem was establishing interface between the medical center and community hospitals. Arkansas, like Illinois and Northern California, was able to establish a neutral location, controlled by all the major treatment centers. This was the Central Arkansas Radiation Therapy Institute (CARTI). It enabled the participants to deal with potentially conflicting issues of domain and served the same purpose as the consortial headquarters did in Illinois and Northern California. CARTI allowed an effective program to develop in Little Rock. However, once it became the headquarters, there were no other hospitals in the region able to treat head and neck cancers, and so the network evolved through interpersonal linkages.

In Wisconsin, an alliance was formed with the other medical school, the Medical College of Wisconsin, and there were several hundreds of miles separating the two. Because this network was so widespread, distance resolved the issue of domain, and contractual relationships established for the head and neck demonstration network were implemented in other areas as a device for ensuring cooperation.

Except, then, for the obvious failure (Mississippi) and the two networks where domain was already established and nonproblematic, all of the networks could be considered fairly effective in terms of domain establishment and/or enhancement. The awarding of funds under the network program provided the applicant medical centers with the resources needed to build or enhance their dominance in cancer research. Over time, status as a network headquarters was parlayed into further cancer control programming and related collaboration, particularly in clinical research. Special status as a headquarters quickly became vital, since more and more cancer patients were being treated in community hospitals (see the discussion in Chapter 3). The biggest payoff came in the form of certification as a comprehensive cancer center since this designation provided access to many other cancer programs.

It is not simply coincidental that the consortial cancer centers established in Illinois and Northern California had as their major focus cancer control and outreach to community hospitals. In Illinois, the individual academic medical institutions built cooperative clinical trials programs using patients from their network hospitals. Clinical research at the comprehensive cancer center was limited to protocols requiring patients that were so scarce that no single institution or network could provide sufficient numbers. In effect, Illinois replicated the cooperative group concept on a regional basis. The Northern California Cancer Program did not become a comprehensive cancer center immediately. However, a regional clinical trials program was implemented with funding from the NCI, and cancer control programs were supported with ad hoc funding. Eventually they received designation and funding as a comprehensive cancer center. Because both centers were consortia, the participating medical centers controlled the research programs that were mounted through the consortium. Research that required institutional facilities were left in the academic centers. As these research programs continued to be funded and conducted at the academic centers, the potential conflict between the consortial centers and their components was minimized.

Thus, on the issue of domain enhancement, Illinois, Northern California, and Wisconsin would be considered highly effective. Among the interpersonal networks, Arkansas was also effective, but in a different way consistent with its particular environment.

The Audience: The Community Hospitals

Finally, the perspective of the community hospitals and the clinical physicians practicing in the community needs to be considered. Our information on this group is much less complete for several reasons. This constituency was the largest group involved in the networks, and also the most amorphous and unstable in commitment and involvement over time, as discussed in Chapter 6. Moreover, because the networks involved the community hospitals in different ways, the data obtained were limited and reported in ways that were consistent only with individual network agendas. Since the NCI did not require any consistent reporting format, these data were of limited comparability. These issues are discussed more thoroughly in Chapter 7.

We have already noted that in the early 1970s the specialty of medical oncology was fairly new, and trained oncologists were scarce. Most of the physicians in that specialty were young, recent graduates from a limited number of medical schools. Although older physicians in the more traditional cancer field of surgery, and to some extent radiation therapy, were of course still treating a significant number of cancer patients, this younger cohort was beginning to make inroads. The professional goals of this group most certainly included gaining access to new drugs that were still considered experimental, and gaining access to new therapies of cancer treatment that might require institutional investment in new technologies. Policy at the National Cancer Institute limited access to experimental drugs to academic medical centers that received research funding. The only route of access to new, experimental treatment was through some afilliation with the academic medical centers. Thus, there were incentives for community-based oncologists to participate in these network programs. Further, the networks provided these community physicians with the desirable backup of a tertiary medical center for treatment of complicated cases. From the point of view of community physicians, then, an effective network program would make new treatment therapies (both drugs and techniques) directly available to community physicians interested in using them.

Facing both a change in population age distributions (with a resultant increase in the number of head and neck cancer patients) and dwindling resource bases to develop new treatment technologies, community hospitals were attracted to the network programs by their potential for providing such resources. Both head and neck specialists and head and neck cancer patients could be attracted to community treatment centers if new facilities and treatment strategies were available there. Furthermore, network affiliation offered the additional advantage of providing valued resources through a university headquarters center, rather than directly through the federal government, which most community providers and institutions would still find problematic.

From the point of view of the target audience, then, the most effective head and neck networks were the interorganizational networks that distributed network resources to community practitioners and/or hospitals: Wisconsin, Northern California, Greater Delaware Valley, and Illinois. There were differences among these four, however, due to the extent to which the networks were built on new or established relationships. In Illinois and Greater Delaware Valley, the head and neck networks were built upon preexisting linkages and established patterns of resource allocation. In Wisconsin and Northern California, these relationships had to be established in order to implement the network program. Thus, there was more pressure on these latter networks to distribute the network resources into community hospitals. As described in Chapter 6, the "common good" needed to be made more tangible in these networks in order to ensure participation. It was clear from the data that the extent of direct involvement by the community hospitals reflected their shared interest and their perception that they were receiving tangible benefits from participation.

Illinois is a good illustration of how the network concept expanded. As we described earlier, at the same time these head and neck networks were being instituted, the NCI initiated cancer control programs for the cooperative groups. This program had an objective similar to the demonstration networks. It was designed to keep these newly trained oncologists linked to the National Cancer Program and, at the same time, recognized that these community oncologists would be treating many of the cancer patients. By the late 1970s it had become clear that as many as half of the cancer patients entered on chemotherapy protocols were coming from community hospitals through these cancer control programs (Begg et al., 1982; McCusker et al., 1982; Murphy, 1981). In Illinois, the same networks that supported the head and neck program also supported the other clinical trials programs. As we have said, the Illinois Cancer Council was a "network of networks," and the cancer center, by bringing together the academic medical centers, obtained access to the community hospitals. Through these links the community oncologists had access to all the available clinical research being conducted in the region and nationally.

The community hospitals participated in the interpersonal networks as components of headquarters. The two interpersonal programs were organized in regions where there were limited resources in the community hospitals and few oncologists in the community outside of the headquarters hospitals. In effect, they confirm the model by revealing that where there was no demand for resources from community hospitals, network linkage did not occur.

To summarize, then, each constituency viewed the network projects as the possible solution to a different set of problems. Thus, performance assessments by each group would undoubtedly stress different factors: dissemination of a particular treatment ideology/approach, the establishment or enhancement of regional dominance, or the direct acquisition of new cancer treatment technologies. An additional complication in assessing network performance is that each of these constituencies is also likely to prefer a different level of analysis. The issue of analytic level in performance assessments is actually a separate concern, to which we now turn.

LEVELS OF ANALYSIS

For the network demonstration projects, performance could be assessed on at least three different levels of analysis: the hospital level, the network or regional level, and finally, the national level. We might expect community physicians and community hospitals in the network regions to prefer that evaluations of network performance be made at the hospital level since the hospital level is closest to their interests. Once again, however, we have the least information about this constituency. Thus, most of our analysis at this level is limited to the process analysis presented in Chapter 6, which looked primarily at factors that influenced participation.

Hospital level changes one might expect as a result of the network programs could occur in a number of ways. For individual hospital members of the networks, there could be changes in the number of head and neck cancer patients seen, the stage of disease progression most frequently seen at member hospitals, referral rates to other hospitals, types of management strategies typically used, the number of patients put onto research protocols, or the morbidity/mortality rates of head and neck cancer patients. How changes in any of these hospital level patterns should be interpreted, however, would depend upon whether the hospital was part of an interorganizational network (i.e., the Illinois, Greater Delaware Valley,

Wisconsin, or California networks) or an affiliated hospital of a physician in an interpersonal network.

Interpretation would also depend upon whether the hospital was a satellite or headquarters institution. For example, increases in the number of patients treated at member hospitals of an interorganizational network could be interpreted as a positive outcome of the network project. However, for hospitals in an interpersonal network, increases in the numbers of head and neck patients treated locally would be considered a negative outcome. Either strategy could be used to increase the overall number of head and neck cancer patients receiving multidisciplinary treatment; thus, hospital-level indicators of performance that focus on patient aggregate measures could be misleading.

Another type of hospital level measure that could be considered would be changes in the level of facilities or staffing relevant to the treatment of head and neck cancer. We could examine changes before and after the network project years in the average number of head-and-neck-cancer-related hospital facilities (as listed by the yearly AHA survey of hospital facilities) for all hospitals in the network regions. Again, however, at the hospital level it is not clear how one should interpret such changes. For any individual hospital, the adoption of such facilities may or may not be directly related to the existence of a network project in the region. Without a control group of nonnetwork hospitals for comparison, network "effects" are not easily determined. Survey measures of structure do not allow for the imputation of any causal effect of network operation on hospital changes in structure. Further, as is the case for patient-based measures, the interpretation of hospital level changes in structure would vary depending upon the form of the network within that region. Hospitals within regions with interorganizational networks would be more likely to exhibit changes in structure that reflect an increased availability of head and neck facilities. The same would not necessarily be true for hospitals within interpersonal network regions.

Clearly, network or regional level measures would be preferable to hospital-level performance measures. As we have seen, hospital level analyses are subject to problems of disaggregation (Hannan, 1971), whether one focuses on structure, process, or outcome measures. Further, no matter how crucial the constituency of community physicians and hospitals, the network programs were designed to affect the delivery of care at the regional level, and the network is itself an aggregate of multiple actors, whether implemented by individuals or by organizations. Thus, in the final analysis, we must ask what those regional or aggregate effects were.

At the regional level, one could theoretically measure the effects of the network programs in terms of all three types of indicators: outcome, process, and structure. However, not all of the three measurement strategies are appropriate, given an understanding of the network program goals, either from the NCI's perspective or from that of the network.

Regionwide outcome measures should ultimately capture the changes in health status, recovery rates, or the survival of head and neck cancer patients in the region as a result of increases in the use of multimodal treatment strategies. Recall, however, our earlier discussion of the status of multidisciplinary treatment in the management of head and neck cancer. Although it had been shown through extensive clinical trials that other diseases responded favorably to multimodal treatment, there was no compelling clinical evidence to claim similar results for head and neck cancer. The effectiveness of the innovation of multidisciplinary treatment had never been demonstrated. Moreover, even if there were strong empirical justification for the multidisciplinary approach, the definition and implementation of this innovation was not completed until the last years of the project. Thus, the data would hardly reflect patient outcomes based on the advocated treatment strategy. Outcome measures based on patient health change are probably premature.

PROCESS MEASURES OF NETWORK PERFORMANCE

The National Cancer Institute's objectives for establishing the network projects were to define and disseminate the state of the art in multidisciplinary care, *not* to prove the strategy's effectiveness. They assumed that these treatments had been demonstrated to be effective and the aims were process-oriented: to ensure that they were uniformly available. The appropriate assessment, then, is the extent of change that occurred in each network in the management of head and neck patients. Our earlier analysis of the diffusion of multidisciplinary teams indicated that each network attempted to diffuse the concept, and that in the interorganizational networks the effort was made to disseminate it to the participating community hospitals. On the basis of this analysis, we argued that different networks had to invest in different strategies depending upon what types of relationships existed between the headquarters and network hospitals. Because there were few preexisting linkages in Northern California and Wisconsin, they had to invest more network resources in building the network than did Illinois and Greater Delaware Valley.

A more direct measurement of change in treatment process at the regional level (and one that would allow the comparison of both interorganizational and interpersonal networks) would be to compare the proportions of head and neck cancer patients who received multimodal treatment before and after network operation. We do have such data, for at least five of the six operative networks, on two of the most frequently occurring types of head and neck cancer, cancer of the larynx and cancer of the oral cavity.* Table 8.2 summaizes those data for the Arkansas, Eastern Great Lakes, Wisconsin, Illinois, and Northern California networks.

Before examining Table 8.2 in detail, however, we should review the obvious problems with these data. As we saw in Chapter 7, data collection was accorded differing levels of importance across the six operative networks, and most of the networks developed their own data-retrieval and collection systems. Thus, we cannot assume that the data summarized in Table 8.2 are truly comparable across networks. Further, not all hospitals where head and neck cancer patients might be treated would have entered data. For example, in Northern California, only a subset of participating hospitals entered data on head and neck cancer patients. This means that there is probably variation across networks in the proportions of head and neck patients actually entered into the individual network data bases.

---

*The Greater Delaware Valley network did not invest much of their resources in data collection because, as noted in Chapter 7, data collection had little relevance to its primary objectives. Consequently, the data are incomplete, and it is not possible to reconstruct the patterns of treatment for these sites before and after the network program.

Table 8.2. Change in Multidisciplinary Treatment[a]
(Pre- and Postnetwork Operation) for Cancers of the Larynx
and Oral Cavity across Networks

	Larynx (Percentage of total cases)			Oral cavity (Percentage of total cases)		
Network	MDT 1st-year data	MDT last-year data	Percentage change	MDT 1st-year data	MDT last-year data	Percentage change
Arkansas (1976–1978)	38[b]	40	+2	38	32	−6
Eastern Great Lakes (1975–1978)	10	17	+7	34	7	−27
Wisconsin (1975–1978)	28	25	−3	27	27	0
Illinois (1975–1979)	27	30	+3	25	25	0
Northern California (1975–1978)	20	26	+6	21	23	+2

[a]Multidisciplinary treatment (MDT) defined as treatment by surgery and radiation; surgery and chemotherapy; chemotherapy and radiation; or surgery, chemotherapy, and radiation.
[b]Numbers represent percent of all laryngeal cancer patients for that year provided with MDT.

Considering the foregoing *caveats*, we now turn to the table. The data show very little change in actual treatment strategies during the period of network funding. Most of the percent changes are quite small and erratic in pattern. Even in the Wisconsin network, where we know a substantial portion of network funds were spent developing and implementing multidisciplinary teams throughout the network region and reviewing the data with the participating network physicians, changes in actual patient treatment strategies are negligible. The only sizable percent change in this table is the 27% decrease in the use of multidisciplinary treatment for cancers of the oral cavity in the Eastern Great Lakes network region. This unexpected decline in multimodal treatment can be attributed to an actual preference in this network for the use of surgery as the primary treatment.

The percentages in Table 8.2 are based on rather small cell frequencies; thus, generalizations are risky. But patterns in treatment do indicate that as the network project progressed, more patients with tumors at all stages received surgery as the only primary treatment. There is very little evidence that combined modality treatment strategies were ever seriously employed.

Of the five networks shown in Table 8.2, only Northern California shows small positive changes toward the use of multidisciplinary treatment for both types of cancers. It is interesting to note, too, that this network devoted considerable effort toward implementing some sort of postnetwork evaluation of the impact of network activities on patient treatment and survival outcomes. The results of that analysis showed very little change in either treatment patterns or outcomes.

In part, this disappointing outcome may be the result of the very short time period over which these data were collected. The data cover a time span of only three years. In our discussion of implementation strategies in Chapter 7, it was clear that the networks spent most of the funding period defining the innovation and developing means of dissemination. The first-year networks that employed guidelines did not even disseminate them until the final year of the contract. Thus, while there may have been some opportunity for changes in the use of multidisciplinary treatment strategies in the headquarters, these institutions were selected because they presumably *already used* state-of-the-art treatment. Diffusion to the community hospitals had only begun when the network funding was terminated.

If the innovation had been ready for diffusion earlier in the demonstration period, the overall time frame would probably still have been too brief to expect any measurable change in practice. Even with rapid diffusion, the literature suggests a minimum of five years between the introduction of an innovation and appreciable diffusion (Rogers, 1983; Warner, 1975). Thus, given the performance period, measurable changes in treatment would be surprising.

It is safe to conclude that no real short-term change in medical process actually occured as a result of any of the network programs. As we showed in Chapter 7, the programs managed to focus physicians' attention on the issue of multidisiplinary treatment for at least a little while, and to persuade them of the importance of considering multidisciplinary approaches to management. But in the end, without evidence from either clinical trials or their own practices to verify the advantage of multidisciplinary treatment, it would appear that no real change in treatment strategies was possible during the brief demonstration period. As Greer has reminded us in her study of Wisconsin physicians (1986), doctors are very conservative in the area of treatment innovation. Greer found these physicians to be particularly sensitive about any efforts to "share" control over patients.

STRUCTURAL MEASURES OF NETWORK PERFORMANCE

Another way of assessing whether the goal of multidisciplinary treatment diffusion was achieved is to examine to what extent the structure in place for treatment of head and neck cancer patients changed or improved after network operation. Although much more indirect as a measure of performance, changes in both medical personnel and hospital facilities that would allow for more multidisciplinary treatment of head and neck cancer patients represents another strategy through which multimodal treatment goals could eventually be reached. We realize, however, that the existence of an appropriate structure or the necessary professionals does not guarantee the actual delivery of multimodal treatment; it does, nonetheless, increase the odds of such treatment's occurring compared with areas where such facilities and personnel are unavailable.

There are, of course, a number of specialists ideally involved in multidisciplinary treatment of head and neck cancer. We are limited, however, in the number of such specialties for which data are available both before and after network operation, aggregated at the network region level. Given the traditional role of the surgeon in cancer treatment, we assumed that an increase in the number of other primary providers in multimodal treatment would increase the odds of that treatment strategy. We have chosen to examine two such specialties: the number of otolaryngologists per thousand population in the network regions, and the number of radiation therapists per thousand population. Radiation therapy, along with surgery and chemotherapy, represents one of the major treatment alternatives for head and neck cancer. Otolaryngologists should ideally be involved in planning both pre- and posttreatment management of head and neck patients, toward the goal of more effective rehabilitation. The numbers of both types of specialists were standardized by population size, in order to control for natural increases in regional growth.

Table 8.3 summarizes the population-based ratios of these two specialties for the six operative networks, before and after network funding. As a baseline against which to judge the changes in the network regions in the availability of these specialists, national figures for the numbers of otolaryngologists and radiologists per 1000 population in 1972 were 0.02 and 0.046, respectively. In other words, across the nation there was on average about 1 otolaryngologist per 50,000 population, and about 2 radiologists per 50,000 people. These ratios remained unchanged at the national level in 1977.

From Table 8.3 we can see that all six of the networks were at the national levels in 1972 for number of otolaryngologists; the Wisconsin and Greater Delaware Valley networks were slightly above the national norm. A similar picture prevailed for the number of radiologists in the network regions in 1972; however, Wisconsin had twice the national level, and both Arkansas and the Greater Delaware Valley were above the national norm. By 1977 all six of the network regions experienced some increase in the numbers of either otolaryngologists or radiologists, and these were increases that did not occur for the nation as a whole. Of course, we cannot claim that these increases were solely the result of network program influences; for example, the largest proportional increases occurred in the Northern California network region, and there are obvious reasons for moving to California, especially if one has the potential for substantial earnings increases. It is important to point out, however, that even those network regions that are not renowned for their attractive climates and trend-setting life-styles evinced substantial proportional changes. Similarly, recall that data on treatment patterns for patients in the Eastern Great Lakes network did not show any trend toward multidisciplinary treatment.

Table 8.3. Change in Regional Availability of Radiologists and Otolaryngologists before and after Network Demonstration Projects[a]

Network	N of otolaryngologists[b] per 1000 population			N of radiologists per 1000 population		
	1972	1977	Percentage change	1972	1977	Percentage change
Arkansas	0.02	0.04	+100	0.06	0.08	+33
Eastern Great Lakes	0.02	0.02	0	0.03	0.05	+66
Wisconsin	0.03	0.04	+33	0.08	0.11	+38
Northern California	0.02	0.04	+100	0.04	0.11	+275
Greater Delaware Valley	0.03	0.04	+33	0.06	0.09	+50
Illinois	0.02	0.03	+50	0.04	0.06	+50

[a]Sources: American Board of Medical Specialists, 1972, 1977; total population from the U.S. Bureau of the Census, 1976, 1980.
[b]The rate of physicians to population was calculated using the number of nonfederal physicians.

Not surprisingly, this network region was the only region to show no change in the number of otolaryngologists per 1000 population. Thus, we suspect that the change in the availability of otolaryngologists and radiologists in these regions might have been at least partially the result of network efforts in that regard.

Another measurable index of structural change toward the adoption of multimodal treatment for head and neck cancer would be change in the hospital facilities available in the network regions. To the extent that area hospitals show an increase in the facilities needed for delivering multimodal treatment, we might assume that the likelihood of such treatment has increased. In Chapter 4 we compared network hospitals' facilities and concluded that there was considerable variation across networks in the supply of hospital facilities at the outset of the network project years. Here we are interested more in the relative degree of change—either a decline or an increase in each network's hospital facilities—by the end of the project period, compared with initial facility levels. Absolute levels of hospital facilities are not of direct concern.

Further, we are not interested in increases in all types of hospital facilities but only in those facilities that would be instrumental in the delivery of multimodal cancer treatment. We have identified 11 such facilities from the American Hospital Association's yearly surveys of hospital facilities for 1973 and 1978, and one type of accreditation (certification by the American College of Surgeons as having an approved cancer program). These 11 facilities and one approval were listed by the AHA in its survey for both the prior network year and the 1978 implementation year. The 11 facilities considered relevant to the management of head and neck cancer were X-ray therapy, cobalt therapy, radium therapy, diagnostic radioisotope facility, therapeutic radioisotope facility, histopathology laboratory, rehabilitation inpatient unit, rehabilitation outpatient unit, social work department, dental services, and speech pathology services.

Table 8.4 summarizes changes in the proportion of network hospitals where such facilities are available. The symbols in Table 8.4 are intended to represent in a general way whether the availability of such facilities remained unchanged (represented by a 0), whether at least 25% of the network's hospitals added or lost such facilities (+ or −), or whether at least 50% of the network's hospitals added or lost such facilities (+ + or − −). Within each network, hospitals are categorized as either headquarters institutions or member hospitals (for interpersonal networks, *member hospitals* refers to hospitals where member physicians practice). This categorization should allow us to determine to what extent these hospital facilities were primarily gained within the university medical centers acting as network headquarters, or whether they were more generally adopted by hospitals throughout the networks.

In general, there is no overwhelming pattern evident in Table 8.4. Very little facility change occurred in the Wisconsin, Northern California, Greater Delaware Valley, and Illinois networks. Whatever change did occur in Wisconsin was consistent with a diffusion pattern. It occurred among the member hospitals: Four member hospitals gained approved cancer programs, and quite a few member hospitals added rehabilitation units. In Northern California, nearly all of the facility change occurred at the four headquarters institutions, and those changes consisted of a loss of one hospital's radiation therapy facilities and the addition in another hospital of histopathology and rehabilitation facilities.

At first glance, it would appear that somewhat higher levels of facility change

Table 8.4. Change in Percent of Network Hospitals with HNC-Related Facilities, 1973–1978[a]

Facility number: Network	7 X-ray therapy	8 Cobalt therapy	9 Radium therapy	10 Diagnostic radioisotope	11 Therapeutic radioisotope	12 Histopathology lab	25 Rehab inpatient	26 Rehab outpatient	36 Social work department	42 Dental services	44 Speech pathology	Approved cancer program
Arkansas												
HQ hospitals (n = 4)	– [b]	– – [b]	– [b]	0	0	0	0	0	+	++	++	0
Member hospitals (n = 18)	+	0	0	0	0	+	0	0	+	0	0	0
Eastern Great Lakes												
HQ hospitals (n = 7)	0	0	0	0	0	0	0	++	0	0	0	0
Member hospitals (n = 2)	– – [c]	0	0	0	++	0	0	++	++	++	++	++ 1 added
Wisconsin												
HQ hospitals (n = 1)	0	0	0	0	0	0	0	0	0	0	0	0
Member hospitals (n = 12)	0	0	0	0	0	0	++	++	0	0	0	+ 4 added
Northern California												
HQ hospitals (n = 4)	–	0	–	0	0	+	–	+	0	0	0	– lost 1
Member hospitals (n = 10)	0	0	0	0	0	0	0	0	0	0	+	0
Greater Delaware Valley												
HQ hospitals (n = 1)	0	0	0	0	0	0	0	0	0	0	–	0
Member hospitals (n = 8)	0	+	0	0	0	0	0	0	0	0	+	0
Illinois												
HQ hospitals (n = 4)	0	0	0	0	0	0	0	0	0	0	0	– lost 1
Member hospitals (n = 17)	–	0	0	0	0	0	0	0	+	0	0	0

[a] Source: AHA Guide to the Health Care Field 1973, 1978.
[b] In Arkansas this resulted from the development of CARTI. This required all medical centers to use the radiation therapy facilities located there.
[c] Facility codes: – – more than 50% decrease, – more than 25% decrease, 0 no change, + more than 25% increase, ++ more than 50% increase.

occurred in the two interpersonal networks, Arkansas and the Eastern Great Lakes, and in some respects this is the proper conclusion. In Arkansas, however, the reduction in radiation therapy facilities among the headquarters institutions represents the implementation of the Central Arkansas Radiation Therapy Institute (CARTI) agreements to centralize radiation facilities there. These were worked out before the network contract was awarded. In addition, the headquarters institution in Arkansas added social work, dental, and speech pathology services, which was in response to the network contract. Finally, most of the facility additions in the Eastern Great Lakes network occurred in one of the two nonheadquarters hospitals and did not reflect changes resulting from the demonstration project.

To summarize, there did not appear to be a noticeable amount of structural change in the network hospitals over the project time period. The change that did occur cannot be clearly attributed to attempts to achieve the diffusion of multimodal treatment for head and neck cancer patients. Possible exceptions might be the Wisconsin network, where four member hospitals obtained cancer program approvals during the project period, and in Arkansas, where the network headquarters added staff consistent with the changes noted by the AHA during the network period.

Admittedly, the new cancer program approvals in Wisconsin could be unrelated to the Wisconsin Head and Neck Cancer Demonstration Project. Nevertheless, they are consistent with the efforts by the University of Wisconsin to obtain certification as a comprehensive cancer research center. Center certification and implementation of multimodal treatment strategies are not incompatible goals. Structural analyses do not permit the direct attribution of added cancer program approvals as the result of actions to achieve either one. It is true, nonetheless, that we have hypothesized that community hospitals would be motivated to participate in such demonstration projects because they provide an opportunity to upgrade their facilities and staff, and attract a larger patient pool and more qualified professionals. The results presented here suggest that, at least in Arkansas and in Wisconsin, these effects occurred in the same time period as the demonstration projects. The fact that these networks both were located in areas of lean resources (see Chapter 4), and that these resources were added in facilities where efforts were being made to increase referrals, is at the least an intriguing outcome that might deserve more investigation.

OUTCOME MEASURES: ONGOING NETWORK STRUCTURES TO SURVIVE

We have indicated elsewhere that outcome measures that focus on patient survival, disease incidence, and mortality are inappropriate because of the time period and the lack of independent evidence that one would expect such outcomes. We have seen that change in treatment, a process objective, did not occur during the network period. These results should not be surprising, given the agendas of these networks and even the agenda of the NCI. At both levels, even though the official objectives were directed toward diffusion of state of the art, multidisciplinary treatment, the *actual agenda* gave priority to program development and domain enhancement.

The NCI had received a congressional mandate to implement cancer control efforts that would result in the dissemination of the results of research into the community. The mandate was broad and included prevention, early detection, and treatment. At the time when these programs were initiated, there was no community-based structure available to the NCI through which these cancer control goals could be achieved. There was no disease control program. Thus, before the mandate could be implemented, the NCI had to develop that structure. The centers program and the early cancer control initiatives were to provide that structure.

From the standpoint of the networks, we have argued that in most cases the headquarters institutions viewed these programs as opportunities to develop regional cancer control programs that would help them meet the requirement that comprehensive cancer centers have cancer control outreach programs. We have tried to demonstrate throughout this book that the likelihood of achieving this goal and the means by which it was approached were conditioned by the environmental context of each network, specifically the organizational environment. Thus, the appropriate outcome measures at this point are not those related to patients' health changes but those that reflect changes in organizational relationships, or *transformations* in interorganizational or interpersonal linkages. Such transformations would result in the survival of the infrastructure desired by both the NCI and the headquarters institutions.

Access to otolaryngologists and radiologists in the network regions (structure) has improved, and the increase in numbers of these specialists did not occur generally across the nation. It could be the case that the network projects attracted enough attention among these medical professionals to signal the utility of locating in the network regions, either because of presumed better access to patients in need of specialized services or because of presumed improved access to specialized facilities. In two networks more hospitals had American College of Surgeons-approved cancer programs. Thus, there may have been some change in the environmental resources of some networks that would support the institutionalization of cancer control programs.

Given that the operant agenda of these networks was to develop a cancer control infrastructure, the next question is: What remains of the network project structures after the cessation of federal funding that will become part of that infrastructure? What happened to the formally created interpersonal or interorganizational linkages once the funding for those exchanges and activities ran out? Under what conditions will these artificially created diffusion networks develop into ongoing channels of resource exchange and communication? To use the second part of this chapter's title, we have already examined the extent of environmental transformation in hospital resources and facilities. We must now turn to the question of network organizational transformation and survival. What vestiges of network structure will survive and become institutionalized as support for the next stages of technology diffusion to support cancer control?

To address these questions we will once again return to the distinction between interpersonal and interorganizational networks. As we have shown elsewhere, each form of network had its own organizational agenda and diffusion strategy, and each had a unique organizational character that was in large measure influenced by its environment. Thus, we would expect that the surviving components would also be conditioned by the environment and by the potential for other cancer control initiatives.

Interpersonal Networks

The salient features of the interpersonal networks were that their focus was on the headquarters, and they encouraged referral to headquarters as their diffusion strategy. As discussion in Chapter 4, there were no hospitals outside of the headquarters institutions that had the facilities to implement complex treatment strategies. The capability for a regional cancer treatment network of community hospitals did not exist. Thus, surviving components of these interpersonal networks are most likely to be those aspects of the network programs that support departmental or institutional agendas of the headquarters.

In Arkansas this is exactly what happened. Certain activities that related to the otolaryngology program at the headquarters or that supported the CARTI program shared by the major hospitals in Little Rock were continued as part of the otolaryngology program. These activities tended to be professional-oriented educational programs for physicians, dentists, public health nurses, and speech pathologists in the region. Certain key staff who were involved in patient management and rehabilitation were put onto the departmental payroll. These staff and facilities included a speech pathologist, a public health nurse, the prosthesis program, a dental operatory, and the cancer detection laboratory.

This outcome is consistent with the interpersonal character of the network, which was dependent upon the willingness of local otolaryngologists to refer oncology patients to the UAMC. Most of the other network features did not survive because they did not support the initial agenda of this network, which was to establish the UAMC and CARTI as a regional referral center for head and neck cancer specifically and radiation therapy more generally.

The principal investigator had the objective of leading a regional cancer center. However, the otolaryngology program and the head and neck network did not appear to be linked to other oncology programs at UAMC. At any event, the network did not evolve into a major cancer program. One explanation for this may be that the level of interconnectedness within the Arkansas network was too loose, or the knowledge of other resource alternatives too incomplete or inadequate to provide a base for continuation. Recalling our analysis of social network linkages based on patient transfers and shared service agreements in Chapter 5, this explanation may be plausible. Linkage density within the network was fairly low, as was the number of external linkages. Boundary spanners within the network may have been inadequately informed or unaware of resources within the network that would absorb other functions under the contract. Linkages outside the network were not strong enough to import new resources into the network that would enable broadening of the program. The absence of a general strategy for cancer management in the region may have contributed to the isolation of this network. What external ties there were linked the network to resources that would underwrite head and neck programs. These included the Junior League of Little Rock and the Little Rock Unit of the American Cancer Society. These connections supported the dental operatory and the early detection laboratory.

A parallel pattern of survival is evident in the SUNYAB component of the Eastern Great Lakes network. The differences between the SUNYAB and Roswell Park components related mainly to the differences in how the program fit with the goals of the sponsoring organization. Unlike the Arkansas network, the Eastern Great Lakes program resulted from the merger of two initially separate programs. At various points in the discussion we have noted that the two programs never fully merged and frequently pursued quite separate paths, such as in data collection. In fact, the activities that survived were those where the integration was most complete, mainly outreach and continuing education. However, even in these areas the integration that occurred was mainly at the policy level, and each unit had its own educational and outreach initiatives.

The network programs were integrated differently at the two sponsoring institutions. Like the situation at UAMC, there was no institutional commitment to a broad cancer program at SUNYAB, and the network demonstration activity was really limited to the otolaryngology department and affiliated residency program. Moreover, there was no apparent interest among the other clinical departments in expanding the cancer-related treatment programs at the university, even though there was other cancer-related research ongoing in epidemiology and basic science. Therefore, the resources available to permit the continuation of the program at SUNYAB had to come from departmental funding.

As a further consequence, continuing support was forthcoming primarily for those activities that would enhance the interests of otolaryngology. The department did find support for the nurse coordinator, and there was at least the intention of continuing to include among her responsibilities coordination of multidisciplinary pretreatment planning. However, as we have noted elsewhere in this chapter, this network was directed by otolaryngologists with a strong preference for surgery, and the pattern evidenced in the SUNYAB data was an increase in patients treated by surgery only. Thus, it was unclear what role this nurse would play in maintaining the innovation at headquarters.

The SUNYAB program did, however, form a liaison with the College of Dentistry and the dental hygienist program. They also developed a community outreach program with the Erie County Dental Society. These components of the program were basically exported and continued in their new locations. Unlike UAMC, the SUNYAB program did not bring into the network resources from participating organizations like the local unit of the American Cancer Society or the Junior League. It did build on some programs sponsored by the regional medical program, but those resources were gone by the conclusion of the network program.

The SUNYAB component did have very good local ties and received referrals from all the local physicians. However, these referral links predated the network formation and merely continued at its conclusion. But these ties were between the chief of otolaryngology and local physicians, similar to the kinds of ties that existed between the principal investigator at Arkansas and the local otolaryngologists. Also, the institutional linkages and access to local resources resembled those in Arkansas: Awareness of resources in the region was also quite low. In the absence of other cancer-related outreach activities sponsored by the medical school, these local referral links could not mature into any kind of a general cancer control program.

The component of the Eastern Great Lakes Network that was located at

Roswell Park Memorial Institute was part of a long-standing cancer treatment program. As described in Chapter 2, RPMI was a free-standing cancer center that had been established by New York State early in the century. RPMI was at the time applying to become a comprehensive cancer center and was among the first group of institutions to receive this designation. However, as with many of those institutions that received early designation, the recognition was related to basic and clinical research and not for community outreach. Also, like the other early cancer centers, RPMI was faced with the need to develop a cancer control program.

What RPMI did within the community was to collaborate with the local unit of the American Cancer Society and offer an extensive program in continuing medical education. Like the other interpersonal units, it developed a model multidisciplinary program at headquarters and invited local practitioners to come and observe and discuss the concepts of multidisciplinary care.

What survived at RPMI were mainly programs that had predated the network. Local clinical outreach beyond the continuing medical education programs was not part of the institutional agenda at RPMI. RPMI viewed clinical research as its primary mission; referral came from all over the state, so it did not have to depend on a local network, as did some of the other comprehensive centers. Moreover, because of its heavy concentration of cancer specialists, it could and did develop local protocols and participated only minimally in the large clinical trials programs.

The one joint effort to survive was the Eastern Great Lakes Head and Neck Oncology Association, which was a loose group of physicians in the area interested in head and neck cancer. By 1979 it had 50 members and had met three times. There was some intention of converting it to a cooperative research group, but that never materialized. It followed the pattern of interactions between community physicians in the area and became a focus for symposia and other continuing medical education programs. In addition it will provide a basis for continuing interaction among professionals interested in head and neck cancer.

In summary, the most successful features of the SUNYAB network appear to be those organized around community and professional education. These programs either were already established parts of the sponsoring institutions or were absorbed by others in the community with direct interest in them, such as the local dentists and dental hygienists. The development of the comprehensive cancer center at RPMI occurred at the same time as the initiation of the head and neck network project, but it seemed to develop on a separate path. Little that was developed by the head and neck network was used to support the emerging cancer control program at RPMI.

As we have said at several points, the head and neck network demonstration projects were envisioned by the NCI as a component of their general effort to establish a cancer control infrastructure. Part of their strategy was to build linkages with community physicians, and through them to diffuse state-of-the-art treatment strategies. The interpersonal networks did this by establishing direct links with primary care providers in the community. There was no institutional commitment to developing a larger cancer control effort at either Arkansas or SUNYAB, and resources were not invested in programs that would build upon the head and neck network programs.

Overall, then, it seems reasonable to conclude that the interpersonal networks did not leave a discernable structure after their termination. At best, some existing programs were enhanced by resources provided by the network. However, it would be hard to identify cancer control programs that continued to exist after funding was withdrawn.

Interorganizational Networks

We turn now to the interorganizational networks. As we have discussed, these networks were introduced into environments where the possibility for both organizational and interpersonal linkages existed. They closely approximated the model that was envisioned by the program staff at the NCI when the concept of the network demonstration programs was introduced. Illinois, Northern California, and Wisconsin had characteristics which made them ideal demonstration sites and which also enhanced the NCI objective of establishing a cancer control infrastructure. These characteristics were (1) interest among leading members of the academic community in relevant disciplines in establishing a comprehensive cancer center, and recognition by these leaders of the need to establish an outreach program, (2) commitment of institutional resources to support establishment of a cancer program, and (3) access to community hospitals with the facilities needed to participate in, and benefit from, a regional cancer program.

Among these three prototypical demonstration programs, similar organizational features persisted after funding was terminated. These were the headquarters organization, a continuing data system that collected patient data from the participating hospitals, and, most important, the linkages with community hospitals. By participating in the network programs, these centers also developed contracting procedures and policies as well as organizational infrastructures that enabled them to continue cooperative research programs with community hospitals.

In two instances, Illinois and Northern California, the consortial arrangements that facilitated the formation of the network were retained as the organizational form for the resulting comprehensive cancer centers. These regional consortia have ultimately become the models for regional cancer control planning at the National Cancer Institute, and new guidelines have recently been published promoting the formation of such centers in other areas of the country. Thus, the form of two of these programs survived as new programs were added.

It is interesting that head and neck cancer became a central cancer control research focus in Illinois through the expansion of the rehabilitation component of the original network program. Rehabilitation ultimately became the channel through which multidisciplinary pretreatment planning for head and neck patients became institutionalized in the region. The speech therapists who organized the network were ultimately supported by their respective otolaryngology departments. When they became permanent staff, they were able to persuade the otolaryngologists and radiation therapists to continue to consider rehabilitation concerns as part of their pretreatment work-up. This initiative was successfully implemented, and gradually, as residents trained in this approach moved into local hospitals, this approach to management became part of standard practice in the region.

Further, under the continuing leadership of the speech therapist at Northwestern University, additional research developed in head and neck rehabilitation. A continuing research program, involving many of the original network hospitals plus investigators from throughout the United States, is still under way, supported by funding from the National Cancer Institute.

In Wisconsin and Northern California, the multidisciplinary pretreatment planning strategies initiated by the network took different forms. In Northern California, a decentralized approach was adopted in which resources and institutions were employed in a synergistic fashion to develop cancer control programs. This strategy, like the "network of networks" in Illinois, avoided competition and duplication of services in the region and allowed the participants to devise a basis for collaboration that was nonthreatening. Geographically, this was a large network, and decentralization was necessary because the headquarters staff could not possibly cover the entire area. Nor could the principal investigator meet with the community physicians, as was done in Wisconsin.

The organizational strategy adopted was to establish community-based cancer councils, called Independent Service Areas (ISA), that would be led by local physicians and could generate local interest. These programs established their own priorities. Programs initiated by the comprehensive center are introduced to these planning councils and they decide whether to participate. These conferences continued because they were organized and structured so that the salaries of the coordinators could be absorbed by the subcontracting organizations that were hired by the network program to implement the conferences.

The Northern California Head and Neck Demonstration Network also brought rehabilitation services to the region. Three maxillofacial prosthodontists were woven into the fabric of cancer treatment in their respective communities. This was done by integrating two into the teaching program at the headquarters, and the third was assisted by the network in establishing a full-time practice in the Sacramento area. In part, their success was assured by the fact that DENTICAL, the state insurance program, and Kaiser, the state's largest HMO, reimbursed for their services.

As in Illinois, the Northern California network enabled the medical schools to develop a consortium that could continue beyond the network program. It enabled them to test organizing strategies and to develop the means by which new programs could be initiated. At about the same time as the network program was initiated, a local clinical trials group became active. It was able to continue well beyond the network and captitalized on the network structure for patient recruitment for protocols.

Geographical distance was also a factor in the transformation and survival of the Wisconsin network. The University of Wisconsin had made a commitment to develop a comprehensive cancer center. Wisconsin had strong programs in basic science and clinical research. It was the headquarters for one of the two largest cooperative clinical research groups, the Eastern Cooperative Clinical Oncology Group (ECOG). However, it had not developed a local outreach program for cancer control, and it used the network as a way of developing such an outreach program. The network also provided contact with many of the large clinics in Wisconsin that ultimately became part of its clinical outreach program funded through ECOG.

Because Wisconsin did not have competing medical schools, and because of the university's physical separation from Milwaukee, there was not the same potential for competition over domain that existed in Illinois, Northern California, and Philadelphia. As a result, a consortium headquarters was not necessary or even possible. The turf issues in Wisconsin were between the university and the free-standing clinics that existed around the state. The network enabled the university to establish interactions with some of these clinics. With others, interaction already existed since many oncologists had trained at the university. In general, the network provided experience and an opportunity to test procedures. The linkages between the network principal investigator and the community physicians remained because they were built on personal ties that predated the network. The headquarters structure was essentially taken over by the cancer center.

Greater Delaware Valley Network was the only one of the four interorganizational networks that did not expand into a comprehensive cancer center. It was superimposed on an existing, larger network established through the cooperative efforts of three medical schools to upgrade radiation therapy in the Delaware Valley region. The major institutional force behind the program was Hahnemann Medical College and Hospital, and the principal investigator was the chief of the Department of Radiotherapy at Hahnemann Hospital. The focus of the program was radiotherapy and head and neck cancer.

Pretreatment planning conferences were a major feature of this network, and by its end the relevant institutions had agreed to employ the individuals critical to organizing these conferences. Thus, for head and neck cancer and for radiation therapy the multidisciplinary planning conference survived. A psychosocial support program, initiated by the network, was sustained via the same mechanism. The participating hospitals, including the community hospitals, found these aspects to be consistent with their agendas and adopted them on an ongoing basis, assuring continuation of some form of multidisciplinary planning and psychosocial support within the region.

This network also established a major oral screening program using local dentists. This program was adopted by the local unit of the American Cancer Society. It had been scaled down in size but was still in place when the network ended.

The Greater Delaware Valley network experience highlights the importance of the organizational environment for the development of the interorganizational networks. It was clearly interorganizational in form. However, it could not evolve into a regional cancer program because environmental constraints in the form of competing organizational linkages limited its capacity for expansion. Moreover, there was no superinstitutional commitment to a broader cancer program either at Hahnemann or elsewhere in the network. Thus, the structure remained but was limited in scope to elements that advanced the delivery of high-quality radiation therapy in the region. Within that framework, it retained the focus on state-of-the-art multidisciplinary care.

In summary, cancer control outreach in some form survived in all four interorganizational networks. The differences between the Greater Delaware Valley and the others was in the relationship of the innovation to the agenda of the sponsoring organization. The Greater Delaware Valley network survived as an extension of a specific program. In this sense it did not differ from the others, which also survived through integration into larger cancer programs. The difference was mainly in the regional and organizational priorities. Collaboration was possible in Illinois and Northern California because all of the major academic units were part of the network, and all were committed to establishing a shared facility. Moreover, establishing the network enabled the participants to institutionalize their "neutral turf," thereby resolving local conflicts over domain.

The importance of institutional and regional support for a network program is clearly evident in the analysis of the interorganizational networks. It is also clear in the analysis of the interpersonal networks, where survival could not occur without a larger agenda tied to the development of a comprehensive cancer center. In the next section we will look briefly at the network that failed, the Mississippi head and neck network demonstration project.

EARLY NETWORK FAILURE: LESSONS LEARNED FROM THE MISSISSIPPI NETWORK

The Mississippi Head and Neck Cancer Control Network did not survive beyond the first implementation year. Our analysis of network performance would be incomplete without an examination of what was different, and, indeed, what was similar to other networks, about the Mississippi case.

The program proposed by the University of Mississippi·reflected the requirements of the NCI request for proposals. It was to be organized around the development of a multidisciplinary approach to all phases of the management of head and neck cancer, including early detection, diagnosis, pretreatment planning, treatment, follow-up care, and rehabilitation. The core of the clinical aspect of the project was to be a multidisciplinary clinic for head and neck cancer patients established by the University of Mississippi Medical Center (UMMC) and the Veterans Administration Center in Jackson, eight months before the application was submitted. The clinic was to be the entry point and patient care center for all head and neck patients seen at these two institutions. It was also to be the planning center for clinical protocols developed by the network staff.

The initial planning year was followed by one year of implementation. After that year, the contract was voluntarily terminated by the contractor. A statement at the beginning of the final report indicated that the principal investigator was voluntarily requesting termination owing to lack of progress in meeting the network objectives. The specific reasons offered by the principal investigator for the failure to attain the program objectives were given in the conclusion to that report. They seem to focus on two areas: lack of environmental resources to support the program objectives, and incompatibility of the program objectives with the interests of the senior staff of the network. We have already examined the resource bases of all of the networks, including Mississippi, and although the area was not rich in medical resources, it was not any worse off than some of the other six networks. How the program objectives were planned and initially implemented warrants closer examination.

The Mississippi network had two stated objectives. The first was to extend the multidisciplinary treatment concepts incorporated into the apparently successful multidisciplinary clinic at the UMMC and the VA center to other network hospitals. The second focus of the program was community and professional health education.

The first objective was to be achieved by setting up the clinic as an area resource, a model for patient management. It was stated by the principal investigator that he hoped to establish the clinic as the tertiary referral center for the region. This was a reasonable expectation since the UMMC was clearly the most well-equipped and centralized treatment center in the region. The participating community hospitals varied greatly in the extent to which they had facilities necessary to introduce multidisciplinary care. Thus, there was an expectation that the UMMC would receive referrals from these outlying hospitals for treatment.

The second objective of providing professional education to primary care physicians, dentists, nurses, and dental hygienists was to be provided by the network staff on the faculty of the university. Lay education was to be aimed at the general population, with some specific orientation to the highest-risk groups, who were also the hardest to reach and the most distrustful of medical professionals. These activities were to be done by participating network units, although the proposal was less specific regarding these responsibilities. There was some indication that other health professionals and maybe the local unit of the American Cancer Society, would assume responsibility for some of these programs.

A data-collection system had been designed to provide two sorts of information: a record of the specific treatment given each patient, and baseline data with which to evaluate the overall impact of the network project. The data system, like the oral screening and lay health education program, were to be subcontracted to participating network institutions.

Despite optimistic intentions and a well-developed plan, the program in Mississippi ended abruptly. Although the principal investigator initiated the termination, it apparently followed what he thought was a rather negative merit peer review. All the network projects were reviewed at that time, using a standard evaluation format based on data compiled by each program. In light of a review of those reports, the situation in Mississippi did not appear to differ greatly from that found in the other networks.

The principal investigator and clinical staff associated with the network were most interested in the clinic and multidisciplinary treatment planning. Though the multidisciplinary clinic was established just eight months prior to the submission of the application, it was expected to be the focal point of the network clinical programs. It was tied to clinical research, and research protocols were to be developed from the experiences of the UMMC clinic and then disseminated to the participating hospitals for implementation. The resulting protocols were to be the Mississippi guidelines.

Since the clinical programs were of primary interest to the network participants, the success of the UMMC clinic as the model of state-of-the-art care was critical to the network's success. It soon became apparent, however, that within the university and within the network there was less than complete support for the principles of multidisciplinary care, as defined by the principal investigator. The lack of support for the clinic is clear in both the summary report prepared for the merit peer review (May 29, 1976) and the final report:

> The nature of the medical practitioner in our network and in our state is such that members function first as private practitioners and secondly as members of the team. For this reason, there is considerable variation in the level of cooperation. . . . The surgical aspects of treatment are generally rendered by individual physicians or groups of physicians, but all surgical members do not participate

in all patients' care. At the present time there is no organized area where all patients are routinely seen by all members of a team in a given institution for the purpose of pretreatment planning and discussion.

Some of the failure of the clinic is blamed on inadequate resources, particularly the availability of radiation therapists and clinic space both at headquarters and in the hospitals. But the underlying theme is the failure of the network leadership to gain the support of other physicians (either in the network or at headquarters) for the concept of multidisciplinary care and the idea of multidisciplinary pretreatment planning. In fact, the principal investigator did not believe that physicians in Mississippi could voluntarily agree on what constituted primary care, nor could they accept any kind of consensus that disagreed with their own views. Even planning conferences, which worked very well in Northern California, Greater Delaware Valley, and Arkansas, were not acceptable to head and neck physicians in Mississippi. This basic frustration was exacerbated by inadequate space, the resignation of one of the three principals in the program, and the inability to hire key staff to conduct some of the programs.

Two critical steps in the progression of failure emerge from these various comments and the changing tone of the network documents. The first step was the inability or refusal of the community physicians to accept multidisciplinary patient management as a way to practice medicine. This lack of acceptance of the innovation led to the dissolution of the UMMC clinic. Since it was to be the model for clinical activity throughout the network region, once it failed there would be no base for stimulating clinical activity and treatment innovation. Because this was the primary focus of the network program, its failure led to a demise of interest in the other network activities. Thus, the second key step in the network's demise was that the principal investigator and the remaining clinician were simply not sufficiently interested in the other network activities to pursue them in the absence of the UMMC clinic. As the principal investigator explained:

> The stress on lay education, training of oral hygienists, data analysis, and oral screening are all important and worthwhile but are not likely to maintain the sustained interest of physicians. As a consequence, interest among faculty members waned with time.

It is interesting to note the perception by the network staff of a shortage of radiation therapists in the region. In fact, an examination of the participating staff at the network hospitals indicated that all but one hospital had a radiation therapist, although most of the institutions outside of Jackson lacked radiation therapy equipment. Implementation of multidisciplinary care at most network hospitals would have been possible only through a referral arrangement. Although some discussion of referral had been included in the initial application, none of the subsequent documents indicated that referrals to support treatment for head and neck cancer had been considered or adopted. Thus, in the network hospitals, as in the headquarters institutions, treatment decisions were apparently defined by the abilities of the individual practitioner and the availability of the particular hospital's resources.

In light of our analysis of successful network programs, several features of the Mississippi network require further comment. First, the resource base of the Mississippi network seemed to be more like that found in the interpersonal networks than in the interorganizational networks. If the implementation of state-of-the-art treatment would have required referral, as was claimed by the network principal investigator, this would clearly indicate that the Mississippi network should have been developed following the interpersonal model. The idea of the clinic at UMMC serving as a model for the regional physicians is also more consistent with the interpersonal than with the interorganizational pattern. The fact that very few network resources were designated for disbursement to the network hospitals also suggests the interpersonal pattern. Thus, one factor may have been inappropriate expectations about what could be done in the hospitals in the network region.

A second observation is the absence of institutional support for the headquarters. There is reference to a lack of space, personnel, and cooperation by some members of the faculty. This problem did not arise in any of the other networks. Without some institutional support and commitment to a headquarters location, it is difficult to mount this type of program.

Third, the investigators appear to have misread the intent of the community physicians. It would appear that the community physicians did not understand or accept what was expected of them, which raises questions about how much prior contact had been made before the proposal was submitted. The successful interpersonal networks were built around long-standing contacts and well-understood relationships in the community. Even where it was understood that local physicians might not refer, the network program reflected that expectation.

In general, the experience of the Mississippi network clearly reveals the importance of the network environment. It demonstrates the effects of lack of fit between organizational form and environmental resources and domain constraints.

NATIONAL POLICY CHANGES AND THE SURVIVAL OF THE NETWORKS

What lasting impact did these network programs have on the way in which the National Cancer Institute pursued its agenda? These networks were the early efforts by the NCI to implement a national cancer control program. They were more or less successful in meeting the agendas established by the local communities in which they were established. Comprehensive cancer centers emerged at four of the six network demonstration sites, and in three of those the network program was instrumental in the implementation of the center. In two the network became the model for the cancer center organization, and that model has since been adopted as an officially designated organizational form for future comprehensive cancer centers. Clearly, one contribution to the national cancer program was an early test of the applicability of the network model for developing disease control programs. The experiences of the Illinois and Northern California programs demonstrate how effective consortia can be in avoiding duplication of resources and implementing amicable resolution of potentially difficult issues regarding organizational domain.

The experiences of these centers also indicate the limitations of such programs. Consortia cannot produce research that requires laboratory or similar facilities. They can provide a resource for field-testing the findings that come from the laboratory. Consortia can only enter areas that are not the domain of a single participant.

In Illinois, when the Illinois Cancer Council was established, the participating universities all had ongoing clinical trials programs, funded through the clinical research program at NCI. Hence arrangements had to be made to ensure that the ICC's clinical activities did not conflict with those at the universities. Representatives of the universities met and reached agreement as to these relationships. Clinical trials sponsored by the ICC were conducted either so they did not conflict with the university research programs or, in some cases, the ICC assumed responsiblity for centralized management of the research activities for all consortium participants. Similar arrangements were made by the Northern California consortium.

The NCI continues to be committed to the network concept. In the aftermath of these projects, the network concept has been implemented in several other programs. These programs have had three forms of network linkage. In one form, the network model developed in the original networks was retained, and community hospitals were linked to academic medical centers. In a second form, the headquarters were large community hospitals that were invited to form consortial or network relationships with smaller local hospitals in their regions. In the third and most recent form, community hospitals were contractually linked directly with the NCI but had to affiliate with some type of academic unit as a research base through which they would have access to research protocols and statistical and data-management support.

Each of these forms retains some features of the original networks, but each represents an attempt to build on the experience and expand the cancer control infrastructure. We will examine each form in more detail.

We noted earlier in this chapter that, at about the same time that the NCI initiated these demonstration network projects, they also initiated a cancer control outreach program through the clinical cooperative groups. This was the Cooperative Group Outreach Program (CGOP). Basically, the Division of Cancer Control and Rehabilitation at the NCI provided funds to the cooperative group programs to enable them to support physicians in community hospitals who wished to enter patients on protocol through an academic-based member institution. This program proved very successful, and eventually about half of the patients on national clinical trials came into them through these network relationships. The rationale for this program was the same as that given for the network demonstration programs: It would provide access to state-of-the-art treatment to patients in community hospitals. It was up to the academic center to ensure the quality of the data from these hospitals, and access to the protocol could be limited to hospitals with the facilities and staff to implement the treatment. In fact, as we have said, in Illinois and Wisconsin, the CGOP program developed in many of the same hospitals that participated in the network demonstration program. Similar experiences occurred with members of the breast demonstration project that paralleled the head and neck networks.

The earliest replications, then, followed the same model as the demonstration networks. However, some lessons have been learned. Greater accountability for data quality was required of the academic centers. Because the CGOPs were research networks, participants were required to follow a single protocol and collect common data that were maintained and evaluated in a data center independent of any participating institution. There was a common research agenda that required strict compliance with common data quality and implementation criteria. These methods, then, avoided the definitional and quality control problems that were experienced by the head and neck networks.

As far as data quality was concerned, it appeared that community physicians who participated through the CGOP network performed as well as, or better than, the academic centers (Begg *et al.*, 1982). They met their obligations to put patients on study because if they did not they risked losing their funding and access to experimental research. Given the research focus, the criteria for performance could be enforced.

The second network initiative was an effort to link community hospitals with other more experienced community hospitals to develop guidelines and community cancer control outreach. There were two such programs: the Community Oncology Program (COP) and the Community Hospital Oncology Program (CHOP). These programs were more directly descended from the network demonstration projects in that they sought to define state of the art in standard care, using the more flexible guideline format instead of the rigid research protocol. Like the network demonstration projects, the CHOPs were initially allowed to define their own data set and to develop evaluation criteria. As the project progressed, however, it became clear that the price of agreement was a very large, cumbersome, and potentially costly data set. The NCI finally stepped in and established a minimal data set that had to be collected and indicated that it would pay only for that set of items. The ultimate result was that the minimal data set became the data set.

The COP program suffered from many of the same problems as the demonstration networks. There was limited control over the physical capabilities of the hospitals to initiate state-of-the-art care. Guidelines were locally developed, and therefore there was no national or uniform definition of standard care, leaving evaluation an open question. However, it did have an effect similar to the network demonstration projects in bringing more community hospitals into the cancer control sphere. By avoiding the requirement that community hospitals enter the network through an academic center, it opened access to cancer control programming to more regions of the country, which was a target of the NCI. Beyond creating awareness and introducing the national cancer program to more physicians, it was impossible to demonstrate any outcome that would indicate modification of treatment practice.

The lessons from these early experiences were finally incorporated into the most recent cancer control outreach program, the Community Clinical Oncology Program (CCOP), which was introduced in 1982. Here, the participating hospitals contract directly with the National Cancer Institute. To be accepted, each applicant hospital must submit a proposal that defines its resources, the institutional commitments, and the quality and experience of the key staff. Evidence of the ability to conduct multidisciplinary treatment is a requirement for a successful applicant. The applicant must affiliate with an academic research base that is responsible for the quality of the research at each of its affiliated community hospitals. However, unlike the CGOP, the CCOPs are eligible to participate more fully in the cooperative groups, including protocol development. They receive their funding directly from the NCI. Because this program has a research focus, all participants are required to use some experimental treatment protocols and to collect a standard data set on patients entered on protocol. The diffusion hypothesis is built into the evaluation of this ongoing program. It is assumed that physicians who put patients on protocol will generally be more sensitive to patterns of care that have been demonstrated to be important for sound treatment. They will be more up-to-date on what is state of the art.

The performance assessment of this program is based on examining specific indicators of what, in the judgment of leading oncologists in the country, constitutes standard care for certain critical kinds of cancer. Data are being abstracted from the records of participating hospitals to define whether these elements are present. Data are also being abstracted from a set of control hospitals to determine whether practices are different in the CCOP hospitals compared with nonparticipating community hospitals. In short, many of the ideas gained from the demonstration networks are being implemented in newer network programs.

A major difficulty with this evaluation is, once again, the time lag. Although the quality of data being obtained in these studies is considerably better (since a common data set was required and collected by a neutral data center), the evaluation is being done after only three years of implementation. It may be too early to see treatment changes, given the conservative nature of physicians in changing treatment patterns.

A final diffusion strategy that has most recently been introduced is the Physician Data Query system. Through this program, information on state-of-the-art management for most tumors, as well as information about experimental treatment protocols, has been incorporated into the National Library of Medicine data base and into two commercial data bases. Physicians can access this system via a personal computer or through their local hospital or medical school library. The information is updated regularly. An evaluation of this program has been initiated.

In summary, the later generations of network programs seem to be addressing many of the problems confronted by their predecessors. In particular, issues of compliance and definition of the state of the art seem to have been addressed. In the latest programs, the environmental and institutional resource pools are specifically taken into account since the qualifications of applicant hospitals are considered. The introduction of a peer review process by which successful applicants are determined also has added to the strength of the program. It remains to be seen whether these latest efforts will really affect diffusion of state of the art in cancer care.

BEYOND CANCER NETWORKS

We began this volume with a two-figure scenario of the diffusion of medical innovation, based primarily on the physician–scientist and the physician–practitioner. We have since traveled through eight chapters full of additional players in the medical innovation game: hospitals, hospital administrators, policymakers, research agencies, advisory panels, the federal government, Congress, the president, community groups, and a smorgasbord of various health professionals. Although our trip has been primarily via the Cancer Turnpike, the road signs we have encountered should apply to the diffusion of innovation in any area of the health sector, and possibly beyond that sector as well.

Organizational networks for innovation diffusion have also surfaced in fields of heart disease, maternal and child health care, neonatal care, and kidney disease. By and large, the assumptions behind the use of the network model are the same as those held by the NCI prior to launching the network demonstration projects: By the linking of medical research centers to community hospitals, innovations travel faster, and "networking" should make possible the ideal of regional care centers, ultimately leading to decreased facility duplication and lower costs. However, our study of the head and neck cancer networks clearly demonstrates that such a simple-minded approach to the complexities of organizational networks is misplaced.

First of all, not all innovations are appropriate (i.e., suitable or ready) for rapid or manipulated dissemination through interorganizational networks, whether in medicine, business, or education. The characteristics of innovations must be well understood prior to diffusion, particularly their trialability, their compatibility with previous procedure, and the extent to which data exist on their performance, either through empirical research or firsthand experience.

In conjunction with the innovation's characteristics, of course, we must consider the characteristics of the targeted organizations. In the case of cancer treatment innovations, not all hospitals are equally well equipped or staffed. In any field, the resource capabilities of targeted organizations must be matched with characteristics and requirements of proposed innovations. When the issue is that of regional dissemination of new technologies, the examination of resource capabilities must expand to an examination of general environmental constraints and opportunities.

Once the innovation itself and the context for targeted adoption are both well understood, then the key players need to be examined: the change agent, the gatekeepers, the influentials, the boundary spanners, and, of course, the audience. Here is where the diffusion process and network channels become particularly interesting and complex. Innovations do not pass through diffusion processes unchanged. They are defined, redefined, reinvented, and transformed in the diffusion process, as part of a negotiated adjustment process between the agendas of change agents and the agendas of targeted organizations and individuals. If the change agent happens to be an agency of the federal government, then that adjustment process can actually involve policy reformulation as the innovation is reinvented. As we saw in the cancer network program, the innovation of multidisciplinary treatment was redefined as either treatment guidelines, pretreatment planning conferences, or multidisciplinary teams, depending upon the perceived performance gaps in the various regions.

Similarly, networks for innovation diffusion become defined and redefined through the diffusion process itself. Network structures develop within social contexts, composed, in part, of preexisting social linkages, social norms, and various definitions of costs and benefits associated with social exchanges. As the innovation is itself redefined to fit local agendas, so are the diffusion channels designed to transmit it.

In essence, what we have described here is a political process of agenda setting, social exchange, and negotiation. But what most clearly illustrates this fact is an attempt to analyze the outcomes and/or performance of these diffusion networks. In this chapter we have examined various conceptualizations of performance, network constituencies, levels of analysis, and types of measures. Diffusion networks can have an impact on several different levels of analysis, from the organizational to the national system level. However, when the innovation itself is not clearly understood or previously tested, and when the diffusion channels are themselves designed to reflect local constraints, the end results are never straightforward. Network outcomes may reflect successful agenda setting and domain enhancement as much as they reflect any actual diffusion of the intended innovation. As was the case examined here, the redefinition of the policies and programs that acted as change agents in initiating these diffusion networks is in fact the most important and far-reaching outcome of the cancer network program.

Appendixes

Site Visit Outline

I. What is a network?

   A. Structure

   B. Function and linkage

   C. Organizational change and the network

II. Description of the network

   A. Initial plan from proposal (first time period)

      1. Context

         a. Characteristics of population

            (1) Sociodemographic
            (2) Medical/health status

         b. Characteristics of physicians and other medical personnel

         c. Characteristics of medical institutions

         d. Overall level of resources

      2. Network staff and resources

         a. Headquarters

            (1) Experience and organization of headquarters as a cancer control operations office
            (2) Staff resources
                (a) Number of staff

       (b) Number of staff in specialties relevant to the care of head and neck cancer patients

       (c) Number of staff involved in the network and their specialties

       (d) Credentials

  (3) Treatment facilities

       (a) Number of facilities

       (b) Number of facilities important to the care of head and neck cancer patients

  (4) Beds

       (a) Number of beds

       (b) Number of beds reserved for head and neck cancer patients

  (5) Patients

       (a) Number of admissions

       (b) Number of admissions of head and neck cancer patients

       (c) Characteristics of head and neck cancer patients

          1. Sociodemographic characteristics

          2. Stage and site of disease

  (6) Other facilities

       (a) Data facilities

       (b) Tumor registry

b. Participating institutions

  (1) Distance to headquarters

  (2) Staff resources

       (a) Number of staff

       (b) Number of staff in specialties relevant to the care of head and neck cancer patients

       (c) Number of staff involved in the network and their specialties

       (d) Credentials

  (3) Treatment facilities

       (a) Number of facilities

       (b) Number of facilities important to the care of head and neck cancer patients

  (4) Beds

       (a) Number of beds

       (b) Number of beds reserved for head and neck cancer patients

  (5) Patients

       (a) Number of admissions

       (b) Number of admissions of head and neck cancer patients

       (c) Characteristics of head and neck cancer patients

          1. Sociodemographic characteristics

          2. Stage and site of disease

(6) Other facilities

    (a) Data facilities

    (b) Tumor registry

3. Network organization

  a. Preexisting general links

    (1) Content of links (registries, residents, therapists, research efforts, shared facilities, overlapping directorates, funds, etc.)

    (2) Those institutions involved in each link

    (3) Form of links

      (a) Multiple or single strand

      (b) Formal or informal

      (c) Mutual or not

      (d) Interinstitutional or interpersonal

  b. Preexisting links related specifically to the treatment of head and neck cancer

    (1) Content of links (registries, residents, therapists, research efforts, shared facilities, funds, etc.)

    (2) Those institutions or bodies involved in each link

    (3) Form of links

      (a) Multiple or single strand

      (b) Formal or informal

      (c) Mutual or not

      (d) Interinstitutional or interpersonal

    (4) Legal and organizational blocks to the formation of links

  c. Establishment of governmental, administrative, or coordinating bodies

    (1) Characterizing tasks of committees

    (2) Number

    (3) Type

    (4) Hierarchical arrangements and power attributes

    (5) Institutions represented on committees

    (6) Frequency of meetings

    (7) Full-time administrative positions

    (8) Constitutions and bylaws created

  d. Establishment of new links

    (1) Content of links (registries, residents, therapists, research efforts, shared facilities, funds, etc.)

    (2) Those institutions or bodies involved in each link

(3) Form of links

    (a) Multiple or single strand

    (b) Formal or informal

    (c) Mutual or not

    (d) Interinstitutional or interpersonal

(4) Legal and organizational blocks to the formation of links

e. Long-range planning for continued operation of the program after termination of contract

(1) Plans for case follow-up and survival analysis

(2) Financial planning for stability

    (a) Institutional commitment

(3) Proposed measures of effect

f. Establishment of new research, study groups, etc., or plans for such endeavors

4. Network procedures

a. Governmental procedures

(1) Primary issues considered for incorporation into the network

    (a) Multidisciplinary plans

    (b) Educational ventures

    (c) Management guidelines

    (d) Other

(2) Ways in which these issues were chosen

(3) Extent to which these choices follow the requirements set forth by the National Cancer Institute (NCI)

    (a) Issues chosen that were not set forth by the NCI

(4) What took place during the national PI meetings

    (a) How did individual networks follow through with the decisions made during the national meetings

(5) Dynamics of the relationships between the networks and the project officer

    (a) Dynamics between the networks themselves

(6) How decisions regarding ongoing policy were made

    (a) Role of staff

    (b) Role of committees

(7) Ways in which decisions were communicated to the staff

    (a) Number of regularly scheduled contacts per month

    (b) Type of contact (tumor boards, etc.)

    (c) Who was involved

b. Case selection

(1) Mechanism for case selection

    (a) Interinstitutional selection procedures

      (b) Who decides criteria for selection

   (2) Patterns of incoming referral

      (a) To whom were the cases referred (which doctor or institution) and by whom

   (3) Rate of accrual

   (4) Mechanism for determining case evaluability

   (5) Quality control mechanism for case selection

      (a) Who evaluated
      (b) What was done
      (c) How often
      (d) To whom were the results of review reported

c. Treatment and rehabilitation

   (1) Routine of multidisciplinary treatment team

      (a) Who sets criteria
      (b) Pretreatment planning (tumor boards)
         1. Who is on tumor board
         2. Number of patients considered
      (c) Steps of treatment
      (d) Points of intervention in patient's treatment
      (e) Who intervened

   (2) Short- and long-term follow-up for survival side effects, and recurrence

   (3) Referral

   (4) Quality control for case management

      (a) Who evaluated
      (b) What was done (audits evaluation of morbidity and mortality data)
      (c) How often
      (d) To whom were the results of review reported

   (5) Communication among staff

      (a) Number of regularly scheduled contacts per month
      (b) Type of contact
      (c) Who was involved

d. Data base management

   (1) Procedures for case registration

   (2) Procedures for completion of forms (data collection and entry)

   (3) Who created forms

   (4) Personnel available for data base activities

   (5) Quality control for data base management

      (a) Who evaluated
      (b) What was done (forms quality maintenance)

          (c) How often

          (d) To whom were the results of review reported

    e. Relationship with the community

      (1) Educational ventures

         (a) With professional community

         (b) With lay community (outreach programs)

      (2) Screening programs

         (a) Organization

         (b) Frequency

         (c) Results

      (3) Community's involvement in, awareness of, and commitment to program

         (a) Local volunteer groups

         (b) Public health agencies and health planning groups

         (c) Other

   f. Initiation of new research or related projects

      (1) Who is involved

      (2) What was initiated

      (3) How project proceeded

  B. Reexamination of network context, resources, organization, and procedures for second time period

III. Comparisons over time

  A. Changes in context

  B. Changes in resources

  C. Changes in organization

  D. Changes in procedure

IV. Assessment of outcomes

  A. Assessment of network effect on interinstitutional collaboration

    1. Internetwork cooperation

  B. Assessment of network effect on multidisciplinary collaboration

  C. Diffusion of information process

    1. Speed of diffusion

   2. Pattern of diffusion (which units followed guidelines first, which followed, when)

   3. Characteristics of the innovation

      a. Did they demand major alterations in management

      b. Did they demand major alterations in resources

      c. Did they demand major reorganization of, or additions to, staff

D. Development of data base

E. Research accomplishments

F. Community impact

   1. Patients

   2. Professional community

   3. Lay community

   4. Knowledge base

G. Educational impact

   1. Professional community

   2. Lay community

   3. Strategies and their effectiveness

H. Impact on nonnetwork organizations in region

 I. Study of comparison between network and nonnetwork experiences

V. Recommendations and conclusions

B

Interview Protocol

For the Principal Investigators

I. Membership and recruitment of new members

1. How is a member of the network defined?

    (probe: by institution, individuals, by whether patients are entered into the data base, by participation in educational programs, other criteria?)

2. Are there different kinds of memberships? How are they defined? How do they affect level and type of participation?

3. Specifically, which of the following can be individual members?

Surgeons	_____
Radiation therapists	_____
Medical oncologists	_____
Pathologists	_____
Oral pathologists	_____
Dentists	_____
Maxillofacial prosthodontists	_____
Speech pathologists	_____
Dieticians	_____
Nurses	_____
Social workers	_____
Epidemiologists	_____
Statisticians	_____
Residents	_____
Lay public	_____

4. Complete charts of membership categories for institutions and individuals.

   a. Must individuals who are members come from institutions that are also defined as being in the network, or can they come from private practice? Can members be just interested individuals without representing any group, agency, or institution?

   b. How does an individual, professional or not, join the network?

   c. Is there a formal memorandum of understanding, contract, letter, etc., that is required before membership is "official"? If yes, get a sample copy.

5. Are there institutional memberships in the network?

   a. Are these defined by any type of formal agreement? Describe, ask for a sample. Who signs for the network? For the institution?

6. How is the institutional membership initiated? Between departments, individuals who are heads of teams, between hospitals and the network?

   a. When a head of a service becomes a participant, do all his/her staff automatically become members? Does each have to apply separately after the institution is accepted as a network member?

   b. Are there minimum requirements for institutional membership, such as:

      Number of patients
      Diversity of staff
      Special facilities
      Evidence of multidisciplinary activity
      Willingness to enter patients in data base
      Participation in educational activities, outreach

   Please describe the minimum requirements.

   c. Have the requirements changed since the initiation of the network?

7. Is there a review process for new members (either institutional or individual)? Describe this process.

   a. Who makes decisions based on the results of this process?

8. Are there provisions by which an institution can terminate its membership? Describe.

   a. Has this ever occurred? Describe the situation.

9. Are there procedures whereby the membership can be revoked? Describe.

   a. Has this ever occurred? Please describe the situation and how it was handled.

For the Principal Investigators

  II. Preexisting and current links

1. Prior to the response to the RFP, what relationships between the participants already existed? (Build on response to RFP.)

2. In the original proposal, institutional linkages and possibilities for the development of those linkages were described that do not appear in the later organization. What kinds of factors promoted or inhibited the maturation of some links and not others?

   a. Some factors that may have been influential are:
   Access to patients
   Institutional policies
   Legal barriers
   Cost, funding

3. Please describe how priorities concerning the network boundaries were established.

4. Where new links were established, on what basis were they made? Was there any prior contact, and, if so, was it between institutions, individuals, etc.?

5. To what extent do the relationships in the network extend beyond the management of head and neck cancers?

   a. Are there residency programs? What institutions and specialties are involved? Did these predate the network?

   b. Is there cooperative research in cancer (ECOG, GOG, RTOG, SOG, other)?

   c. Were there any other forms of cooperative research?

   d. Were there cancer control programs? Educational outreach programs?

   e. Please describe the referral patterns that existed between the participating institutions. For example, did senior staff have students who were located at an institution other than his/her own? Have the patterns changed since the establishment of the network?

6. To what extent are nonmedical, cancer-related agencies such as ACS, Candlelighters, laryngectomy clubs, etc., integrated in the network?

   a. Do such agencies hold positions on committees? If so, which ones and what types of responsibilities do they have? How much power do they have?

   b. Are links with these types of organizations established through various educational programs? If so, what programs and what organizations? Please describe the extent of involvement.

   c. Do the links with these agencies take the form of funding?

   d. Are these agencies involved in rehabilitation and treatment programs sponsored by the network? Do these agencies sponsor such programs in which network patients participate?

e. Do these sorts of organizations hold any type of membership in the network?

f. To what extent is local government (state or municipal) involved and/or committed to the head and neck program?

g. Are any lay groups that are not necessarily cancer-related involved? For example, do volunteer groups or youth groups donate time or funds to the program?

h. If other forms of support of, or involvement in, your program developed during the history of the network, please describe briefly.

For the Principal Investigators

III. Patient Management Guidelines/Protocols

1. Were any treatment protocols developed at this network?

   a. Were these specifically related to the development of the guidelines?

   b. Which network participants were involved in the development of these treatment protocols?

2. Although the guidelines have not as yet been introduced formally, in 1977 a trial set was widely disseminated. Were they adopted in this network? With what effect? Were there any procedures for obtaining feedback regarding their utility and acceptability?

   a. What aspects of the guidelines were implemented locally?

   b. Is there any systematic procedure for monitoring the implementation of guidelines or treatment procedures?

   c. See chart on participation of individuals in treatment procedures.

   d. Were any meetings held in which network participants were introduced to the guidelines?

3. Were nonphysicians ever involved in the preparation of the guidelines?

   a. Which guideline sites received attention from nonphysicians?

   b. Which specialties were involved?

   c. What were the institutions represented by this involvement? Where were they?

For the Principal Investigators

IV. A. Research Activities

1. Was there any effort to establish intranetwork collaboration for research and publications?

2. Were protocols for research developed?

    a. Who were the investigators? With what institution were they affiliated? What was their degree?

    b. What is the title of the study?

3. Were any proposals submitted for funding?

    a. Who submitted the proposals? With what institution were they affiliated? What was their degree?

    b. What is the title of the study?

    c. What is the title of the funding agency?

4. Were there any publications or new prosthetic devices that resulted from the program?

    a. Reprint?

    b. Who is the author? What is his/her degree? With what institution was he/she affiliated?

    c. What is the title of the paper or the type of device?

5. Were data on which these publications were based from the data base?

6. Please list any other collaborative research projects or publications.

For the Educational Coordinator or Committee

IV. B. Educational and Outreach Programs

1. Is there a list of programs and speakers?

2. What attendance was experienced?

3. Were target groups for such programs defined?

    a. How were they defined? Professional, lay?

4. Was a single person designated as the education/outreach coordinator?

    a. When was this person designated?

    b. What are his/her qualifications, professional degrees, etc.?

5. Did this person coordinate all educational activities?

    a. How was the scope of responsibility defined?

6. How was he/she paid?

7. Was there an educational program coordinator at each participating institution?

    a. Who were these coordinators? What were their degrees?

    b. What activities did they conduct?

    c. Were these people network members?

8. Was there a committee or a preexisting organization (continuing education program, etc.) that either assisted or directed the educational activities?

9. Did educational activities focus on certain areas?
   a. What are these areas?
   b. Who chose them?

10. Did educational activities interface with other educational efforts, such as CME, ACS, other? Please describe.
    a. Was this interface a result of systematic planning?
    b. Who was responsible for the planning?
    c. Were there any meetings? Are there records of meetings?

11. Was there a written report summarizing each educational program?

12. Were there workshops for new ideas and concepts in care and management?
    a. Please describe these symposia.
    b. How were they initiated?
    c. Were they evaluated? How?

13. What written and/or visual educational materials were developed?
    a. How were they evaluated? By whom?
    b. Were they disseminated?

14. What materials or activities were particularly popular? Useful? Well received?

15. What was the mix of old materials and new materials?

16. Was there any cross-network educational activity (i.e., between projects)?
    a. Who participated in this activity?
    b. What were their degrees, titles?
    c. What was the topic for the program?

For the Financial Administrator

V. A. Management for financial affairs

1. How is the annual budget prepared?

2. Who reviews it?

3. Who has responsibility for reports, etc.?

    4. Is there a central project office and/or a project manager? Project manager (CV) request.

For the Principal Investigators and Administrator

  V. B. Committee Structure and Network Governance

    1. Are there bylaws that define the structure of the network? If we do not have a copy, request one.

    2. Is there a committee structure for the governance of the network?

    3. What are the major committees? What are their responsibilities? For example, is there an executive committee?

      a. Who are the members of each committee?

      b. How often do they meet?

      c. Dates of last meetings?

      d. Are minutes of these meetings available? Ask for sets.

      e. Are there records of attendance?

    4. Must committee members have institutional affiliations or can any member of the network serve on a committee?

    5. Must someone be a committee member to have the authority to include cases in the data base?

    6. Are representatives of any other agencies, such as the ACS, laryngectomy societies, etc., on any committees? Which ones?

  C. Please provide a staff roster if you haven't done so already.

For the Principal Investigators

  VI. A. Data System and Patient Registration Objectives

    1. What are the objectives of the data collection at this network?

      a. How were these objectives determined?

      b. Are they consistent with the overall objectives determined?

      c. By whom were these objectives determined?

      d. How important was data collection considered compared with other tasks of the network?

    2. Who designed the data forms?

      a. How were the forms devised to incorporate the objectives?

3. Were any departures in the data-collection protocol made at this network?

   a. Why were these departures made?

   b. Who decided to make them?

   c. Were they discussed with the project officer and other network principals?

4. Data use

   a. To what uses were the data supposed to be put?

   b. What local uses have been made of the data? Did publications, protocols, or research procedures arise out of the data? (Get list)

   c. Are there plans for such endeavors?

For Network Coordinators, Data Coordinators, Principal Investigators

VI. B. Data System and Patient Registration Procedures

1. Are all head and neck patients at each institution entered into the data set?

   a. If not, what criteria were established to define eligibility? How were these criteria established? Are disease type and location of the institution included in the criteria?

   b. If so, are there procedures that ensure that all cases are in fact entered? How were these procedures established, and what are they?

2. Was there a single data-collection center?

   a. How many head and neck staff are located there?

3. Who decides that a particular case is eligible for inclusion in the network?

4. Who completes the initial registration form?

   a. Who is responsible for subsequent forms on the same patient?

   b. Who is responsible for patient follow-up data?

   c. What procedures are used?

   d. Are forms logged? Is there a system for case review for timeliness, etc.?

5. How are data transferred from forms to data base?

   a. What type of person does this coding?

   b. Does the same person enter the coded data?

6. Are data forms spot-checked for completeness and consistency?

   a. Who does the spot-checking?

   b. Is this checking a routine part of the data entry process?

   c. Are data systematically rechecked against records for accuracy?

7. Were data ever reviewed by a central committee of network PIs to assure quality?

8. Is there unevenness in the data?

   a. Are there procedures for returning to the data sources for more detailed information?

   b. Describe how and for what reasons these procedures have been followed.

9. To what extent is the data base linked to the registries at the participating hospitals?

10. Does the patient have to consent to inclusion in the data base and/or the network?

For the Principal Investigators

The original request for proposals for the network demonstration project listed six objectives to be achieved. The attached list describes them. We would like to know how these objectives are currently perceived and the strategies for pursuing them. Please rank the objectives in order of importance and answer the following questions for the two or three most important and the least important ones.

VII. A. General Objectives

1. What approach have you utilized to achieve this objective?

2. What conditions or special aspects of your network's situation have affected the way in which this objective is being, or has been, pursued? Are there any particular strengths or needs in the current situation that have encouraged pursuit of this objective in this way?

3. In your opinion, after all is considered, how well has this network met this goal? Can you point out what has led you to perceive the network's development in this way?

4. If you were organizing a program such as this again, would this remain a major objective? Would there be ways that you would change the manner in which this activity was organized and/or pursued?

5. If changes in this objective had been made, ask:

   a. How was this change decided? Within the network—by committee, by staff, necessitated by the situation?

   b. Was it discussed with the other principal investigators of other networks? Why or why not?

c. Was it discussed with the network project officer? How did this change affect the scope of work in your contract and the budget?

Objectives of the cancer network demonstration projects

1. Delivery of standardized, modern, multidisciplinary, health care methods to all head and neck patients in each geographic area served by one of the network programs.

2. Development of management guidelines.

3. Establishment and implementation of a standard data system.

4. Conduct of regional, professional, and public educational programs dealing with the detection and management of head and neck cancer.

5. Provision of a vehicle for sharing specialized personnel and facilities to effect the highest-quality and most economical health care delivery to head and neck cancer patients in the region served.

6. The conduct of evaluation of the project in terms of activity, process, and impact prescribed by the NCI program evaluation guidelines.

VII. B. General Objectives Not Included in the RFP

1. Have any objectives not originally covered by these seven been added to the program?

2. How was the decision to pursue this objective made? By committee, PI, staff?

3. Did this additional objective affect your ability to meet the objectives already discussed? Did it supplement or build upon them?

4. Was the scope of work modified with the addition of this objective? Were other network PIs consulted? Was this objective discussed with the project officer?

For the Principal Investigators, Administrator, and Network Coordinator

VIII. Long-Term Planning

1. What are the long-term plans for funding?

2. What are the long-term plans for continued implementation of programs and collaborative relationships?

a. Are there plans for the follow-up of cases entered into the data base after the funding terminates? If so, what plans have been developed?

3. To what extent will the program be affected by reduced or loss of NCI funding?

4. Are new programs building on the network project? Describe both plans and funding status.

   a. Has this network developed any formal plans to measure or evaluate the impact of network activities on the quality of care provided for head and neck cancer patients? Please describe these plans.

5. Are there plans for publication of local data?

C

CEO Cover Letter and Questionnaire

Dear _____:

As you may know, your hospital is a participant in the _____ Head and Neck Cancer Network. Six such networks were established in 1973–1974 across the country for the purpose of improving and coordinating the screening, treatment, and rehabilitation of patients with head and neck cancer.

In 1979 the National Cancer Institute contracted with the Illinois Cancer Council to produce a monograph describing the network experience in the management of head and neck cancer. As part of our efforts to document that experience we are contacting all network-affiliated hospitals to help us obtain various information about the resources available to the network through the hospitals that participate. We are also interested in collaboration or sharing relationships between hospitals in any area of patient service or research. In order to complete this project meaningfully, it is necessary to obtain this information in a standard format. Therefore, we are asking each network-affiliated hospital to complete the enclosed brief questionnaire and return it to us as soon as possible in the enclosed stamped envelope.

If you should have any questions concerning the questionnaire or the monograph project, please feel free to call us collect at (312) 996-6129. We realize that people in your position get many questionnaires but we hope that you will help us with this one. Thank you in advance for your cooperation.

Sincerely,

_____
Network Principal Investigator

_____
Richard B. Warnecke, Ph.D.
Associate Director and
    Principal Investigator

Enclosure

1. How long have you been Chief Executive Officer of this hospital?

_____ Number of years

2. How many beds does this hospital currently operate? _____

3. Are any beds in this hospital currently reserved for the care of patients with head and neck cancer? _____ Yes . . . If yes: Number _____

_____ No

3a. Has there been any change in the number of beds in this hospital reserved for patients with head and neck cancer during the past five (5) years?

_____ Yes . . . If yes: 3b. Has the number of these beds:

_____ Significantly increased?
_____ Increased slightly?
_____ Decreased slightly?
_____ Significantly decreased?

_____ No

4. Approximately how far in miles is this hospital from (network headquarters)?

_____ Number of miles

5. Does this hospital have its own tumor registry?

_____ Yes . . . If yes: Is it computerized?
_____ Yes
_____ No

_____ No . . . If no: Does this hospital share with
_____ Another hospital; please name _____
_____ A university; please name _____
_____ Contract for tumor registration with a private company;
Please name _____

6. Does this hospital have an active tumor board?

_____ Yes . . . 6a. How often does it meet? _____

6b. When was this board formed? _____ (year)

6c. Who are its members? (list names if possible):

_____
_____
_____

6d. Does the tumor board follow a formalized protocol or set of procedures for the review of cases?
_____ Yes
_____ No

6e. Approximately what percentage of all head and neck cancer patients seen at this hospital are reviewed by the tumor board?

_____%

_____ No tumor board

7. Does your office have a current list of all physicians and their specialties who have staff privileges at this hospital?

_____ Yes . . . If yes: Please attach list to this questionnaire

_____ No . . . If no: Please indicate the name of someone in your office whom we can contact to obtain this information:

_____

8. How many members currently serve on your hospital governing board?

_____ Number of members

9. How many members have full voting privileges?   _____ members

10. Is the chief executive officer the chairman of the governing board?

_____ Yes

_____ No . . . If no: Who is the chairman?   (Specify by title):

_____

11. Do the hospital bylaws stipulate how often the governing board must meet?

_____ Yes

_____ No

12. How often does the board meet each year? _____number of meetings per year.

13. Is the governing board responsible for other non-health-care-related institutions linked with the hospital, such as schools, churches, and so forth?

_____ Yes

_____ No

14. Is your governing board responsible for more than one hospital?

_____ Yes . . . If yes: How many hospitals? _____

Please name: _____

_____

_____

_____

_____

_____ No

15. Is the hospital governing board responsible to a higher board or organizational authority?

            _____ Yes . . . If yes: Please indicate which higher authority?

                                    _____ The board of a religious order or organization

                                    _____ The board of a not-for-profit multi-institutional system

                                    _____ The board of a university or college

                                    _____ The board of a corporation

                                    _____ A unit of state, county, or local government

                                    _____ Other (Please specify) _____

_____ No

16. How many hospital board members also serve on the board of other hospitals that are *totally independent* of your institution? (Enter 0 if none)

      _____ Number of individuals

17. Does your hospital currently maintain an office or staff for the coordination and/or planning of interhospital relations?

            _____ Yes . . . If yes: How many staff (full and parttime) work in this office?

                                      _____ Number of staff

                          When was this office established? _____ Year

                          Approximately what percentage of the total hospital operating budget is specified for the operation of that office?

                                    _____ %

_____ No

18. Shared services

Shared services are defined as those clinical or administrative functions which are common to two or more health care institutions, which are used jointly or cooperatively by them in some manner for the purpose of improving patient service, containing costs, and/or effecting economies of scale.

Does your hospital participate in any shared services with another hospital?

      _____ Yes

      _____ No

If your hospital does participate in any shared service programs, please review the following list and check those *shared services* that are applicable to your hospital. Please also indicate in the space provided the YEAR in which the shared service was initiated and the INSTITUTION with which the sharing arrangement exists.

Service	Year	Sharing institution
— Ambulatory care facilities	——	_____
— Biomedical engineering	——	_____
— Blood bank	——	_____
— Burn care unit	——	_____
— Credit and collections	——	_____
— Diagnostic radiology	——	_____
— Education and training (residents, interns, undergraduate, nursing)	——	_____
— Electrocardiology	——	_____
— Computer services	——	_____
— Trauma center, emergency medical service	——	_____
— Facilities engineering	——	_____
— Financial management	——	_____
— Food service	——	_____
— Hospital management services	——	_____
— Home health care	——	_____
— Insurance programs	——	_____
— Cardiac intensive care	——	_____
— Other intensive care	——	_____
— Laboratory services	——	_____
— Laundry and linen	——	_____
— Management engineering	——	_____
— Microfilm	——	_____
— Obstetrics	——	_____
— Open-heart surgery	——	_____
— Pediatrics	——	_____
— Personnel services	——	_____
— Pharmacy services	——	_____
— Printing and duplicating	——	_____
— Purchasing	——	_____
— Psychiatric care	——	_____
— Quality assurance program	——	_____
— Rehabilitation	——	_____
— Renal dialysis	——	_____
— Respiratory care	——	_____
— Safety programs	——	_____
— Security	——	_____
— Social services	——	_____
— Therapeutic radiology	——	_____

Service	Year	Sharing institution
__ Tumor registry	___	_____
__ Tumor board	___	_____
__ Other, please specify	___	_____
_____	___	_____
_____	___	_____

Shared staff

We are also interested in personnel that might be shared or referred. Here we are mainly interested in head-and-neck-related professionals. For each type of professional listed would you indicate in the appropriate column the number on your hospital's staff, the number of these professionals who regularly relate to head and neck patients, whether the person is shared through cross-appointment with another institution, or whether you refer to another institution for this service.

Specialty area	(A) Number on staff	(B) Number who treat head and neck	Number of (B) shared with another institution	Name of institution	Check here if you refer to another institution (√)	Name of institution
Surgeon	___	___	___	_____	___	_____
Oral surgeon	___	___	___	_____	___	_____
Head and neck surgeon	___	___	___	_____	___	_____
Radiologist	___	___	___	_____	___	_____
Medical oncologist	___	___	___	_____	___	_____
Oncology nurse	___	___	___	_____	___	_____
Social worker	___	___	___	_____	___	_____
Dentist	___	___	___	_____	___	_____
Speech pathologist	___	___	___	_____	___	_____
Maxillofacial prosthodontist	___	___	___	_____	___	_____
Pathologist	___	___	___	_____	___	_____
Oral pathologist	___	___	___	_____	___	_____
Other (please list)	___	___	___	_____	___	_____

19. Medical staff organization policies

The following is a list of the hospitals in the head and neck cancer control network in your area. Please CIRCLE the number that best describes the procedures by which staff privileges are extended between your hospital and *each hospital listed*. Please indicate the year in which the staff privilege arrangement was initiated when applicable.

1. Both hospitals have separate medical staffs and no privileges are extended.
2. Both hospitals have separate medical staffs but the bylaws provide for automatic extension of privileges to physicians at the other hospital.

3. Both hospitals have separate medical staffs but the bylaws provide for automatic extension of privileges to physicians at the other hospital.
4. Both hospitals have separate medical staffs, provision is made in the bylaws for automatic extension or privileges and for a liaison committee to discuss mutual interests and problems.
5. There is a single staff for both hospitals.

Network hospital	Separate staff/no privileges extended 1	Separate staff/ privileges extended on request 2	Separate staff/ automatic bylaws 3	Separate staff/ bylaws provide automatic privileges and liaison 4	Combined staff 5	Year
_____	1	2	3	4	5	___
_____	1	2	3	4	5	___
_____	1	2	3	4	5	___
_____	1	2	3	4	5	___
_____	1	2	3	4	5	___
_____	1	2	3	4	5	___
_____	1	2	3	4	5	___
_____	1	2	3	4	5	___
_____	1	2	3	4	5	___
_____	1	2	3	4	5	___

20. Patient transfers. We are interested in determining the extent to which patients are transferred between the network hospitals. Please CIRCLE the number that best describes the frequency with which patients are transferred for the treatment of head-and-neck-cancer-related problems *from your hospital to each hospital listed* in the following chart.

Name of hospital	Frequency of transfer			
	Frequent	Periodic	Seldom	Never
_____	1	2	3	4
_____	1	2	3	4
_____	1	2	3	4
_____	1	2	3	4
_____	1	2	3	4
_____	1	2	3	4
_____	1	2	3	4
_____	1	2	3	4
_____	1	2	3	4
_____	1	2	3	4

21. Now please CIRCLE the number that best describes the frequency with which patients are transferred for treatment of head-and-neck-cancer-related problems *to your hospital from each hospital listed* in the following chart.

	Frequency of transfer			
Name of hospital	Frequent	Periodic	Seldom	Never
_____	1	2	3	4
_____	1	2	3	4
_____	1	2	3	4
_____	1	2	3	4
_____	1	2	3	4
_____	1	2	3	4
_____	1	2	3	4
_____	1	2	3	4
_____	1	2	3	4
_____	1	2	3	4

22. During 1979, did any member of your active medical staff conduct funded research projects?

_____ Yes . . . If yes: Please estimate the number of staff funded for research projects:

_____

If yes: Please estimate the number of research projects involving a collaboration of two or more of your active medical staff:

_____

If yes: Please estimate the number of research projects involving a collaboration of at least one of your active medical staff with medical staff from another hospital:

_____

_____ No

Thank you very much for your cooperation. Please return this questionnaire in the enclosed stamped envelope.

References

Aiken, M., and Hage, J. (1968). Organizational interdependence and intraorganizational structure. *American Sociological Review, 33,* 912–929.

Aiken, M., Dewar, R., DiTomaso, N., Hage, J., and Zeitz, G. (1975). *Coordinating Human Services.* San Francisco: Jossey-Bass.

Aldrich, H. E. (1979). *Organizations and Environments.* Englewood Cliffs, NJ: Prentice-Hall.

Aldrich, H. E., and Pfeffer, J. (1976). Environments of organization. *Annual Review of Sociology, 2,* 79–105.

Aldrich, H. E., and Whetten, D. (1981). Organization-sets, action-sets and networks: Making the most of simplicity. In P. C. Nystrom and W. H. Starbuck (Eds.), *Handbook of Organizational Design* (Vol. 1, pp. 385–408). London: Oxford University Press.

Alford, E. M. (1976). Shared services. *Topics in Health Care Financing, 2,* 13–23.

American Board of Medical Specialists. (1972). *Directory of Medical Specialists* (14th ed.). Chicago: Marquis Who's Who.

American Board of Medical Specialists. (1973). *Directory of Medical Specialists* (15th ed.). Chicago: Marquis Who's Who.

American Board of Medical Specialists. (1975). *Directory of Medical Specialists* (16th ed.). Chicago: Marquis Who's Who.

American Board of Medical Specialists. (1977). *Directory of Medical Specialists* (17th ed.). Chicago: Marquis Who's Who.

American Hospital Association. (1973). *American Hospital Association Guide to the Health Care Field.* Chicago: Author.

American Hospital Association. (1974). *Hospital Statistics.* Chicago: Author.

American Hospital Association. (1975). *Hospital Statistics.* Chicago: Author.

American Hospital Association. (1980). *Hospital Statistics.* Chicago: Author.

American Medical Association. (1974). *Directory of Physicians in the United States, Puerto Rico, Virgin Islands, Certain Pacific Islands and U.S. Physicians Temporarily Located in Foreign Countries* (24th ed.). Chicago: Author.

American Medical Association. (1975). *Directory of Physicians in the United States, Puerto Rico, Virgin Islands, Certain Pacific Islands and U.S. Physicians Temporarily Located in Foreign Countries* (25th ed.). Chicago: Author.

American Medical Association. (1979). *Directory of Physicians in the United States, Puerto Rico, Virgin Islands, Certain Pacific Islands and U.S. Physicians Temporarily Located in Foreign Countries* (26th ed.). Chicago: Author.

Andersen, R., and Anderson, O. W. (1979). Patterns of use of health services. In H. E.

Freeman, S. Levine, and L. G. Reeder (Eds.), *Handbook of Medical Sociology* (3rd ed., pp. 371–391). Englewood Cliffs, NJ: Prentice-Hall.

Arabie, P., Boorman, S., and Levitt, P. (1978). Constructing blockmodels: How and why. *Journal of Mathematical Psychology, 17,* 21–63.

Astolfi, A. A., and Matti, L. B. (1972). Survey profiles shared services. *Hospitals, 46,* 61–65.

Barnes, J. (1954). Class and committees in a Norwegian island parish. *Human Relation, 7,* 39–58.

Becker, M. H. (1970). Factors affecting diffusion of innovations among health professionals. *American Journal of Public Health, 60,* 294–305.

Begg, C., Carbone, P., Elson, M., and Zelen, M. (1982). Participation of community hospitals in clinical trials. *New England Journal of Medicine, 306,* 1076–1080.

Benson, K. J. (1975). The interorganizational network as a political economy. *Administative Science Quarterly, 20,* 229–249.

Beyer, J. M., and Trice, H. M. (1978). *Implementing Change.* New York: Free Press.

Boje, D. M., and Whetten, D. A. (1981). Effects of organizational strategies and contextual constraints on centrality and attributions of influence in interorganizational networks. *Administrative Science Quarterly, 26,* 378–395.

Bonacich, P., and McConaghy, M. (1979). The algebra of blockmodeling. In K. Schuessler (Ed.), *Sociological Methodology* (pp. 489–532). San Francisco: Jossey-Bass.

Boorman, S., and White, H. (1976). Social structure from multiple networks II, Role structure. *American Journal of Sociology, 81,* 1384–1446.

Breslow, L. (1977). Policy assessment of preventive health practice. *Preventive Medicine, 6,* 242–251.

Carbone, P., Davis, T., Zelen, M., and Lavin, P. (1978). Eastern cooperative oncology group: Progress report of activities and plans. *Cancer Clinical Trials, 1,* 65–75.

Cohen, M. D., March, J. G., and Olsen, J. P. (1972). A garbage-can model of organizational choice. *Administrative Science Quarterly, 17,* 1–25.

Coleman, J., Katz, E., and Menzel, H. (1966). *Medical Innovation: A Diffusion Study.* New York: Bobbs-Merrill.

Cook, K. S. (1977). Exchange and power in interorganizational networks. *Sociological Quarterly, 18,* 62–82.

Crane, D. (1972). *Invisible Colleges.* Chicago: University of Chicago Press.

Cromwell, J., and Kanak, J. R. (1982). The effects of prospective reimbursement programs on hospital adoption and science sharing. *Health Care Financing Review, 4,* 67–88.

Daft, R. L. (1978). A dual-core model of organizational innovation. *Academy of Management Journal, 21,* 193–210.

DeVries, R. A. (1978). Strength in numbers. *Hospitals, 52,* 81–84.

DiMaggio, P., and Powell, W. (1983). The iron cage revisited: Institutional isomorphism and collective rationality in organizational fields. *American Sociological Review, 48,* 147–160.

Downs, G., and Mohr, L. (1976). Conceptual issues in the study of innovations. *Administrative Science Quarterly, 21,* 700–714.

Dunbar, R. L., and Wasilewski, N. (1985). Regulating external threats in the cigarette industry. *Administrative Science Quarterly, 30,* 540–559.

Emerson, R. M. (1962). Power-dependence relations. *American Sociological Review, 27,* 31–40.

Evan, W. H. (1966). The organization set: Toward a theory of interorganizational relations. In J. D. Thompson (Ed.), *Approaches to Organizational Design* (pp. 173–191). Pittsburgh: University of Pittsburgh Press.

Feldstein, M., and Taylor, A. (1977). The rapid rise of hospital costs. *Report of the President's Council on Wage and Price Stability.*

Feldstein, P. J. (1979). *Health Care Economics.* New York: Wiley.

Fennell, M. L. (1980). The effects of environmental characteristics on the structure of hospital clusters. *Administrative Science Quarterly, 25,* 484–510.

Fennell, M. L. (1982). Context in organizational groups: The case of hospital clusters. *Journal of Health and Social Behavior, 23,* 65–83.

Fennell, M. L. (1984). Synergy, influence and information in the adoption of administrative innovations. *Academy of Management Journal, 27,* 113–129.

Fennell, M. L., and Alexander, J. A. (1987). Organizational boundary spanning in institutionalized environments. *Academy of Management Journal, 30,* 456–476.

Fennell, M. L., Ross, C. O., and Warnecke, R. B. (1987). Organizational environment and network structure. In S. Bacharach and N. DiTomaso (Eds.), *Research in the Sociology of Organizations* (Vol. 5, pp. 311–340). Greenwich, CT: JAI Press.

Flexner, A. (1910). *Medical Education in the United States and Canada.* Washington: Science and Health Publications.

Galaskiewicz, J. (1979). *Exchange Networks and Community Politics.* Beverly Hills: Sage.

Gibbs, J. P., and Poston, D. L. (1975). Division of labor—Conceptualization and related measures. *Social Forces, 53,* 468–476.

Gluckman, M. (1955). *The Judicial Process among the Barotse of Northern Rhodesia.* Manchester, England: Manchester University Press.

Greenfield, H. (1975). *Accountability in Health Facilities.* New York: Praeger.

Greer, A. L. (1977). Advances in the study of diffusion of innovation in health care organizations. *Milbank Memorial Fund Quarterly/Health and Society, 55,* 505–532.

Greer, A. L. (1984). Medical technology and professional dominance theory. *Social Science and Medicine, 18,* 809–817.

Greer, A. L. (1986). Medical conservatism and technological acquisitiveness: The paradox of hospital technology adoptions. In J. A. Roth and S. B. Ruzek (Eds.), *The Social Impact of Medical Technology, Vol. 4: Research in the Sociology of Health Care* (pp. 185–235). Greenwich, CT: JAI Press.

Hage, J., and Aiken, M. (1967). Program change and organizational properties: A comparative analysis. *American Journal of Sociology, 72,* 503–519.

Hall, R. M. (1963). The concept of bureaucracy: An empirical assessment. *American Journal of Sociology, 69,* 32–40.

Hall, R. M. (1986). Interorganizational or interprofessional relationships: A case of mistaken identity? In W. R. Scott and B. L. Black (Eds.), *The Organization of Mental Health Services* (pp. 147–158). Beverly Hills: Sage.

Hannan, M. T. (1971). *Aggregation and Disaggregation in Sociology.* Lexington, KY: Heath Lexington.

Hannan, M. T., and Freeman, J. (1977). The population ecology of organizations. *American Journal of Sociology, 82,* 929–964.

Hirschman, A. O. (1970). *Exit, Voice and Loyalty.* Cambridge: Harvard University Press.

Jacobs, D. (1974). Dependency and vulnerability: An exchange approach to the control of organizations. *Administrative Science Quarterly, 19,* 45–59.

Jesse, R. (1981). The head and neck oncologic surgeon: Self-evaluation. *American Journal of Surgery, 142,* 428–430.

Joskow, P. O. (1982). *Controlling Hospital Costs: The Role of Government Regulation.* Cambridge: M.I.T. Press.

Kaiser, R. F. (1955). Some results of the cancer teaching program. *Journal of Medical Education, 30,* 643–645.

Kaluzny, A. D. (1974). Innovation in health services: Theoretical framework and review of research. *Health Services Research, 9,* 101–120.

Kaluzny, A. D., and Hernandez, S. R. (1983). Managing change in health care organizations. *Medical Care Review, 40,* 161–203.

Kaluzny, A. D., Veney, J. E., Smith, D. B., and Elliot, W. (1976). Predicting two types of hospital innovation. *Hospital and Health Service Administration, 21,* 24–43.

Kanter, R. M., and Brinkerhoff, D. (1981). Organizational performance: Recent developments in measurement. *Annual Review of Sociology, 7,* 321–349.

Katz, E., and Lazarsfeld, P. F. (1955). *Personal Influence: The Part Played by People in the Flow of Mass Communications.* New York: Free Press.

Kimberly, J. R. (1978). Hospital adoption of innovation: The role of integration into external informational environments. *Journal of Health and Social Behavior, 19,* 361–373.

Kimberly, J. R. (1981). Managerial innovation. In P. C. Nystrom and W. H. Starbuck (Eds.), *Handbook of Organizational Design* (Vol. 1, pp. 84–104). London: Oxford University Press.

Kimberly, J. R., and Evanisko, M. J. (1981). Organizational innovation: The influence of individual, organizational, and contextual factors on hospital adoption of technological and administrative innovations. *Academy of Management Journal, 24,* 689–713.

Kimberly, J. R., and Miles, R. H. (1980). *The Organizational Life Cycle.* San Francisco: Jossey-Bass.

Kornhauser, W. (1962). *Scientists in Industry: Conflict and Accommodation.* Berkeley: University of California Press.

Kuhn, T. S. (1962). *The Structure of Scientific Revolutions.* Chicago: University of Chicago Press.

Lawrence, P. R., and Lorsch, J. W. (1967). *Organization and Environment: Managing Differentiation and Integration.* Boston: Graduate School of Business Administration, Harvard University.

Lazarsfeld, P. F., and Menzel, H. (1961). On the relation between individual and collective properties. In A. Etzioni and E. W. Lehman (Eds.), *A Sociological Reader on Complex Organizations* (pp. 508–521). New York: Holt, Rinehart & Winston.

Lehman, E. (1975). *Coordinating Health Care.* Beverly Hills: Sage.

Light, J. M., and Mullins, N. C. (1979). A primer on blockmodeling procedure. In P. W. Holland and S. Leinhardt (Eds.), *Perspectives on Social Network Research* (pp. 85–118). New York: Academic Press.

Lincoln, J. R., and McBride, K. (1985). Resources, homophily, and dependence: Organizational attributes and asymmetric ties in human service networks. *Social Science Research, 14,* 1–30.

Mansfield, R. (1973). Bureaucracy and centralization: An examination of organizational structure. *Administrative Science Quarterly, 18,* 477–488.

March, J. G. (1981). Footnotes to organizational change. *Administrative Science Quarterly, 26,* 563–577.

March, J. G., and Simon, H. A. (1958). *Organizations.* New York: Wiley.

Marrett, C. (1971). On the specification of interorganizational dimensions. *Sociology and Social Research, 56,* 83–99.

McCusker, J., Wax, A., Bennett, J. (1982). Cancer patient accessions into clinical trials: A pilot investigation into some patient and physician determinants of entry. *American Journal of Clinical Trials, 5,* 227–236.

Meyer, J. W. (1978). Strategies for further research: Varieties of environmental variation. In M. W. Meyer (Ed.), *Environments and Organizations* (pp. 352–368). San Francisco: Jossey-Bass.

Meyer, J. W., and Rowan, B. (1977). Institutionalized organizations: Formal structure as myth and ceremony. *American Journal of Sociology, 83,* 340–363.

Meyer, M. W. (1979). Organizational structure as signaling. *Pacific Sociological Review, 22,* 481–500.

Miles, R. H., and Cameron, K. (1982). *Coffin Nails and Corporate Strategies.* Englewood Cliffs, NJ: Prentice-Hall.

Mindlin, S. E., and Aldrich, H. (1975). Interorganizational dependence: A review of the concept and a reexamination of the findings of the Aston Group. *Administrative Science Quarterly, 20,* 382–391.

Mitchell, J. C. (1969). The concept and use of social networks. In J. C. Mitchell (Ed.), *Social*

Networks in Urban Situations (pp. 1–29). Manchester, England: Manchester University Press.

Mizruchi, M., and Koenig, T. (1986). Economic sources of corporate political consensus: An examination of interindustry relations. *American Sociological Review, 51,* 482–491.

Moch, M. K., and Morse, E. V. (1977). Size, centralization and organizational adoption of innovations. *American Sociological Review, 42,* 716–725.

Mohr, L. B. (1969). Determinants of innovation in organizations. *American Political Science Review, 63,* 111–126.

Mohr, L. B. (1971). Organizational technology and organizational structures. *Administrative Science Quarterly, 16,* 444–459.

Mueller, J. H., Schussler, K. F., and Costner, H. L. (1970). *Statistical Reasoning in Sociology* (2nd ed.). Boston: Houghton Mifflin.

Mullins, N., Hargens, L., Hecht, P., and Kick, E. (1977). The group structure of cocitation clusters: A comparison study. *American Sociological Review, 42,* 552–562.

Mullner, R., Byre, C. S., and Kubal, J. D. (1981). Multihospital systems in the United States: A geographical overview. *Social Science and Medicine, 15,* 353–359.

Murphy, J. (1981). Conducting clinical trials with practicing community oncologists. *Controlled Clinical Trials, 2,* 115–122.

Olson, M. (1975). *The Logic of Collective Action.* Cambridge: Harvard University Press.

Palmer, D., Friedland, R., and Singh, J. V. (1986). The ties that bind: Organizational and class bases of stability in a corporate interlock network. *American Sociological Review, 51,* 781–796.

Pelz, D. G., and Andrews, F. M. (1966). *Scientists in Organizations: Productive Climates for Research and Development.* New York: Wiley.

Pennings, J. (1975). The relevance of the structural-contingency model for organizational effectiveness. *Administrative Science Quarterly, 30,* 393–410.

Perrow, C. (1961). The analysis of goals in complex organizations. *American Sociological Review, 26,* 845–866.

Perrow, C. (1965). Hospitals: Technology, structure, and goals. In J. March (Ed.), *The Handbook of Organizations* (pp. 910–971). Chicago: Rand McNally.

Perrow, C. (1967). A framework for the comparative analysis of organizations. *American Sociological Review, 32,* 194–208.

Pfeffer, J. (1972). Size and composition of corporate boards of directors. *Administrative Science Quarterly, 17,* 218–228.

Pfeffer, J. (1973). Size, composition, and function of hospital boards of directors: A study of organization-environment linkage. *Administrative Science Quarterly, 18,* 349–364.

Pfeffer, J. (1981). *Power in Organizations.* Marshfield, MA: Pitman.

Pfeffer, J., and Salancik, G. R. (1978). *The External Control of Organizations: A Resource Dependence Perspective.* New York: Harper & Row.

Pugh, D. S., Hickson, D. J., Hinings, C. R., and Turner, C. (1968). Dimensions of organization structure. *Administrative Science Quarterly, 13,* 65–105.

Pugh, D., Hickson, D., and Hinings, C. R. (1969). The context of organizational structures. *Administrative Science Quarterly, 14,* 91–114.

Rogers, E. M. (1983). *Diffusion of Innovations* (3rd ed.). New York: Free Press.

Rogers, E. M., and Shoemaker, F. F. (1971). *Communication of Innovations.* New York: Free Press.

Roman, P. M. (1980). *Barriers to the initiation of employee alcoholism programs.* Presented at the Research Conference on Occupational Alcoholism, Reston, Virginia, May 22–24, 1980.

Rowe, L. A., and Boise, W. B. (1974). Organizational innovation: Current research and evolving concepts. *Public Administration Review, 34,* 284–392.

Rushing, W. A. (1971). Public policy, community constraints, and distribution of medical resources. *Social Problems, 19,* 21–36.

Salomon, J. W. (1984). Organizing medical care for profit. In J. B. McKinlay (Ed.), *Issues in the Political Economy of Health Care* (pp. 143–186). New York: Tavistock.

Schoonhoven, C. B. (1981). Problems with contingency theory: Testing assumptions hidden within the language of contingency "theory." *Administrative Science Quarterly, 26,* 349–377.

Scott, W. R. (1977). The effectiveness of organizational effectiveness studies. In P. S. Goodman and J. M. Pennings (Eds.), *New Perspectives on Organizational Effectiveness* (pp. 63–95). San Francisco: Jossey-Bass.

Scott, W. R. (1987). *Organizations: Rational, Natural, and Open Systems* (2nd ed.). Englewood Cliffs, NJ: Prentice-Hall.

Scott, W. R., and Shortell, S. M. (1983). Organizational performance: Managing for efficiency and effectiveness. In S. M. Shortell and A. Kaluzny (Eds.), *Health Care Management: A Text in Organization Theory and Behavior* (pp. 418–456). New York: Wiley.

Selznick, P. (1949). *TVA and the Grass Roots.* Berkeley: University of California Press.

Smart, C. (1981). Progress in cancer patient management in community hospitals. *Bulletin of the American College of Surgeons, 66,* 5–13.

Starkweather, D., and Cook, K. S. (1983). Organization-environment relations. In S. M. Shortell and A. D. Kaluzny (Eds.), *Health Care Management: A Text in Organization Theory and Behavior* (pp. 333–377). New York: Wiley.

Starkweather, D., and Kirsch, A. (1971). A model of the life cycle dynamics of health service organizations. In M. Arnold, L. V. Blankenship, and J. M. Hess (Eds.), *Administering Health Systems* (pp. 307–329). Chicago: Aldine-Atherton Press.

Starr, P. (1982). *The Social Transformation of American Medicine.* New York: Basic Books.

Steers, R. M. (1975). Problems in the measurement of organizational effectiveness. *Administrative Science Quarterly, 20,* 546–559.

Taylor, E. (1977). Participation in shared service programs up sharply, AHA survey discloses. *Hospitals, 51,* 192–193.

Teece, D. J. (1980). The diffusion of an administrative innovation. *Management Science, 26,* 464–470.

Thompson, J. D. (1967). *Organizations in Action.* New York: McGraw-Hill.

Tilson, D., Reader, J. W., and Morrison, R. J. (1975). The federal interest. In G. Gordon and G. L. Fisher (Eds.), *The Diffusion of Medical Technology.* Cambridge, MA: Ballinger.

Tolbert, P., and Zucker, L. (1983). Institutional sources of change in the formal structure of organizations: The diffusion of civil service reform, 1880–1935. *Administrative Science Quarterly, 28,* 22–39.

U.S. Bureau of the Census. (1976). Estimates of the population of counties: July 1, 1973 and 1974. In *Current Population Reports,* Series P-25, No. 620. Washington: U.S. Government Printing Office.

U.S. Bureau of the Census. (1977). Estimates of the population of counties and metropolitan areas: July 1, 1974 and 1975. In *Current Population Reports,* Series P-25, No. 709. Washington: U.S. Government Printing Office.

U.S. Bureau of the Census. (1978). Population estimates and projections. In *Current Population Reports,* Series P-25, No. 727. Washington: U.S. Government Printing Office.

U.S. Department of Health, Education, and Welfare: National Center for Health Statistics. (1975). *Vital Statistics of the United States, Vol. II, Parts A and B: Mortality.* Washington: U.S. Government Printing Office.

U.S. Department of Health, Education, and Welfare: National Center for Health Statistics. (1976). *Vital Statistics of the United States, Vol. II, Parts A and B: Mortality.* Washington: U.S. Government Printing Office.

U.S. Department of Health, Education, and Welfare: National Institutes of Health, National Cancer Institute. (1973). *National Cancer Control Program Planning Conference, Report of Panel 9: Treatment.* Washington: U.S. Government Printing Office.

U.S. Department of Health, Education, and Welfare: National Institutes of Health, National Cancer Institute. (1979). *Management Guidelines for Head and Neck Cancer*, NIH Publication No. 80-2037. Washington: U.S. Government Printing Office.

VandeVen, A. H., and Drazin, R. (1985). The concept of fit in contingency theory. In L. L. Cummings and B. M. Staw (Eds.), *Research in Organizational Behavior* (pp. 333–365). Greenwich, CT: JAI Press.

Warnecke, R. B., Mosher, W., Graham, S., and Montgomery, E. B. (1976). Health guides as influentials in central Buffalo. *Journal of Health and Social Behavior, 17*, 22–34.

Warner, K. E. (1975). A "desperation-reaction" model of medical diffusion. *Health Services Research, 10*, 369–383.

Warren, R. L. (1967). The interorganizational field as a focus for investigation. *Administrative Science Quarterly, 12*, 369–419.

Weick, K. (1976). Educational organizations as loosely coupled systems. *Administrative Science Quarterly, 21*, 1–19.

White, H., Boorman, S., and Breiger, R. (1976). Social structure and multiple networks; Blockmodels of roles and positions. *American Journal of Sociology, 81*, 730–780.

Yuchtman, E., and Seashore, S. E. (1967). A system resource approach to organizational effectiveness. *American Sociological Review, 32*, 891–903.

Zald, M. N., and Hair, F. D. (1972). The social control of general hospitals. In B. S. Georgopoulos (Ed.), *Organization Research on Health Institutions* (pp. 51–82). Ann Arbor: Institute for Social Research, University of Michigan.

Zaltman, G., Duncan, R., and Holbek, J. (1973). *Innovations and Organizations*. New York: Wiley.

Zey-Ferrell, M. (1979). *Dimensions of Organizations: Environment, Context, Structure, Process, and Performance*. Santa Monica: Goodyear.

Zuckerman, H. S. (1979). Multi-institutional systems: Promise and performance. *Inquiry, 16*, 291–314.

Index